11th ANNUAL MEETING OF THE EBMT

(European Cooperative Group for Bone Marrow Transplantation)

Bad Hofgastein (Salzburg). Austria   January 28 - 30. 1985

PATRONAGE

Doz. Dr. Heinz FISCHER
Federal Minister of Science and Research

Dr. Kurt STEYRER
Federal Minister of Health and Environmental Protection

Dr. Wilfried HASLAUER
Governor of Salzburg

Adolf WEBER
Mayor of Bad Hofgastein

HONORARY PRESIDENT

Prof. A. J. BARRETT, M. D.
President of EBMT

ORGANIZING COMMITTEE

Prof. Dr. Dr. h. c. E. DEUTSCH
President

Doz. Dr. W. HINTERBERGER
Secretary

SECRETARIAT

INTERCONVENTION
P. O. Box 80, A-1107 Vienna, Austria
Phone: (222) 57 63 05, 57 62 88, 57 64 50
Cable: intecon wien
Telex: 11 12 10

ISBN 978-3-662-39399-4   ISBN 978-3-662-40457-7 (eBook)
DOI 10.1007/ 978-3-662-40457-7

IV

INFECTIONS AFTER BMT

IMMUNOLOGIC RECONSTITUTION AND DIAGNOSIS OF ACUTE GVH-D

Lymphocyte Reconstitution

The Skin in GVH-D

PREVENTION OF GRAFT VERSUS HOST DISEASE II

CHRONIC GVH-D

CLINICAL MANAGEMENT

T-CELL DEPLETION

List of authors

(Paper Number bold faced – 1st author)

Leukemia I

Exp. Hematol. (suppl. 17) 13: 1–2 (1985)
© International Society for Experimental Hematology

Intensified Induction and Consolidation Chemotherapy with or without Monthly Maintenance for Adult AML: A Multicenter Study

Th. Büchner

Medizinische Universitätsklinik Münster, D-4400 Münster, Federal Republic of Germany, for the AML Cooperative Group

By the present report the AML Cooperative Group in Germany wants to contribute data on response, long-term remission duration and -survival, their correlations to treatment modalities and possible prognostic factors.

Patients and protocols: A total of 712 evaluable patients at a median age of 50 (range 15-80) years entered the 1978 pilot study and the 1982 randomised study. For remission induction patients uniformly received 1-2 courses of TAD9, a nine day combination of 6-thioguanine with ARA-C and daunorubicin, designed on a cell kinetic basis (1). After achieving complete remission (CR) patients in the 1978 pilot study, differently at the different centers, received either monthly CALGB type 5 day maintenance chemotherapy or induction type consolidation by 1-2 courses or both consolidation plus maintenance. A fourth group remained without therapy in remission for reasons of too early relapse (1/3) or medical and patients personal reasons (2/3). CR patients in the 1982 randomised study were randomly assigned to receive consolidation with or without subsequent monthly maintenance. A part of the patients in the 1982 randomised study entered a trial on immunotherapy and are included only in the data on response to induction.

Results: 63% of all patients achieved a CR within a median of 33 (range 17-180) days. In the 1978 pilot study the probability of continuous CR (CCR) after 5 years is 17% and 30 patients are in CCR for 18 to 66 months. Patients receiving any type of treatment in CR show a 22% long-term CCR rate without significant differences between the treatment groups vs 0% for the non-treatment group (p=0.01) (2). Patients < 40 years in the 1978 pilot study achieving CR within one month show a 37% probability of CCR at 5 years and 43% when considering only those with a remission duration of at least 6 months (fig. 1). A prognostic factors analysis in the Münster part of the 1978 pilot study revealed long-term remission of >3 years to be significantly correlated with Auer rods (p=0.043), days to CR < median (p=0.032) and LDH in serum on day 15 of therapy < median (p=0.032).

In the 1982 randomised study the rate of CCR at 30-36 months is 31% in the maintenance and 17% in the non-maintenance arm (p=0.011). Patients < 40 years show a 38% probability of survival after 36 months and 43% when considering only those with a survival of at least 6 months (fig. 2). Patients < 40 yrs with a CR of at least 6 months show a 48% probability of survival at 30 months.

Conclusions: The data from both the 1978 pilot and the 1982 randomised study strongly suggest that myelosuppressive chemotherapy of AML in CR has an impor-

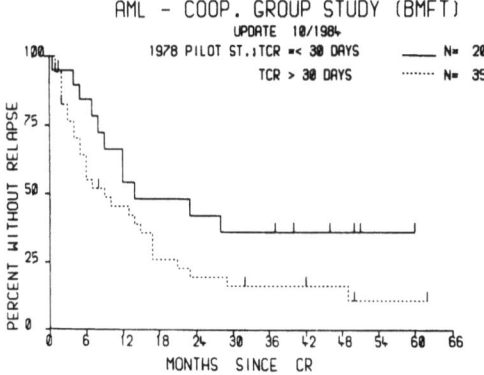

Figure 1: Kaplan-Meier plot of CR duration for patients < 40 years in the 1978 pilot study for two groups according to time to CR (TCR).

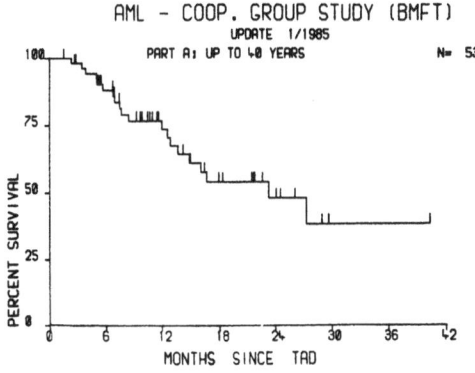

Figure 2: Kaplan Meier plot of survival for patients < 40 years in the 1982 randomised study.

tant impact on remission duration. Factors predicting for long-term CR may be found among early response parameters rather than among pretherapeutic characteristics. Younger patients - especially in favourable subgroups - may have a long-term survival and - CCR rate by chemotherapy in the same range as by BMT. Further prospective studies have to compare the validity of both therapeutic alternatives and have to define patients with a favourable prognosis by chemotherapy, too.

References:
1. Büchner, Th., Urbanitz, D., Emmerich, B. et al. for the AML Coop. Group: Multicentre study on intensified remission induction therapy for acute myeloid leukemia. Leukemia Research 6:827 (1982)
2. Büchner, Th., Urbanitz, D., Fischer, J. et al.for the AML Coop. Group: Longterm remission in acute myelogenous leukemia. Lancet I, 571 (1984).

Exp. Hematol. (suppl. 17) 13:3–5 (1985)
© International Society for Experimental Hematology

Bone Marrow Transplantation for Leukemia in Europe: Factors Influencing the Possibility of Long-Term Leukemia-Free Survival

F. E. Zwaan[1], J. Hermans[2], and A. Lyklema[2]

[1] Department of Hematology-Bone Marrow Transplantat Unit, [2] Department of Medical Statistics, University Medical Center, Leiden, The Netherlands

INTRODUCTION

Bone marrow transplantation (BMT) has been increasingly used for patients with acute leukemia and chronic myeloid leukemia (1,2,3). In 1979, the Leukaemia Working Party of the European Cooperative Group for Bone Marrow Transplantation (EGBMT) was instituted to analyse existing data and compare results with a view to developing common protocols. The previous results have been published (4,5,6) and two detailed surveys on acute myeloblastic leukemia (ANLL) and lymphoblastic leukemia (ALL) have been reported in 1984 (7,8). Although the early results after BMT are promising, some doubts have been raised about the probability of long-term survival, viz. longer than 2 years after BMT. This survey reports the results of 34 European teams, giving data on patients with acute leukemia and chronic myeloid leukemia (CML), grafted in remission, or in chronic or accelerated phase of the disease between 1979 and December 31, 1984. We hope that this study will help to determine prognostic factors of long-term leukemia-free survival after BMT and establish the most effective pretransplant regimen for the European group.

PATIENTS AND METHODS

A questionnaire was sent to all EBMT members, asking for complete reporting on every consecutively transplanted patient. Thirty-four participating teams gave details of over 1100 patients. Included in this study were 434 patients with ANLL, 395 with ALL and 265 with CML. Various details about the handling of patients data were previously reported (7,8). Factors studied for prognostic value with respect to survival and leukemia-free survival were: age (recipient/donor), sex (recipient/donor), cytogenetic abnormalities at diagnosis, splenectomy before BMT, phase of the disease, various irradiation parameters, type of GVHD prevention, acute and chronic GVHD, and leukemic subtypes.

STATISTICAL ANALYSIS

The closing data for this analysis was December 31, 1984. In univariate analysis, chi-square analysis was used to test for differences between percentages and student's t-test for differences between groups when a continuous variable was studied. Time from transplantation to transplant failure was studied with survival analysis. The differences between survival curves were studied with the Lee-Desu test, available in the SPSS-software package (9). After that, multivariate analyses were carried out using the Cox regression model for studying various potential prognostic factors, as is available in the program BMDP-2L (10).

RESULTS

A. Acute nonlymphoblastic leukemia (ANLL). 434 patients were transplanted; the majority had FAB-M2 classification. 222 (52%) were male and 212 (48%) female. 348 patients (80.2%) were grafted during first remission; 81 (18.7%) in second remission and 5 patients (1.2%) in third remission. Prevention of acute GVHD was carried out with MTX in 226 (52.1%) of them, with cyclosporin-A in 118 (27.7%), with bone marrow pretreatment for T-cell removal in 14 (3.2%), and with a combination of various approaches in 76 (17.5%) patients. Acute GVHD was absent in 169 (39%) patients, mild in 93 (22%), moderate in 80 (20%), and severe in 77 (19%). Chronic GVHD was observed in 96 patients (23%), 67 (68%) of whom suffered from limited disease. Interstitial pneumonitis was observed in 105 (24%) patients and relapse after BMT in 56 (13%) patients. Life-table analysis revealed a 44% actuarial survival at 4 years for patients grafted in first remission, and a 30% survival for second or higher remission patients (p=0.07) (Fig. 1).

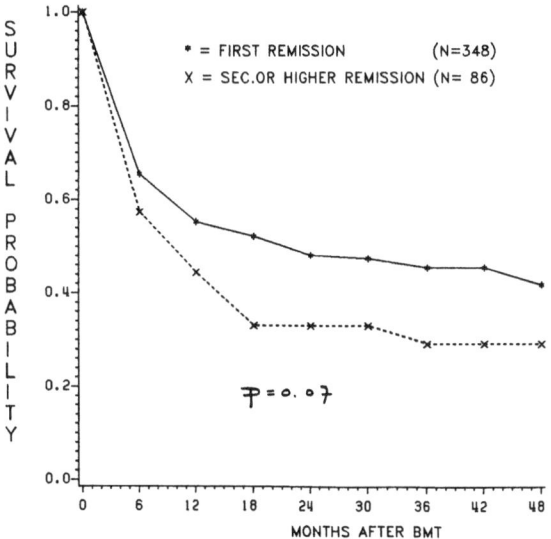

Fig. 1: Probability of survival of patients with ANLL grafted in first or second remission. The difference in survival is not significant (p=0.07).

Patients with subtypes M1, M2, M3 showed a better survival (50% at 4 years) than patients with subtypes M4-M5 (p=0.04). This was caused by a higher relapse incidence in the latter group (40% versus 20%; p=0.006). A higher actuarial relapse incidence was also observed in patients grafted in second or higher remission, compared to first remission grafts (40% versus 20%, respectively; p=0.01).
Patients on cyclosporin-A prophylaxis did significantly better than patients on MTX prophylaxis (p=0.006) (Fig. 2). This was also the case for patients transplanted with HLA-identical siblings compared to identical twins (44% at 4 years and 20%, respectively; p=0.03).
As previously reported, age (≤ 20 years) of the patient and/or donor had a beneficial effect on survival (p=0.01 and p=0.001, respectively).

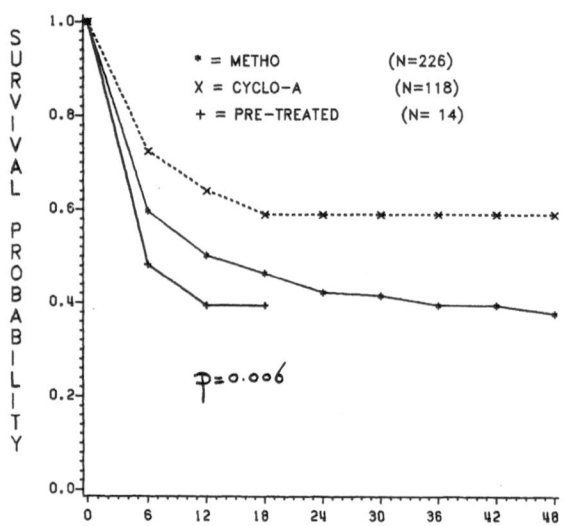

Fig. 2: Probability of survival of patients with ANLL on prophylaxis with methotrexate, cyclosporin-A or bone marrow depletion of T cells. The difference in survival is significant (p=0.006).

B. Acute lymphoblastic leukemia (ALL). 395 patients were transplanted, most of them of the common-ALL type. 256 were male (64%) and 139 female (36%). 155 patients (39.2%) were transplanted in first remission, 178 (45.1%) in second remission, 51 (12.9%) in third remission and 11 patients (2.9%) in fourth or higher remission.
Prevention of acute GVHD was carried out with MTX in 130 patients (32.9%), with cyclosporin-A in 163 (41.3%), with bone marrow pretreatment in 16 (4.1%) and with a combination of approaches in 86 (21.8%) patients. Therefore, compared to ANLL, more patients received cyclosporin-A prophylaxis than MTX.
The incidence and severity of acute GVHD was not significantly different as described for ANLL (p=0.18). The same holds good for the incidence and severity of chronic GVHD (p=0.34), although chronic GVHD resolved more often in ALL than in ANLL or in CML (p=0.03). Interstitial pneumonitis was observed less frequently in ALL (15.2%) than in ANLL (p=0.004). More relapses, however, were observed in ALL (23.8%; p=0.0001) compared to ANLL.
Life-table analysis revealed a 40% actuarial survival at 4 years, irrespective of the remission state in which the patients were transplanted (Fig. 3). The reason is that a high actuarial incidence of relapse

is observed in all remission groups (approximately (40-60%; p=n.s.).
However, it seems that patients with B- or T-cell type ALL did somewhat better than other types of ALL (54% and 38% survival at 4 years, respectively; p=0.03). As was also the case for ANLL, patients on cyclosporin-A prophylaxis did somewhat better than the patients on MTX prophylaxis; the effect, however, was marginal (p=0.02). Again, the age of the patient and/or the donor was of importance (p=0.05 and p=0.0006, respectively).

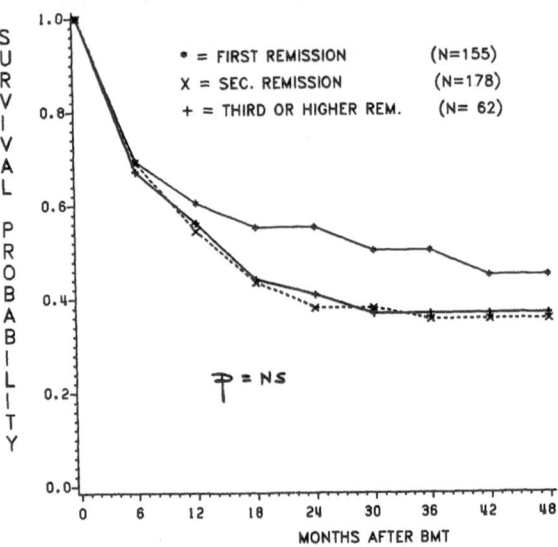

Fig. 3: Probability of survival of patients with ALL grafted in first, second, and third or higher remission. The difference in survival is not significant.

C. Chronic myeloid leukemia. 265 patients were grafted: 188 (70%) in first chronic phase, 63 (24%) in accelerated phase and 14 (6%) in second chronic phase. 143 were male (54%) and 122 female (46%). Cytogenetic abnormalities at diagnosis were found in 232 (88%) patients; they were absent in 16 patients (6%) and unknown in 17 (6%).
The majority of patients (48.3%) received cyclosporin A prophylaxis.
The incidence and severity of acute and chronic GVHD was not significantly different from that observed in ANLL (p=0.62). The same holds good for interstitial pneumonitis (56 patients; 21.2%) and relapse after BMT (24 patients; 9.1%).
Life-table analysis revealed a 4-year actuarial survival of 58% for patients grafted in first chronic phase and 24% for patients grafted in accelerated or second chronic phase, respectively (Fig. 4).
Although these differences are impressive, statistically, they were only borderline "significant" (p=0.08).
It is to be expected that a significant difference will develop in time, due to the higher actuarial relapse incidence (40% at 4 years) in the accelerated phase group, compared to the first chronic phase group (20% at 4 years; p=0.0001). An important observation is that splenectomy before BMT did not result in a better survival, nor in a difference in acute GVHD or relapse, compared to patients who did not undergo splenectomy.
In CML again, cyclosporin-A prophylaxis resulted in a marginally better survival (p=0.07) compared to patients on MTX prophylaxis. As was the case in acute

leukemia, the age of the patient and/or the donor was of importance (p=0.03 and p=0.02, respectively). The sex of the donor too seems to influence survival (an advantage for patients with a female donor, p=0.03).

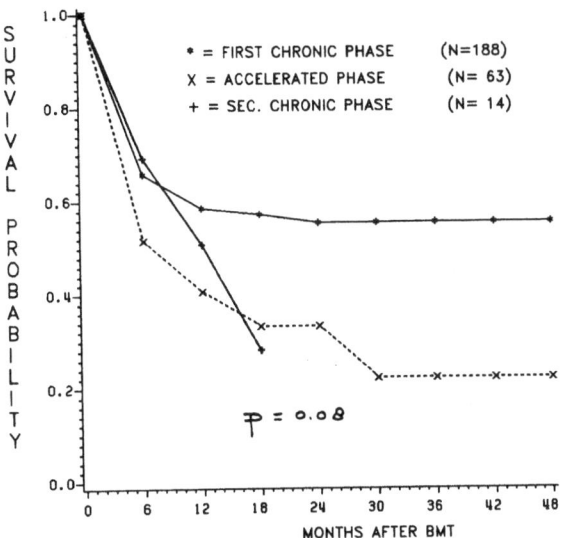

Fig. 4: Probability of survival of patients with CML grafts in first chronic, accelerated, or second chronic phase. The difference in survival is not significant (p=0.08).

Multivariate analysis was performed to sort out factors that had a favorable influence on long-term survival. In all three diagnosis categories, young age of the patient was an important factor.
For ANLL: a) the FAB subtypes M1, M2 and M3 had a much better survival than M4 and M5 (p=0.02).
b) Secondly, patients on cyclosporin-A prophylaxis did considerably better than patients on MTX prophylaxis (p=0.04). For ALL, apart from age, the most important factor for a good survival was B- or T-cell subtype (p=0.04). For CML, the phase in which the graft was performed (e.g. first chronic phase) was the most important in multivariate analysis (p=0.04).

ACKNOWLEDGEMENTS
The authors gratefully acknowledge the secretarial assistance from Ms J. Kooreman.

The authors would like to thank the physicians of the following institutions for their cooperation in this report: University Hospital, Vienna, Austria; Cliniques universitaires St.-Luc, Brussels, Belgium; St.-Raphael Hospital, Louvain, Belgium; The Finsen Institute, Copenhagen, Denmark; Bloomsbury Transplant Group, London, England; Royal Free Hospital Hospital, London, England; Royal Postgraduate Medical School, London, England; Westminster Hospital, London, England; Children's Hospital, University of Helsinki, Finland; Department of Medicine, University of Helsinki, Finland; University of Turku, Finland; Centre de transfusion sanguine, Besançon, France; Centre hospitalier et universitaire de Bordeaux, France; Centre hospitalier régional et universitaire de Caen, France; Hôpital Mondor, Créteil, France; Centre hospitalier régional de Nancy, France; Hôpital St.-Louis, Paris, France; Hôpital Bellevue, St. Etienne, France; University of Essen, West Germany; University of Tübingen, West Germany; University of Ulm, West Germany, San Martino Hospital, Genova, Italy; Bone Marrow Transplantation Centre, Hospital of Pesaro, Italy; University of Rome, Italy; Department of Pediatrics, University of Leiden, The Netherlands; Isolation Ward, University of Leiden, The Netherlands; Rotterdam Radiotherapy Institute, Rotterdam, The Netherlands; University of Nijmegen, The Netherlands; University of Utrecht, The Netherlands; Royal Infirmary of Edinburgh, Scotland; University of Barcelona, Spain; University Hospital, Huddinge, Sweden; Kantonsspital, Basle, Switzerland; Hôpital cantonal universitaire, Geneva, Switzerland.

REFERENCES

1. Zwaan FE & Jansen J: Bone marrow transplantation in acute nonlymphoblastic leukemia. Semin Hematol 21:36-42, 1984.

2. Buckner CD & Clift RA: Bone marrow transplantation for acute lymphoblastic leukemia. Semin Hematol 21:43-48, 1984.

3. Speck B, Gratwohl A, Osterwalder B, & Nissen C: Bone marrow transplantation for chronic myeloid leukemia. Semin Hematol 21:48-52, 1984.

4. Zwaan FE: Bone marrow transplantation for acute leukemia in remission - European results. Blut 41:208-213, 1980.

5. Zwaan FE: Bone marrow transplantation for acute leukemia in remission - European results. *Bone Marrow Transplantation in Europe II* (eds. Touraine JL, Gluckman E, & Griscelli C), Excerpta Medica, Amsterdam, pp. 63-71, 1981.

6. Zwaan FE & Hermans J (for the EBMT Leukaemia Working Party): Allogeneic bone marrow transplantation for leukemia: European results in 264 cases. Exp Hematol 10 (suppl. 12): 96-106, 1982.

7. Zwaan FE, Hermans J, Barrett AJ, & Speck B: Bone marrow transplantation for acute nonlymphoblastic leukaemia: a survey of the European Group for Bone Marrow Transplamtation (E.G.B.M.T.). Brit J Haematol 56:645-653, 1984.

8. Zwaan FE, Hermans J, Barrett AJ, & Speck B: Bone marrow transplantation for acute lymphoblastic leukaemia: a survey of the European Group for Bone Marrow Transplantation (E.G.B.M.T.). Brit J Haematol 58:33-42, 1984.

9. Hull CH & Nie NH: SPSS - update 7-9. MacGraw Hill, New York, 1981.

10. Dixon WJ, Brown MB, et al.: BMDP - statistical software 1981. University of California Press, Berkeley, CA, USA, 1981.

Exp. Hematol. (suppl. 17) 13:6–8 (1985)

Marrow Grafting for Leukemia

R. Storb

Seattle Bone Marrow Transplant Team, Seattle, Washington, USA

Until 1975, marrow grafting following high-dose chemotherapy combined with total body irradiation (TBI) was considered only for patients with acute leukemia in advanced relapse when all other therapy had failed. 110 such patients were given marrow grafts from HLA-identical siblings in Seattle, and 10% are alive in unmaintained remission between 9 and 14 years without further treatment (1). Even though many patients died from graft-versus-host disease (GVHD), interstitial pneumonias and other infections, it was clear that leukemic relapse was a major complication after marrow grafting, occurring at an actuarial rate of 75% (2). As far as could be determined, leukemic recurrences usually originated from host cells which were apparently resistant to the high-dose chemoradiotherapy used to prepare the patients for transplantation. This was true both for patients with acute lymphoblastic (ALL) and acute non-lymphoblastic leukemia (ANL) in advanced relapse.

A more recent study showed that results in patients with ANL could be improved when transplants were carried out early in first relapse, before chemotherapy reinduction (3). Projected survival in these patients was 25%, compared to only 10% in patients who received reinduction therapy but failed to respond. Of interest was that survival of patients with ANL transplanted in second remission was no better than that of patients transplanted early in first relapse. In all three groups recurrent leukemia continued to be a major problem.

In early 1976, the Seattle Transplant Team decided to treat patients with ANL by marrow grafting in first remission and those with ALL in second or subsequent remission. The conditioning regimen for transplantation continued to be cyclophosphamide (CY), 60 mg/kg on each of two successive days, followed by TBI. Initially, TBI was used as a single dose of 9.2 to 10 Gy, and as of 1977 fractionated-dose TBI was employed.

Twelve of the first 22 patients with ANL transplanted in first remission are alive between 6 and 7.5 years after marrow grafting (4). These encouraging results continue to be seen with larger numbers of patients transplanted in Seattle. Overall, it appears that over 50% of patients with ANL grafted in first remission can be cured of their disease. This figure is approximately 70% for patients below the age of 20 years, 50% between 21 and 30 years, and 40% in patients above the age of 30. The leukemic recurrence rate has been on the order of 25%, with relapses occurring as late as 4 years after transplantation.

From May 1977 to July 1982, a prospective study was carried out comparing the outcome of continued chemotherapy with that of marrow transplantation for adult patients (18-55 years of age) with ANL who achieved a first remission (5). One hundred eleven consecutive patients with newly-diagnosed ANL were treated with chemotherapy consisting of daunorubicin, cytosine arabinoside, 6-thioguanine, vincristine and prednisone, with 90 of these (81%) entering complete remission. Forty-four of the 90 patients had an HLA-identical sibling and were offered the option of marrow grafting. Of these 44, 11 refused transplantation and 33 were transplanted. Forty-six of the 90 patients did not have HLA-identical sibling donors, and were given continued chemotherapy. Kaplan-Meyer estimates with 95% confidence limits of 5-year disease-free survival (measured from complete remission) were 49 + 18% for marrow graft recipients, and 20 + 13% for chemotherapy patients. This demonstrates that marrow grafting results in a significantly greater chance for long-term disease-free survival than continued chemotherapy.

The curve showing disease-free survival among the first 51 patients with ALL transplanted in second to sixth remission has a plateau at 25%, 5.5 to 8 years after transplantation (6,7).

Between October 1976 and April 1980, 55 children between the ages of one and 17 with ALL relapsed in the bone marrow on maintenance chemotherapy and then reentered remission. They were enrolled into a study comparing the results of marrow grafting to those of continued chemotherapy (8). Specifically, we compared the progress of 24 children given CY, TBI and an HLA-identical marrow transplantation to that of 21 children treated with conventional chemotherapy according to one of the Children's Cancer Group Study protocols. All 21 children in the chemotherapy arm have died within 3.5 years of entering the study, with a median survival of 1.5 years. In contrast, 8 of the 24 children undergoing marrow transplantation are enjoying disease-free survival between 4.5 and 8 years after transplantation. The major cause of failure in both groups was relapse. The study demonstrates that marrow graft currently offers the best chance of long-term disease-free survival for a child with ALL who has had a relapse in the bone marrow. Results of marrow grafting can be further improved if satisfactory conditioning regimens are developed to increase the killing of malignant cells, thereby decreasing the risk of leukemic relapse.

Patients with chronic myelocytic leukemia (CML) maintained on chemotherapy and conventional care have median survivals reported to range from 1 to 3.5 years. Chemotherapy has not been able to significantly influence survival. It seemed logical, therefore, to attempt treating patients with CML by CY, TBI, and HLA-identical sibling marrow grafts. At first, in analogy to the approach taken in patients with acute leukemia, marrow grafting was attempted only when patients had entered blast crisis. Not surprisingly, results in blast crisis have been comparable to those in patients with acute leukemia in advanced relapse, with projected survival at 3 years not better than 15% (reviewed in reference 9). Similarly, when transplants were attempted in the accelerated phase of the disease, survival was at 15% at 3 years. However, the marrow in surviving patients shows absence of the Philadelphia chromosome, suggesting cure of the disease, a unique and impressive result.

Marrow grafting early in the course of CML promised to improve these results. Eight of twelve patients with CML in chronic phase given syngeneic marrow grafts are alive in unmaintained remission without the Philadelphia chromosome 4-8 years later (10). This result has encouraged allogeneic marrow grafts from HLA-identical siblings. Six of the first ten patients with CML in chronic phase given HLA-identical sibling transplants are alive, with the longest survivor close to 6 years (11). These results have been continued to be observed with 67 patients transplanted at the end of 1983. It is probably too early to comment on the leukemic recurrence in patients with CML in chronic phase. However, it appears that it will be in excess of 20%.

In patients with ANL grafted in first remission and CML grafted in chronic phase, interstitial pneumonia and GVHD associated complications have been major problems. Two randomized trials have evaluated the usefulness of cyclosporine in preventing acute GVHD as compared to methotrexate (12,13). While there was a trend toward a lesser probability of developing acute GVHD, at least in patients with ANL, overall survival was identical in methotrexate and cyclosporine treated patients. Currently, a combination of a short course of methotrexate plus six months of cyclosporine is being evaluated for better prevention of acute GVHD. Pilot studies have explored the usefulness of in vitro depletion of T cells in donor marrow for prevention of acute GVHD, using a combination of monoclonal antibodies and complement (14). While this has led to a reduction in the incidence of acute GVHD, a number of patients have shown late failure of marrow engraftment, suggesting a role of lymphocytes in facilitating sustained engraftment after HLA-identical marrow transplantation. Thus, despite a decreased incidence of GVHD, survival was not improved in these patients. It remains to be determined whether changes in the pre- or post-transplant regimens can decrease the graft failure associated with T cell depletion of the marrow.

139 patients with malignant disease received marrow grafts from HLA-nonidentical family members (16). Donors and recipients possessed genotypic identity for one HLA haplotype, and some degree of similarity for the other, or they were phenotypically identical for all HLA antigens. Patients who received marrow from HLA phenotypically identical family members had an acute GVHD rate not different from that seen in HLA-identical siblings, while patients differing for one, two or three antigens on the second haplotype had significantly increased probability of acute GVHD, ranging from 55 to 75%. Analyses of survival showed that patients receiving transplants from donors mismatched for only one antigen on the second haplotype was not significantly different from that of HLA-identical siblings, while patients differing for two or three antigens had significantly worse survival. It remains to be seen whether more effective conditioning regimens combined with marrow purging for T cells will improve these results.

REFERENCES

1. Thomas ED, Buckner CD, Banaji M, et al. One hundred patients with acute leukemia treated by chemotherapy, total body irradiation, and allogeneic marrow transplantation. Blood 49: 511-533, 1977.

2. Thomas ED, Flournoy N, Buckner CD, et al. Cure of leukemia by marrow transplantation. Leukemia Research 1: 67-70, 1977.

3. Appelbaum FR, Clift RA, Buckner CD, et al. Allogeneic marrow transplantation for acute nonlymphoblastic leukemia after first relapse. Blood 61: 949-953, 1983.

4. Thomas ED, Buckner CD, Clift RA, et al. Marrow transplantation for acute nonlymphoblastic leukemia in first remission. N Engl J Med 301: 597-599, 1979.

5. Appelbaum FR, Dahlberg S, Thomas ED, et al. Bone marrow transplantation or chemotherapy after remission induction for adults with acute nonlymphoblastic leukemia - A prospective comparison. Ann Intern Med 101: 581-588, 1984.

6. Thomas ED, Sanders JE, Flournoy N, et al. Marrow transplantation for patients with acute lymphoblastic leukemia in remission. Blood 54: 468-476, 1979.

7. Sanders JE, Flournoy N, Thomas ED, et al. Marrow transplant experience in children with acute lymphoblastic leukemia: An analysis of factors associated with survival, relapse and graft-versus-host disease. Med Pediatr Oncol, in press.

8. Johnson FL, Thomas ED, Clark BS, et al. A comparison of marrow transplantation to chemotherapy for children with acute lymphoblastic leukemia in second or subsequent remission. N Engl J Med 305: 846-851, 1981.

9. Storb R. Marrow transplantation for the treatment of malignant diseases. In: Progress in Transplantation, Vol. 1, Morris PJ, Tilney N (eds). London: Churchill Livingstone, 1984, pp 46-70.

10. Fefer A, Cheever MA, Greenberg PD, et al. Treatment of chronic granulocytic leukemia with chemoradiotherapy and transplantation of marrow from identical twins. N Engl J Med 306: 63-68, 1982.

11. Clift RA, Buckner CD, Thomas ED, et al. The treatment of chronic granulocytic leukaemia in chronic phase by allogeneic marrow transplantation. Lancet 2: 227-228, 1982.

12. Deeg HJ, Storb R, Thomas ED, et al. Cyclosporine as prophylaxis for graft-versus-host disease: A randomized study in patients undergoing marrow transplantation for acute nonlymphoblastic leukemia. Blood, 1984, in press.

8

13. Storb R, Deeg HJ, Thomas ED, et al. Marrow transplantation for chronic myelocytic leukemia: A controlled trial of cyclosporine versus methotrexate for prophylaxis of graft-versus-host disease. Blood, in press.

14. Martin PJ, Hansen JA, Storb R, et al. A clinical trial of in vitro depletion of T cells in donor marrow for prevention of acute graft-versus-host disease (GVHD). Transplant Proc, in press.

15. Clift RA, Beatty PG, Thomas ED, et al. Marrow transplantation from mismatched donors for the treatment of malignancy. Transplant Proc, in press.

16. Clift RA, Hansen JA, Thomas ED, et al. Marrow transplantation from donors other than HLA-identical siblings. Transplantation 28: 235-242, 1979.

This work was supported in part by grants CA 18029, CA 18221, CA 15704 from the National Cancer Institute DHHS. We would like to thank Dr. D. Winter, Sandoz Inc., for his support and for supplying cyclosporine.

Exp. Hematol. (suppl. 17) 13:9–10 (1985)
© International Society for Experimental Hematology

Factors Determining Relapse and Survival

A. J. Barrett

Department of Haematology, Westminster Hospital, London SW1, Great Britain

INTRODUCTION

Between 1979 and 1983 we have treated 63 adults and children with ALL by allogeneic BMT either in first remission for poor risk patients or as a rescue procedure for patients who have relapsed after adequate chemotherapy. While the transplant procedure was relatively well tolerated, the major problem had been relapse of leukaemia. The characteristics of relapse after BMT for ALL, its prediction from prognostic factors and the results of leukaemia reinduction treatment are described.

PATIENTS AND METHOD

The transplant procedure has been described in full previously (1). All patients received a combination chemotherapy pre-irradiation schedule which included Vincristine and Prednisolone and either Daunorubicin 50mg/m^2 x 2, Cytosine arabinoside 300mg/m^2 twice daily x 4 and VM26 200mg/m^2 x 2 (VRAPID), or Cyclophosphamide 60mg/Kg x 2 (VIPER). Whole body irradiation was given to a total dose of 9.5Gy delivered by a linear accelerator or a cobalt source at a dose rate of less than 3cGy/min.

RESULTS

Overall survival
Of the sixty-three patients transplanted, twelve (19%) died from complications associated with BMT - seven before 75d after BMT and five between 75d and 706d after BMT. Twenty-one patients (33%) relapsed of whom sixteen (25%) are dead. The remainder are well and leading a full life although three continue on treatment for chronic GVHD affecting the mouth and skin. The actuarial survival for the whole group is 38% at five years after BMT.

Factors predicting relapse
The effect on relapse of standard prognostic features and other variables was studied. The method of Kaplan and Meier was used to determine the relapse risk and significant differences between predicted survivals was tested by log rank analysis.

Remission status
A third of patients transplanted in second or subsequent remission had prognostic features at diagnosis similar to the (poor risk) first remission transplant group. These patients had a higher relapse risk than those grafted in first remission (P = < 0.05). Conversely, a group of "good prognosis" patients transplanted in second remission fared better than patients transplanted in first remission. The relapse probability of the good and poor risk second and subsequent remission transplant groups also differed significantly (P = < 0.05). (Table 1)

TABLE 1

Standard prognostic features at diagnosis demonstrating poor risk features of first CR patients

Poor prognostic factor	Score	First remission patients (16) Percent of group	Other remission patients (38 Percent of group
Male sex	1	81%	63%
Age > 14 at diagnosis	1	69%	24%
Presenting WBC > 30 x 10^9/l	1	37%	26%
Cell type Not C-ALL	1	69%	7%
"Good" score 0 - 1		0%	68%
"Bad" score 2 - 4		100%	32%

10

Relapse in second and subsequent remission BMT
Twenty-one patients with "slow disease" (diagnosis
to relapse interval greater than 2 years) had a 31%
relapse probability compared with a relapse
probability of 79% in twenty patients with "fast
disease" (diagnosis to relapse interval less than 2
years) (P = < 0.001). The difference was even
greater when comparing actuarial survival of the two
groups: slow disease patients had a survival
probability of 81% compared with 15% for fast
disease patients (P = < 0.0001). This was due to
the continued survival of four slow disease patients
who had relapsed after their graft and subsequently
achieved sustained remission (Fig.1)
Other factors
No effect of treatment schedule (VIPER or VRAPID) or
GVHD on relapse risk was found.

Treatment of relapsed patients
Nineteen of twenty-one relapsed patients received
Vincristine, Prednisolone and other agents including
daunorubicin, VM26, Cytosine Arabinoside, and
Vindesine. Patients with CNS disease received
weekly methotrexate alternating with cytosine
arabinoside by lumbar puncture or via an Omaya
reservoir. Testicular relapse was treated by
orchidectomy at diagnosis or by 12Gy radiation to
both testes (2 patients). Fourteen patients,
including two who achieved a partial remission,
ultimately died of complications associated with
relapsed leukaemia. Seven patients achieved a
sustained remission with relative ease. They
supported induction treatment well with
pancytopenias of normal duration following
chemotherapy. BMT was attempted in two of these
patients. One patient died in remission of
infection associated with severe gastrointestinal
mucositis from intermediate dose cytosine
arabinoside, one day before BMT. The second
patient was given a BMT from her original donor
following melphalan 180mg/m². She died in
remission of severe acute gastrointestinal and liver
GVHD on day 27 after BMT. Five patients survive in
remission. Two have stopped maintenance treatment.

DISCUSSION

The analysis highlights several important
considerations for evaluating treatment studies and
for selecting appropriate treatment for ALL.

1. Prognostic features at diagnosis and those
   associated with pace of disease transcend other
   variables in determining relapse risk. Any
   analysis comparing treatment schedules in
   grafted or non-grafted ALL patients must take
   these prognostic criteria into account if valid
   comparative studies are to be made.

2. Patients with poor prognosis disease at
   diagnosis should ideally receive BMT in first
   remission.

3. Treatment of patients in second or subsequent
   remission should be selected by the pace of the
   disease: fast disease patients (patients
   relapsing on maintenance treatment) have poor
   prognosis with chemotherapy (2). One
   comparative study has shown that BMT is
   superior to chemotherapy in this patient group
   (3). The results of BMT in our study are
   disappointing. These patients might therefore
   benefit from more intensive chemoradiotherapy
   BMT schedules.

4. Slow disease patients have a low risk of
   relapse after BMT and comparative studies of
   chemotherapy vs. BMT for this patient group are
   indicated.

It is possible to identify a group of post BMT
relapsed ALL patients who should receive further
treatment since they are likely to achieve long
remissions. They are in general patients with a
diagnosis to first relapse interval of greater than
two years, "slow disease" who have solitary
relapses, either in the bone marrow or testes and
have a disease free interval after BMT of over 500
days. Remission was reinduced using conventional
chemotherapy and their prolonged survival after BMT
relapse discourages retransplantation in such
patients who achieve remission.

Prospective study: in the light of these results,
the pre-graft regimen has been modified to attempt
to reduce the relapse incidence of ALL patients
after BMT. Low relapse risk patients now receive
V-RAPID using 10.5Gy TBI in a single fraction while
high risk patients receive V-RAPID with 13.5Gy TBI
given in two fractions. Since 3 out of 37 males
had isolated testicular relapses after BMT they now
receive testicular irradiation to 12Gy prior to BMT.
Preliminary results of this approach are
encouraging.

FIG.1

Prognostic score at
presentation
< 0.05

Blast cell count
at presentation
< 0.05

Disease pace
< 0.001

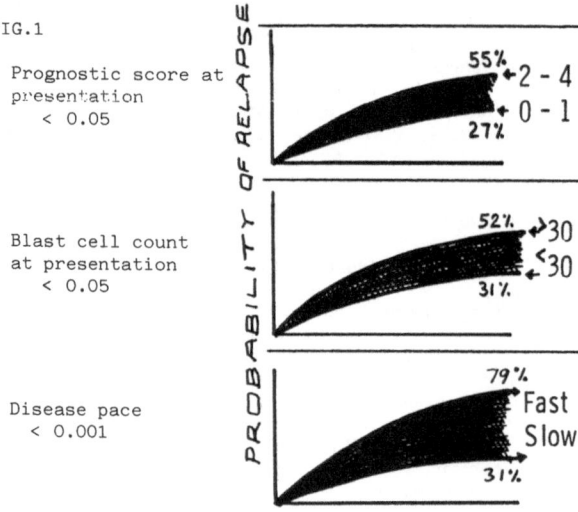

REFERENCES

1. BARRETT, A.J., KENDRA, J.R., LUCAS, C.F., JOSS,
   D.V., JOSHI, R., DESAI, M., HUGH-JONES, K.,
   PHILLIPS, R.H., ROGERS, T.R., TABARA, S.,
   WILLIAMSON, S., HOBBS, J.R. (1982) Bone marrow
   transplantation for acute lymphoblastic
   leukaemia. British Journal of Haematology 52,
   181-188

2. CHESSELLS, J.M., CORNBLEET, M. (1979)
   Combination chemotherapy for bone marrow
   relapse in childhood lymphoblastic leukaemia.
   Medical and Pediatric Oncology 6(4), 359-365.

3. JOHNSON, F.L., THOMAS, E.D., CLARK, B.S.,
   CHARD, R.L. HARTMANN, J.R., STORB, R. (1981) A
   comparison of marrow transplantation with
   chemotherapy for children with acute
   lymphoblastic leukaemia in second or subsequent
   remission. New England Journal of Medicine,
   305, 846-854.

Exp. Hematol. (suppl. 17) 13:11 (1985)
© International Society for Experimental Hematology

High Dose ARA-C and VP-16 as Preconditioning for Marrow Transplantation before Cyclophosphamide and Total Body Irradiation for Patients with Acute Lymphocytic Leukemia

A. Gratwohl, B. Osterwalder, A. Lori, C. Nissen, and B. Speck

Division of Hematology, Department of Internal Medicine, University Clinic, Kantonsspital Basel, Switzerland

Relapse remains the major problem following bone marrow transplantation for acute lymphocytic leukemia (ALL). Better ideas are needed and include changes in the conditioning regimen, fractionated radiotherapy and/or posttransplant chemotherapy. Increased chemotherapy so far has invariably augmented transplant related mortality, e.g. interstitial pneumonia, GvHD and infections. In an attempt to bypass this increased toxicity we tested the following protocol in a pilot study.

All patients with ALL and high risk for relapse were entered into this protocol, using High dose Ara-C (HdAra-C) and VP-16. HdAra-C was given $3g/m^2$ as a 1-hour infusion q 12 hours for 6 days (12 doses, day 1-6) and VP-16 was given as a continuous infusion $100 \ mg/m^2$ per day for 5 days (day 1-5). As soon as patients begun to recover their white blood cell count after the nadir, they were transferred to the transplant unit and the conditioning with Cy (2x60 mg/kg) and total body irradiation (10Gy) was started, if possible the first day of a total white blood cell count $>1x10^9/1$. All were given Cy-A as prophylaxis against GvHD and all were nursed in steril units as reported.

7 patients were treated (table). All tolerated HdAra-C + VP-16 with acceptable toxicity. Nausea occured in all, generalized skin rash and exanthema in 3 and moderate conjunctivitis despite prophylaxis in 3. One patient suffered severe, 3 mild CNS toxicity. All 4 recovered completely. 5 patients had fever, clearly associated with the HdAra-C but 3 of them developed in addition proven septicemia. Aplasia was profound in all patients with a nadir of 0 total white blood cell count in all patients. All recovered and showed no signs of toxicity at the day of the first dose of Cyclophosphamide.

Patient	204	208	212	220	226	228	237
Age	37y	16y	8y	7y	17y	24y	14y
Sex	m	m	f	m	m	f	f
Type of ALL	O	C	C	T	B	C	C
Status	2drr	2drr*	2dr*	1CR	1CR	1CR	2dr
BM blasts							
pre Ara-C	+	+	+	-	-	-	+
post Ara-C	+	-	-	-	-	-	-
days							
AraC-Cy	24	25	28	28	27	30	30
outcome	✝	a/w	a/w	a/w	✝	a/w	✝
cause	relapse	-	-	-	GvHD/aspergillus	-	B.subtilis sepsis
days	260	+354	+306	+217	114	+67	6

r	relapse
rr	relapse, refractory to reinduction
*	prior CNS relapse
a/w	alive and well
CR	complete remission

The posttransplant course was complicated in two patients. Patient 237 developed fulminant septicemia with B. subtilis and died of acute intracerebral hemorrhage on day 6. Patient 226 developed pericarditis at 1 week (infection, Cyclophosphamide?), and intestinal GvHD, pancytopenia and aplasia at 3 months. He died in aplasia with intestinal GvHD and aspergillus enteritis. One patient relapsed. 4 patients are well and alive with no signs of leukemia.

This study shows that intensive chemotherapy can be given before marrow transplantation with acceptable morbidity when some time is allowed to regenerate the tissues although the death in patient 237 could be due to the previous aplasia. One patient relapsed. However, he as well as the two subsequent patients had refractory leukemia, resistant to reinduction chemotherapy. All 3 went into remission and patients 208 and 212 remain in remission. This result suggests some optimism, but should be further tested in a prospective study.

Speck B, Gratwohl A, Nissen C, Osterwalder B, Signer E, Jeannet M Knochenmarktransplantation bei Leukämie und aplastischer Anämie Schweiz med Wschr 113, 622 - 629 (1983)

Exp. Hematol. (suppl. 17) 13: 12–13 (1985)
© International Society for Experimental Hematology

Melphalan plus Total Body Irradiation Versus Cyclophosphamide plus Total Body Irradiation prior to Bone Marrow Transplant in Acute Myeloid Leukemia in First Remission

G. D. Goss[1], R. L. Powles[1], Ann Barrett[1], J. Millar[1], M. Gore[1], F. Porta[2], P. Pimentel[1], S. Bagnulo[1], and F. Hernandez[1]

[1] The Royal Marsden Hospital, Downs Road, Sutton, Surrey SM2 5PT, Great Britain
[2] Clinica Pediatrica, Universita di Pavia, Pavia, Italy

A major factor influencing long-term survival in patients with acute leukaemia undergoing bone marrow transplant (BMT) is relapse of their leukaemia following transplant. A relapse rate of 12-25% has been reported for patients with acute myeloid leukaemia transplanted in first remission.[1,2] A number of attempts to increase the anti-leukaemic action of the 'conditioning' have been made, either by increasing the effective dose of total body irradiation (TBI) and/or chemotherapy.[3,7] In a prospective randomised trial we compared cyclophosphamide (CY) plus TBI with melphalan plus TBI as conditioning prior to transplant. This is an ongoing trial and we report here the preliminary results of this trial.

METHOD

Between June 1981 and January 1985, 54 patients with acute myeloid leukaemia in first remission with HLA matched donors were entered into a prospective randomised study. This study compared CY 1.8 g/m^2 intravenously given on two consecutive days followed 36 hours later by 10 Gy TBI given as a single dose, at a rate of 2.5 rads/min with a single dose of melphalan 110 mg/m^2 intravenously followed 12-18 hours later by 10 Gy TBI given as a single dose at a rate of 2.5 rads/min, as conditioning therapy prior to transplant. Patients receiving melphalan plus TBI were given a small 'priming' dose of CY 300 mg/m^2 intravenously seven days prior to the melphalan. Thirty-four patients have received CY plus TBI, whereas 20 patients have received melphalan plus TBI. The different numbers in the two arms of the study are because patients who had ABO blood group mismatched donors were not entered into the melphalan/TBI arm. The reason for this is that patients receiving a priming dose of CY maintained high levels of anti-A and/or anti-B antibody levels despite plasmaphoresis and three patients in a pilot study had a severe haemolytic crisis (data to be published) following donor marrow infusion. All patients were nursed in protective isolation in cubicles with filtered positive-pressure ventilation, received sterile food and were given non-absorbable anti-microbial drugs by mouth for intestinal decontamination. All patients received systemic antibiotics as required for infections. Platelets were given prophylactically when the platelet count fell below 20,000/mm^3. All patients received cyclosporin A (CYA) as prophylaxis against GVHD.

RESULTS

One of 20 patients receiving melphalan/TBI has relapsed compared with 5 of 34 receiving CY/TBI as conditioning therapy. Eleven of 20 patients who received melphalan/TBI are alive and well, compared with 21 of 34 in the CY/TBI group from 12-182 weeks post transplant.

Of the 9 deaths in the melphalan/TBI group, 4 were initiated by the development of renal failure (44%) compared with none out of the 13 deaths in the CY/TBI group. In the melphalan/TBI group 8 out of 20 patients developed renal failure. Dividing the melphalan/TBI groups into 2 cohorts (the first 10 and the second 10 transplanted patients) 7 out of 10 in the first cohort compared with one out of 10 in the second cohort developed renal failure.

The overall disease-free survival from 12-182 weeks post-transplant is 55% and 58% (11 out of 20; 20 out of 34) for the melphalan/TBI and CY/TBI groups respectively.

DISCUSSION

A number of transplant centres have tried to decrease the incidence of leukaemic relapse following bone marrow transplant, by increasing the anti-leukaemic effect of the conditioning regimen.[3,4] This has to a large extent been offset by an unacceptable increase in the toxicity of the conditioning regimen and consequently there has been no overall improvement in survival. The decision to use melphalan as a conditioning agent was based on the fact that melphalan is a stem cell poison and consequently has good anti-leukaemia potential.[5]

The results, although not statistically significant, suggest that melphalan may have a better anti-leukaemia action, with only one patient in the melphalan/TBI group relapsing. Unfortunately, the overall survival for the melphalan/TBI group as compared with the CY/TBI group has not improved and if anything at this time appears to be worse. If, however, the cause of death in the two groups are considered, 4 out of 9 (44%) in the melphalan/TBI group were due to renal failure, wheras none in the CY/TBI group were due to renal failure. There are a number of factors in these patients that could contribute to the renal failure, viz, aminoglycosides, amphotericin, irradiation, sepsis and CYA. All these factors, however, are operative in both the melphalan/TBI plus the CY/TBI groups, and we know from our experience in autologous transplantation that melphalan is nephrotoxic. Therefore, it must be the melphalan that is the responsible agent. In an attempt to decrease the toxicity of melphalan, we are now carefully monitoring drug levels in our patients (in particular aminoglycoside levels) ensuring adequate hydration, and have decreased the dose of CYA from CYA 25 mg/kg/day intravenously for 5 days followed by 8 mg/kg/day orally to CYA 8 mg/kg/day orally. Dividing the melphalan/TBI group into two cohorts it can be seen that the first cohort of 10 patients had 7 episodes of renal failure and 4 of these 7 patients died as a result of this initial renal failure. In the second cohort of 10 patients only one patient developed renal failure, and this patient is alive and well. Clearly our ability to use melphalan has improved.

This ability to use melphalan whilst limiting its toxicity should result in a decrease in the mortality rate in the immediate post-transplant period. This, together with the potential anti-leukaemia action of melphalan should in time be translated into an increase in the overall disease-free survival.

REFERENCES

1. Powles RL, Clink HM, Bandini G, et al.The place of bone marrow transplantation in acute myelogenous leukaemia. Lancet i: 1047-1050, 1980.

2. Zwaan FE, Hermans J, Barrett AJ, et al. Bone marrow transplantation for acute non-lymphoblastic leukaemia: A survey of the European Group for Bone Marrow Transplantation. (EGBMT). Br J Haematol 56: 645-653, 1984.

3. Thomas ED, Appelbaum FR, Buckner CD, et al. Marrow transplantation for acute nonlymphocytic leukaemia. (Ed. Gale RP) Recent Advances in Bone Marrow Transplantation. Pub. Alan R Liss Inc, New York 1983, pp, 61-70.

4. Santos GW, Tutschka PJ, Brookmeyer R, et al. Marrow transplantation for acute non-lymphocytic leukaemia after treatment with busulfan and cyclophosphamide. NEJM 309: 22; 1347-1353.

5. Bergsagel DE. An assessment of massive dose chemotherapy for malignant disease. Canad Med Assoc J 104: 31-36, 1971.

Leukemia II

Exp. Hematol. (suppl. 17) 13: 14–15 (1985)
© International Society for Experimental Hematology

Bone Marrow Transplantation for Patients in the Chronic Phase of Chronic Granulocytic Leukaemia: Apparent Low Incidence of Relapse within the First Two Years Post-BMT

J. M. Goldman, J. F. Apperley, R. E. Marcus, J. Hows, E. C. Gordon-Smith, C. D. Reid, D. Catovsky, and D. A. G. Galton

Hammersmith Hospital and Royal Postgraduate Medical School, London and Northwick Park Hospital, Harrow, Great Britain

SUMMARY

Of 50 patients transplanted in the chronic phase of chronic granulocytic leukaemia (CGL), 38 (76%) survive without evidence of leukaemia. One of these patients had Ph'+ve marrow metaphases one year post-transplant that have now disappeared. The actuarial 3-year survival for these patients is 72%. This contrasts with results of transplanting 18 patients in later phases of CGL: only 6 survive and the actuarial 3-year survival is 24%.

INTRODUCTION

We began in 1981 to treat patients in the chronic phase of chronic granulocytic leukaemia (CGL) by high dose chemoradiotherapy and allogeneic bone marrow transplantation (BMT) using HLA-identical sibs as marrow donors. The preliminary results of this programme are summarized in this paper.

PATIENTS AND METHODS

Between March 1981 and December 1984 we treated 52 patients with CGL in the chronic phase (51 Ph'+ve, 1 Ph'-ve) by high dose chemotherapy followed by fractionated total body irradiation (2Gy x 5 or 6) followed by transfusion of bone marrow cells collected from their HLA-identical sibs (1). Patients who retained their spleens at the time of BMT received in addition splenic irradiation (5Gy x 2). All but 5 patients received cyclosporine in an attempt to prevent or mitigate the severity of graft-versus-host disease. The 17 patients treated most recently received marrow that had been T-cell depleted by incubation ex vivo with monoclonal antibodies (Campath-1, n=15; MBG6 + RFT8, n=2). Graft-versus-host disease was classified by criteria established in Seattle. Survival was analysed on 31st December 1984. Results were compared inter alia with those achieved by treating simultaneously a group of 18 patients classified before BMT as blastic transformation (n=3), accelerated phase (n=9), second chronic phase (n=4) or secondary chronic phase (n=2).

RESULTS

From the 52 patients transplanted in chronic phase, 2 were excluded from further analysis because they proved difficult to classify. One of these patients relapsed 4 months after BMT in obvious blastic transformation; review of her pre-BMT haematological findings showed that she had undoubtedly been erroneously classified as chronic phase. The second patient was transplanted with T-depleted marrow which failed to engraft. She was then 'rescued' with cryopreserved autologous stem cells and restored to chronic phase CGL. Thus she is no longer at risk for dying of BMT-related causes, nor can she correctly be classified as a leukaemic relapse.

Thirty-eight of these 50 patients are alive and free of evidence of leukaemia at the date of analysis; one patient had cytogenetic evidence of leukaemic relapse one year post-BMT but is now cytogenetically normal. He has been classified as a leukaemic relapse even though his prospects for long-term survival seem good. The actuarial 3-year survival for these patients is 72% (Figure). Of the 18 patients transplanted in later phases of their disease, 6 survived at the date of analysis and the actuarial three year survival is 24%. The difference between these two groups of patients is of course highly significant (p<0.001).

DISCUSSION

The incidence and severity of graft-versus-host disease in this group of patients seems to us to be very similar to what might have been observed in a group of patients of comparable age transplanted for acute myeloid leukaemia. Likewise the incidence of CMV pneumonitis and of idiopathic interstitial pneumonitis seems not to be greatly different from what might have been expected in other transplant series. We have however been impressed by the relatively low incidence of relapse within the first two years of BMT in the patients transplanted in chronic phase. Our own results seem to run parallel to those report from the International Bone Marrow Transplant Registry (2), though the Registry of course includes data on some of the patients reported in this paper. Because of the potentially slow evolution of CGL it is too early to make any prediction about the incidence of relapse in the first say 10 years after BMT.

We can define a number of problems which cannot yet be resolved: (1) We have difficulty defining relapse in this group of patients because the finding of Ph'+ve metaphases post-BMT does not necessarily mean that leukaemia will inexorably recur (see above); (2) We cannot yet recommend a definite upper age limit for BMT because we hope that the introduction of T-cell depletion may make BMT safer for those in the age range 40-50; (3) We do not know what measures are necessary for handling the spleen at the time of BMT - splenectomy, splenic irradiation or nothing; and most important (4) We are not yet able safely to perform transplants using partially mis-matched family members or phenotypically matched unrelated individuals as donors.

REFERENCES

(1) Goldman JM, Baughan ASJ, McCarthy DM et al (1982): Marrow transplantation for patientsin the chronic phase of chronic granulocytic leukaemia. Lancet 1. 623-625.

(2) Speck B, Bortin MM, Champlin R et al (1984): Allogeneic bone marrow transplantation for chronic myelogenous leukaemia. Lancet 1. 665-668.

FIGURE

Actuarial survival from date of BMT for 50 patients with CGL in chronic phase transplanted with HLA-identical sib marrow according to status of disease at BMT.

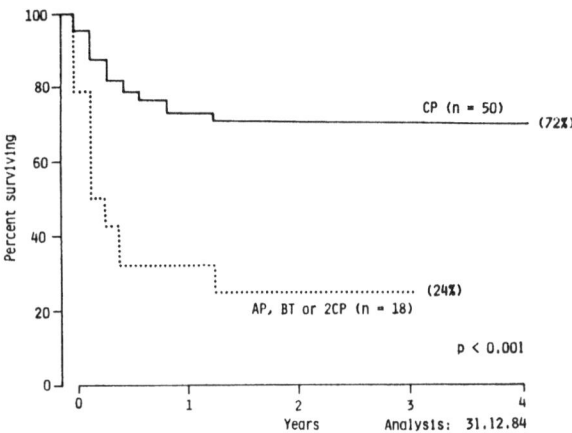

CP=chronic phase, AP=accelerated phase, BT=blastic transformation, 2CP=second or secondary chronic phase. The median follow-up period for all survivors is 22 months, range 1 to 44 monnths. Date of analysis: 31.12.84.

Exp. Hematol. (suppl. 17) 13:16 (1985)
© International Society for Experimental Hematology

Serial Chromosome Studies in Transplanted Ph1 + CML Patients

Sporadic Observation of Ph1+ Cells after BMT

Alfonso Zaccaria [1], Gianantonio Rosti [1], Nicoletta Testoni [1], Paolo Ricci [1], Cristina Guardigli [1], Simona Rizzi [1], Michele Cavo [1], Enza Barbieri [2], and Sante Tura [1]

[1] Centro di Genetica e Citogenetica oncologica, Istituto di Ematologia "Lorenzo e Ariosto Seràgnoli" dell'Università degli Studi di Bologna, Bologna, Italy
[2] Istituto del Radio "Luigi Galvani" dell'Università degli Studi di Bologna, Bologna, Italy

The cytogenetic follow-up of patients with chronic myeloid leukemia (CML) submitted to bone marrow transplantation (BMT) is particularly useful since this disease is marked by a specific chromosome aberration, the Philadelphia chromosome (Ph1) and residual leukemic cells may be easily detected. We report on the sporadic observation of Ph1+ cells after BMT, without signs of relapse of the disease.

PATIENTS AND METHODS

Fifteen patients with Ph1 + CML were submitted to BMT. Age varied between 19 and 47 years.

Conditioning treatment consisted of Daunorubicin 2 mg/kg on day − 6, Cyclophosphamide 60 mg/kg on days − 5 and − 4, followed, on day − 1 by total body irradiation, 10 Gy from a single ^{60}Co source, in a single fraction at a dose-rate ranging between 2.8 and 5 rads/min. In addition, 1 patient in accelerated phase received Arabinosyl Cytosine and 1, in blastic phase, Busulfan.

The karyotypes were performed after 24 hrs culture and were banded with trypsin and quinacrine mustard.

RESULTS

Seventyseven chromosome studies were performed in the 15 patients and 2.133 metaphases were scored.

In 3 patients sporadic Ph1+ cells were observed (Table 1). Ph1+ metaphases were observed after 11 and 28 days from BMT in patient n. 1, after 123 days in patient n. 2 and after 54 days in patient n. 3. The patients are in clinical, hematological and cytogenetical complete remission 368, 302 and 272 days after BMT.

DISCUSSION

These data indicate that neoplastic cells may survive and be detected up to several weeks after BMT without evidence of persisting or recurring leukemia. Moreover, sequential chromosome studies have not allowed to observe neoplastic cells any more up to 70-200 days after their detection. Lawler et Al. demonstrated that recipient cells may still be detected in the bone marrow some weeks after BMT for acute leukemia, without signs of relapse (1). We think that mechanisms other than cell destruction (immunological? cell-to-cell competition?, etc.) may be involved in reducing the leukemic clone under the level of detection. Chromosome studies may be very useful in understanding the behaviour of recipient and donor cells after BMT.

The knowledge of the mechanisms involved in controlling the residual disease could be usefully employed to prevent the recurrence of leukemia.

REFERENCES

1) Lawler SD et Al. - Cytogenetic studies on recipient of allogeneic bone marrow using the sex chromosomes as markers of cellular origin. Br J Haematol, 56, 431, 1984.

Table 1.

Case age/sex	Day	Karyotype	Clinical status	Donor's karyotype
1. M.G. 39,F	− 298	46,XX,Ph1+	CML, diagn.	
	− 9	46,XX,Ph1+	Before BMT	46,XX
	+ 11	46,XX(58)/ 46,XX,Ph1+(2)	Engraftment	
	+ 28	46,XX(99)/ 46,XX,Ph1+(1)	CR	
	+ 68	46,XX(30)	CR	
	+ 95	46,XX(40)	CR	
	+ 236	46,XX(30)	CR	
2. M.A. 24,M	− 84	46,XY,Ph1+	CML, diagn.	
	− 21	46,XY,Ph1+(3)/ 46,XY,Ph1+, +8(7)	Before BMT	46,XX
	+ 11	46,XX(36)	Engraftment	
	+ 60	46,XX(25)	CR	
	+ 123	46,XX(16)/ 46,XY,Ph1+(1)	CR	
	+ 178	46,XX(52)	CR	
	+ 200	46,XX(50)	CR	
3. P.G. 27,M	− 112	47,XY,Ph1+,+Ph1	CML, diagn.	
	− 11	47,XY,Ph1+,+Ph1	Before BMT	46,XX
	+ 11	46,XX(30)	Engraftment	
	+ 54	46,XX(99)/ 47,XY,Ph1+,+Ph1(1)	CR	
	+ 157	46,XX(10)	CR	
	+ 193	46,XX(50)	CR	

This study was supported by C.N.R., Rome, Progetto Finalizzato Oncologia, contracts n. 84.00834.44 and 84.00613.44.

Exp. Hematol. (suppl. 17) 13:17 (1985)
© International Society for Experimental Hematology

Bone Marrow Transplantation in Multiple Myeloma

Sante Tura, Michele Cavo, Michele Baccarani, Paolo Ricci, Giuseppe Bandini, Daniela Belletti, Loretta Leardini, and GianPiero Frezza

Institute of Hematology "Lorenzo & Ariosto Seràgnoli", S. Orsola's University Hospital, Bologna, Italy

The shortcomings of the drugs currently available for the treatment of multiple myeloma (MM) and, in particular, their inability to achieve cures have encouraged in the last years the search for different therapeutic approaches to the disease. Based on the high sensitiveness of the myeloma clone to both ionizing radiation and alkylating agents bone marrow transplantation (BMT) has been proposed in selected patients with an HLA compatible donor. Therapeutic results are, however, still preliminary and conflicting: thus, we wish to report an additonal case we have carried out one year ago.

The patient, a caucasion woman aged 35, had a 3 year history of MM, IgG/K type, stage III A. Diagnosis was made on the basis of more than 80°/o plasma cells in the bone marrow and a high serum M protein concentration (9.7 g/dl). She received six montly 4-day courses of high-dose melphalan and prednisone (MP), as described elsewhere (1), until remission occurred. Remission lasted unmaintained for 9 months, after which the disease relapsed. Cyclic MP were resumed and again induced a marked decrease in tumour mass.

In January 1984, i.e. 5 months after the relapse, BMT was performed from the patient's HLA-identical, MLC-negative, sister. At this time laboratory features showed a low serum M protein concentration (1.8 g/dl) and about 10°/o monoclonal plasma cells in the bone marrow. Skeletal x-ray survey was negative for osteolytic lesions. Conditioning treatment consisted of oral melphalan (1 mg/Kg/day from Day – 9 to Day – 5), cyclophosphamide (60 mg/Kg/day i.v. on Days – 4 and – 3) and TBI (1000 rads in a single fraction at a dose rate of 3.2 rads/min on Day – 1), followed by the infusion of 5.2 x 10^8 marrow cells/Kg. Engraftment was prompt and on day 20 white cell and platelet counts exceeded 3 x 10^9/l and 50 x 10^9/l, respectively. Bone marrow aspiration, performed on Day 18, revealed normal myelopoiesis and less than 5°/o polyclonal plasma cells. Disappearance of monoclonal protein at serum electrophoresis and immunoelectrophoresis was recorded within 47 days after BMT. Cyclosporin A, as described elsewhere (2), and acycloguanosine (5 mg/Kg/day i.v. from Day – 1 to Day 12) were given as prophylaxis against GVHD and herpes virus infections. The early post transplant course was uneventful and the patient was discharged on Day 23. Genital herpes simplex, without costitutional symptoms, developed on Day 33 and was successfully treated with topical idoxuridine. On day 45 the patient was again admitted with symptoms and signs of meningoencephalitis. A cerebrospinal fluid sample showed 300 lymphocytes/μl and was negative for viruses; antiviral antibody titers didn't evidence any significant change. Treatment consisted of high-dose acycloguanosine (30 mg/Kg/day i.v. for 9 days) and dexamethasone (0.5 mg/Kg/day i.v. for 9 days) and within 7 days a complete disappearance of the neurological picture was observed. At the time of writing (Day 365) the patient is in good health and is haematologically normal.

Both the present case and those previously reported in the literature (3,4) appear to suggest the potential usefulness of BMT in MM. We believe that this procedure deserves strong consideration in young patients, given the disappointingly slow progresses in the conventional treatment of MM and the ominous prognosis of the disease.

REFERENCES

1. Cavo M., Baccarani M., Gobbi M., Tura S. (1983) - High-dose melphalan for multiple myeloma. Lancet ii: 1194.

2. Bandini G., Ricci P., Rosti G., et al. (1984) - Cyclosporin A (Cy-A) prophylaxis of graft versus host disease (GVHD) in allogeneic bone marrow transplantation. Exp. Hematol. 12 (Suppl. 15): 74.

3. Osserman EF., DiRe LB., DiRe J., et al. (1982) - Identical twin marrow transplantation in multiple myeloma. Acta Haemat. 68: 215.

4. Higby DJ., Brass C., Fitzpatrick J., Henderson ES. (1982) - Bone marrow transplantation in multiple myeloma: a case report with protein studies. Proc of ASCO C-747: 192.

ACKNOWLEDGMENTS

This investigation was supported by grant 84.00834.44 from the C.N.R., Rome, Italy.

Autologous BMT I

ABMT without Marrow Purging

Exp. Hematol. (suppl. 17) 13:18–19 (1985)
© International Society for Experimental Hematology

Autologous Bone Marrow Transplantation for Acute Leukemia in Remission: Second European Survey

N. C. Gorin, P. Aegerter, and Y. Parlier

For the working party on autologous bone marrow transplantation (President: J. Goldman) of the European bone marrow transplantation group

Autologous bone marrow transplantation (ABMT) is now extensively used to consolidate patients in remission of acute leukemia, both with cleansed or non cleansed marrow, in an effort to prolong disease free survival and hopefully increase the cure rate. It has been one of the major goals of the working party on ABMT of the European bone marrow transplantation group (EBMTG) to collect all available data in Europe and provide a computerized analysis leading to recommendations for further evaluation. The 1983 survey on a total of 135 patients showed that ABMT at time of relapse was associated with poor survival (< 10% at 2 years). In contrast, in a series of 28 patients with ANLL autografted in first complete remission (CR), 10 were disease free with a long term follow up greater than 1 year, including 6 long term survivors (> 2 years). Therefore the 1984 survey was restricted to ABMT delivered in the consolidation mode. Results of this survey are presented here.

I - MATERIAL AND METHODS.

A - QUESTIONNAIRE :

Computer forms approved at the 1983 EBMTG meeting were sent to all transplant teams in May and October 1984. All information collected before January 1st 1985 was taken into account and the data were analized up to October 31st 1984. Questions raised included : - Age and sex. - Classification of leukemia by cytological examination (FAB) and immunotyping. - Presence of poor risk criteria such as
1) leucocyte count > 100.10^9/l at presentation
2) acute leukemia secondary to previous malignancies
3) previous extramedullary localization including CNS
4) presence of a Philadelphia chromosome.
Patients were defined as having standard risk leukemia in the absence of all precited characteristics, or high risk leukemia otherwise. - Status of the patient at time of marrow collection, and ABMT.
- Details of high dose regimen preceeding ABMT including for total body irradiation : total dose delivered or fractionnated, organ shielding, dose rate at the source and estimated mean dose rate. - Dose of marrow infused in nucleated cells/kg and CFUGM/kg. - If used details on marrow cleansing procedure including, for treatment with cyclophosphamide derivatives, the precise dose per number of treated cells. - Course and follow-up including the status of the patient in relation to leukemia, infectious complications, cause of death.

B - POPULATION OF PATIENTS :

148 charts from 15 European institutions were collected. 5 institutions reported more than 10 patients. The median age of patients submitted to ABMT was 26 years, 22 y in ALL (range 2 - 55) and 32 Y in ANLL (2 - 53). The sex ratio M/F was 86/62. Of 65 patients with ALL, 30 were autografted in first CR, 27 in second CR and 8 either in a subsequent CR or in partial remission (PR). Of 77 patients with ANLL, 58 were in CR1, 17 in CR2, 2 in PR. The median time from CR to marrow collection was 3 months in patients with ALL and 4 months in ANLL. The median time from CR to ABMT was 4 months in ALL and 5 months in ANLL. The median time from marrow collection to ABMT was 1 month both in ALL and ANLL. 70 patients were autografted with non treated marrow (27 ALL, 41 ANLL, 2 unclassified). 62 patients had their marrow cleansed by 4 HC (6) or ASTA Z (56)(23 ALL, 35 ANLL, 4 unclassified). According to results of phase 1 studies and specifications furnished by various teams, we defined optimal conditions for marrow cleansing by cyclophosphamide derivatives as corresponding to a dose > 50 ug/2.10^7 nucleated cells, and an incubation at 37 dgC for 37 mn. These conditions were reached in 47 cases (76%). Monoclonal antibodies were used in 14 ALL and 1 ANLL. One patient with T ALL had his marrow treated with deoxycoformycin + deoxyadenosine. The high dose consolidation regimen delivered prior to ABMT consisted of TBI, single dose (35 ALL, 32 ANLL, 5 unclassified) or fractionnated (FTBI)(16 ALL, 7 ANLL), the BACT or TACC regimen (2 ALL, 17 ANLL), the UCH regimen (11 ALL, 12 ANLL) and other combinations (9 ANLL), in a total of 146 analyzable charts.

C - ANALYSIS OF RESULTS :

All data were entered in an IBM X T microcomputer (capacity 10 megabytes). Curves plotted to show the distribution of disease free survival (DFS) and survival times for groups of patients were calculated by the method of Kaplan and Meier. Differences between distributions were determined by means of the Logrank test.

II - RESULTS.

A - GLOBAL ANALYSIS :

* DFS from ABMT in the whole population of patients with acute leukemia (ALL+ANLL) was 52.6% at 560 days with a plateau untill day 1365 (132 patients).
* In term of survival :
- there was no difference in the group of patients engrafted in CR1, whether they received purged (42 patients) or non purged (47 patients) marrow.
- On the other hand, patients in CR2 engrafted with purged marrow (23 patients) had a better survival than those receiving non purged marrow (20 patients) (68% VS 18% at 547 days).
Indeed, as will appear further, this advantage for purging in CR2 was essentially due to patients with ALL.

* Relapse following ABMT was associated with a very

poor survival : 41 patients, median survival at 90 days, 11% surviving at 730 days.

B - ALL (65 PATIENTS) :

* Age may be a prognostic factor with patients below 30 years having a better survival. However, the difference was not statistically significant (p < .1).

* The DFS was similar in patients engrafted in CR1 (28 pts) and in CR2 (25 pts) with a plateau at 52% and 60% respectively from day 365 to day 800. Similarly, there was no difference between these 2 groups in term of survival (60% at 583 days for patients in CR1 VS 49% at 346 days for patients in CR2).

* The value of marrow purging was not demonstrated by DFS analysis neither in CR1 nor in CR2. In contrast, by survival analysis, there seems to be an advantage for marrow purging in the group of patients grafted in CR2 : 80% survival with purged marrow (16 patients) versus 30% with non purged marrow (11 patients) at 547 days (not statistically significant). Marrow purging with cyclophosphamide derivatives at dosages we defined previously as "optimal"(16 patients) was statistically better (DFS 75% at 466 days) than all other purging procedures combined (44 patients, DFS : 41%)(p < 0.05).

* TBI was associated with the best survival over chemotherapy alone (TBI : 33 patients, 62% survival at 583 days - chemotherapy : 13 patients, 30% survival at 346 days. p < .05).

C - ANLL (77 PATIENTS) :

* There was a major advantage both in term of DFS and survival for patients autografted in 1st CR (51) over those autografted in second CR (16)(DFS : 73% with a plateau from day 547 to day 1277 versus 0% on day 255 p < .001 ; survival 47% on day 1152 versus 0% on day 803 p < .01).

* Marrow cleansing was not associated with improvement both from DFS and survival analysis, neither in CR1 nor in CR2. Although the difference is not statistically significant, there seems to be a trend in favour of autografting with non purged marrow in patients in CR1.

* TBI may be associated with a better DFS than chemotherapy alone (78% versus 48% at 730 days) (p < .1)(not statistically significant).

D - COMPARISON BETWEEN ALL AND ANLL :

By DFS analysis, results were significantly better for ANLL (79% versus 50%, on day 560 with a plateau untill day 887 for both. p < .01).

E - VALUE OF AN ESTIMATED OPTIMAL MANAGEMENT :

We selected 17 patients for the following reasons:
- All were consolidated in first CR
- The consolidation regimen used was heavy :
  TBI
  TACC or BACT
  UCH regimen
- All received marrow purged by ASTA Z 7557 or 4 HC at dosages considered to be high or "optimal" (> 50 ug/2.10^{7}nucleated cells)
- Also, as a consequence of the precited criteria, all these patients were treated by teams reporting more than 10 ABMT.
In this particular hyperselected group, the DFS was 80% at 547 days.

III - CONCLUSION.

1) 148 patients have been consolidated in remission of AL : 65 ALL, 77 ANLL, 6 others.
2) ABMT was done with non treated marrow in 70 cases, with cleansed marrow in 78 cases. A majority of treated marrows was cleansed by Cyclophosphamide derivatives (62).
3) Globally, there is a plateau of disease free survival (DFS) at 50% from day 547 to day 1365, and some indication that marrow purging is associated with a better survival only in patients consolidated in second CR.
4) In patients with ALL, the disease free survival is 55% both for CR1 and CR2.
TBI is associated with better results than chemotherapy alone.
In CR2, patients grafted with purged marrow may have a better survival than patients grafted with non purged marrow. Cleansing with cyclophosphamide derivatives at proper dosage is superior to other procedures.
5) In patients with ANLL autografted in CR1, there is a plateau of DFS at 70% from day 547 to day 1277. In contrast patients autografted in CR2 do poorly (30% DFS at 182 days).
There is a slight trend in favour of TBI over chemotherapy.
There is no detectable advantage of marrow purging.
6) Patients with standard risk AL in CR1 consolidated by TBI, TACC,BACT or UCH regimen followed by ABMT with marrow cleansed by Cyclophosphamide derivatives at high (optimal ?) dosage have the best disease free survival : 80% at 547 days (17 patients).

IV SUGGESTION.

1) Patients with ALL may be autografted in CR1 or CR2. Patients with ANLL should not be autografted beyond CR1.
2) Although marrow purging may improve the results for patients with ALL in CR2, there is yet no definitive conclusion. Therefore at present time both cleansed and non cleansed marrow may be used.
3) Give preference :
- to patients with standard risk leukemia in CR1
- to TBI
- to optimal cleansing with ASTA Z 7557 at appropriate dosage.

AUTOLOGOUS BONE MARROW TRANSPLANTATION IN EUROPE : PATIENTS WITH ACUTE LEUKEMIA IN REMISSION.

TEAM	COORDINATOR	NUMBER OF PATIENTS
BESANCON	HERVE	35
ST ANTOINE	GORIN	25
BLOOMSBURY	GOLDSTONE	23
GLASGOW	BURNETT	11
LEIPZIG	HELBIG	11
ROMA	MELONI	8
UTRECHT	VERDONCK	8
PARMA	RIZZOLI	7
NANTES	HAROUSSEAU	6
GENOVA	CARELLA	5
BERNE	BRUN DEL RE	3
PARMA + GENOVA	RIZZOLI + CARELLA	2
ROYAL FREE HOSP.	PRENTICE	2
BORDEAUX	J REIFFERS	1
ST ETIENNE	FREYCON	1
TOTAL		148

Data from Centre Paoli-Calmettes, Marseille (Dr Maraninchi) and from Katholieke Universiteit Nijmegen, the Netherlands (Dr De Witte) were communicated too late for inclusion in this study. They will appear in the next survey.

Exp. Hematol. (suppl. 17) 13:20–21 (1985)
© International Society for Experimental Hematology

Autologous Bone Marrow Transplantation for Lymphoma in Europe

A. H. Goldstone and L. D. Dones

For the EBMT Group, Department of Haematology, University College Hospital, London WC1, Great Britain

Computer Analysis by Leanne D. Dones, Clinical Operational Research Unit, University College, London, Great Britain

A computerised registry has now been established to collect European data on ABMT in non-Hodgkin's lymphoma and Hodgkin's disease. 9 centres have reported a total of 111 cases for computer analysis. NHL: 81 cases; HD: 29 cases.

Age and Sex Distribution

	NHL	HD
1 year	1	0
1-15	3	1
15-30	32	19
30-45	33	8
45-60	12	1
Males	54	20
Females	25	9

Histology

Histology	Status at ABMT:					
	D.	CR	PR	A	B	Total
HD NS gd. prog.				1	9	10
HD NS bd. prog.				2	7	9
HD LP						0
HD LD				1		1
HD MC			1	1	7	9
NHL int. grd.	3	4	1	1	7	16
NHL Brk. h.grd.	2		2			4
NHL lym. h.grd.	1	11	4	4	9	29
NHL oth. h.grd.	8	7	5	1	11	32
	14	22	13	10	51	110

(D=diagnosis, A=responding relapse, B=resistant relapse)

Immunology

	Unknown	34
(NHL only)	T-cell	20
	B-cell	16
	Null	3
	True histiocytic	8

Conditioning
Chemotherapy: HD 28 NHL 62
Chemo & DXR: HD 1 NHL 19

Purging
10/110 had marrow purged
    1   with T monoclonal
    2   with 4 HC
    7   with Asta 7

Results
Haemopoietic recovery is shown in relation to dose in Table 1.

Table 1. NHL & HD (110)

Nucl. cells	Mean time for neuts to recover (DAYS)	Mean time for leucs to recover (DAYS)	Mean Time for plates to recover (DAYS)
0 → 0.99	17.1(8)	19.9(9)	30.8(9)
1 → 1.99	16.9(36)	15.3(39)	24.2(37)
> 2	15.3(39)	14.7(39)	22.1(39)
Overall	16.2(83)	15.5(87)	23.9(85)

Haemopoietic recovery following ABMT to neutrophils $>0.5 \times 10^9/1$, leucocytes $>1.0 \times 10^9/1$, platelets $>50 \times 10^9/1$. ( )= number of observations in each category.
Results according to status at ABMT are shown in Tables 2 & 3 and Graphs 1 & 2.

Table 2. The effect of ABMT on NHL patients of differing status at time of graft.

	Status at ABMT:					
	D.	CR	PR	A	B	Total
Achieved CR	11	22	8	4	14	59
Toxic death	-	1	3	-	1	5
A&W in CR	8	15	3	-	4	30
Rlps. or prog. disease	6	6	6	6	21	45
Totals	14	22	12	6	27	81

Table 3. The effect of ABMT on HD patients of differing status at time of graft.

	Status at ABMT:					
	D.	CR	PR	A	B	Total
Achieved CR	-	-	-	2	14	16
Toxic death	-	-	-	1	5	6
A&W in CR	-	-	(1)	1	11	12
Rlps. or prog. disease	-	-	-	1	7	8
Totals	-	-	1	4	24	28(+ 1 lost to follow-up)

Graph 1.

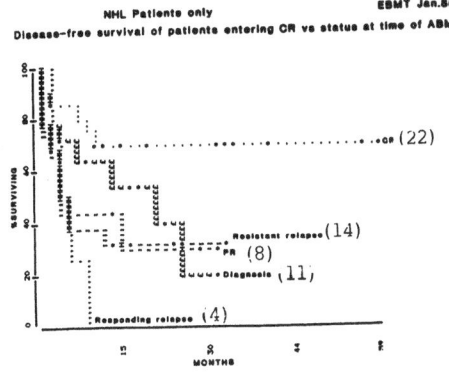

Graph 2.

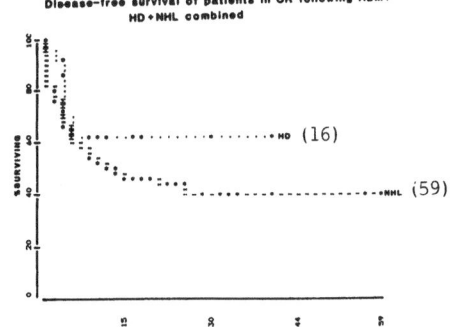

The effect of purging
Graph 3.

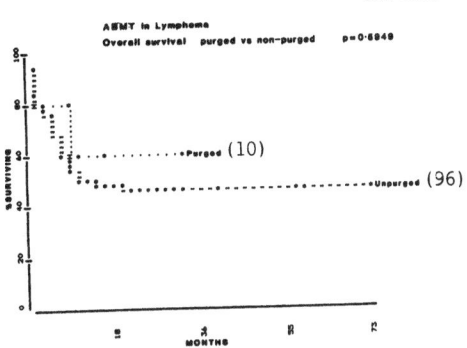

Post-graft consolidation
Graph 4. NHL & HD combined. Effect of post-graft consolidation of patients entering CR following ABMT.

Overall Survival

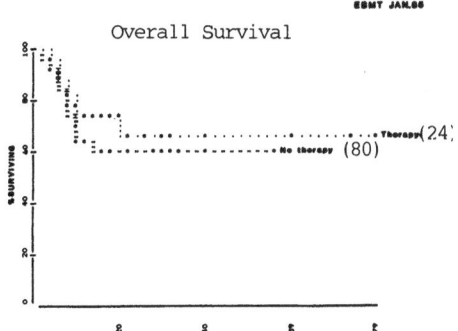

Early death was related to dose infused. Death < 30 days post ABMT (11) mean dose 1.087×10^8 nucleated cells/kg, others (86) 1.967×10^8/kg p < 0.01. Relapse occurred at a median of 126 days in NHL and 127 days in HD. Relapse tends to occur in sites of previous disease.

CONCLUSIONS

1. Several of our initial collaborating centres have not filled in computer forms. On the computer now very few children (5/111) and very few cases in 'responding relapse' (10/110).
2. In NHL patients, CR is achieved in a high percentage of patients (73%) whilst procedure-related death is low (6%). However, 55% of the total either have progressive disease or relapse after CR. The best results are obtained in patients autografted in CR (68% remaining alive and well) but these may have had a good result on conventional chemotherapy anyway.
3. In NHL there is a trend towards lymphoblastic histology cases and T cell cases doing better after ABMT, but this has no statistical validity.
4. In HD, CR is also achieved in a high percentage of cases (57%). Procedure-related death is higher than in NHL (21% vs 6%) and might be related to advanced status of disease at autograft (96% HD in relapse vs 41% NHL in relapse). However, since 50% with HD remain alive and well in CR and only 28% are in relapse or have progressive disease, the overall picture of ABMT in HD might be more encouraging than in NHL.
5. Unhappily post-graft consolidation after CR does not at the moment appear to be of value. Relapse occurs early and at a similar time in both NHL and HD. Nothing can be said about the value of purging the marrow at the moment.
6. The best results occur in CR patients who might have an excellent prognosis on conventional therapy. Poor prognosis disease needs to be identified in CR.

LIST OF CONTRIBUTING CENTRES AND NUMBER OF PATIENTS REPORTED FOR ANALYSIS

MARSEILLES:	Dr D. Maraninchi	15
PARIS: (St Antoine)	Dr N.C. Gorin	13
GENOVA:	Drs Carella & Marmont	19
LONDON: (Bloomsbury)	Drs Goldstone,Souhami & Linch	17
UTRECHT:	Dr G.C. Gast	14
BOLOGNA:	Dr Ricci	22
PARMA:	Dr V. Rizzoli	8
VIENNA:	Dr W. Hinterberger	1
ROME:	Dr F. Mandelli	2

TOTAL NUMBER OF PATIENTS 111

Exp. Hematol. (suppl. 17) 13:22 (1985)
© International Society for Experimental Hematology

Superintensive Therapy and Autologous Bone Marrow Transplantation (ABMT) in Malignant Lymphomas (Bologna Experience)

P. Ricci, P. Mazza, G. Visani, M. R. Motta, F. Gherlinzoni, G. Bandini, L. Leardini, D. Belletti, C. Finelli, M. Fiacchini, and S. Tura

Institute of Haematology, Bologna University, Bologna, Italy

23 pts with lymphomas underwent intensive therapy and ABMT as hematological rescue (Table 1). NHL received BAVC[1] regimen (16 pts) or CTX and TBI (pt. N. 13), followed by the reinfusion of the previously cryopreserved marrow. HL were treated with CTX, 3500 mg/m², BCNU, 500 mg/m², and VBL, 15 mg/m², administered over a 4 hour period and received 24 hours later the autologous marrow stored at + 4 °C for 36 hours (6 pts). The clinical course after ABMT was uneventful in all but pt N. 17, and complete hematological recostitution was promptly achieved in all cases. The therapeutic response and current status of the pts are summarized in the Table. Complete remission occurred in 11 pts with NHL and in 8 cases further consolidation with radio and/or chemotherapy was administered. The experience in NHL suggests that untreated patients can tolerate well a high-dose regimen and that marrow cells harvested before chemotherapy permit a fast hematological recovery. BAVC regimen is sufficient to induce complete remissions: these pts should then receive, we feel, consolidation chemotherapy/ radiotherapy. However, in pts with lymphoblastic/immunoblastic histology or with very extensive disease the BAVC/ABMT regimen should not be used as the initial treatment.

In HL our preliminary data don't allow to draw conclusions on the role of ABMT. A wider experience should be obtained before proposing such therapy as consolidation phase in pts with poor prognostic factors.

Table - Clinical details of patients transplanted, therapeutic response and current status.

Pat. N. age/sex	Histology	Disease status at: Harvesting	Reinfusion	Antitumor Response (ms)	Outcome (ms)
1. 24/M	Centroblastic*(NHL)	Diagnosis (II)⁰	idem	CR[1] (37+)	Alive & Well Ned[3] (37+)
2. 26/M	Centroblastic*	Diagnosis (III)	idem	CR (4)	BM Involvement (20)
3. 35/M	Histiocytic	Diagnosis (II)⁰	idem	CR (26)	Alive with lymphoma (32+)
4. 18/F	Lymphoblastic	Diagnosis (IV)⁰	idem	PR[2]	CNS Involvement (7)
5. 23/F	Lymphoblastic	Ist Remission	2nd relapse	PR	Progression IP[4] (3)
6. 44/M	Centroblastic	1st Relapse⁰	idem	CR (27+)	Alive & Well Ned (27+)
7. 27/M	Centroblastic*	Diagnosis (II$_E$)	idem	CR (24+)	Alive & Well Ned (24+)
8. 26/M	Immunoblastic	Diagnosis (IV)⁰	idem	PR	BM Involvement (1.5)
9. 36/M	Histiocytic	Diagnosis (IV)⁰	idem	PR	Progression BM Involvement (4)
10. 45/M	Lymphoblastic	Diagnosis (IV)⁰	1st relapse	CR (3)	BM Involvement (8)
11. 37/M	Histiocytic	Diagnosis (II)⁰	Resistance	CR (18+)	Alive & Well Ned (18+)
12. 34/F	Histiocytic	Diagnosis (IV)⁰	idem	CR (17+)	Alive & Well Ned (17+)
13. 47/M	Lymphoblastic	Diagnosis (IV)⁰	idem	CR (16+)	Alive & Well Ned (16+)
14. 39/M	Histiocytic	Diagnosis (II)⁰	idem	PR	Progression (6.5)
15. 20/F	Histiocytic	Diagnosis (II)	idem	CR (11+)	Alive & Well Ned (11+)
16. 20/F	Lymphoblastic	Diagnosis (I)⁰	idem	CR (7+)	Alive & Well Ned (7+)
17. 28/F	Immunoblastic	Diagnosis (II)⁰	Resistance	NE**	Alive with infective problem (2+)
18. 29/M	NS (HL)	3rd resistent Relapse		CR (19+)	Alive & Well Ned (19+)
19. 21/M	NS	2nd resistent Relapse		CR (6)	Alive with Lymphoma (13+)
20. 28/M	NS	3rd resistent Relapse		CR (4)	Alive with progressive lymphoma (7+)
21. 22/M	NS	4rd resistent Relapse		CR (9.5+)	Alive & Well Ned (9.5+)
22. 33/F	MC	3rd resistent Relapse		PR	Progression (3)
23. 25/M	NS	4rd resistent Relapse		CR (5.5+)	Alive & Well Ned (5.5+)

1 = Complete response; 2 = Partial response; 3 = No evidence of disease; 4 = Interstitial pneumonitis; * = Polymorphous; ⁰ = With Bulky disease; ** = Not evaluable.

1: BCNU 200 mg/m², ARA-C 1200 mg/m², VP 16-213 1200 mg/m², and CTX 180 mg/Kg, administered over a 4 day period.

* Supported in part by Grant "Ministero Pubblica Istruzione - (40%)", by C.N.R., Finalized Project for Control of Tumor Growth, Contract N. 83.00969.96 and by C.N.R. Finalized Project "Oncologia".

Exp. Hematol. (suppl. 17) 13:23–24 (1985)
© International Society for Experimental Hematology

High Dose Chemotherapy (HDC) and Non Frozen ABMT in Refractory Hodgkin's Disease (HD)

A. M. Carella [1], G. Santini [1], F. Frassoni [1], A. Santoro [2], P. Coser [3], M. Martinengo [1], A. Congiu [1], S. Nati [1], D. Giordano [1], and A. M. Marmont [1]

[1] Division of Hematology, Genova, Italy
[2] National Cancer Institute, Milan, Italy
[3] Division of Hematology, Bozen, Italy

The optimal management of patients who develop progressive or recurrent disease after primary chemotherapy remains to be established. New salvage regimens have been shown to be able to control the disease in many relapsed patients. There is, however, a sizable group of truly malignant patients who either fail to achieve a remission or relapse after few months and respond poorly even to powerful salvage regimens such as CEP (CCNU+Etoposide+prednimustine). In all these cases, survival is extremely poor. For such patients new hope seems to come from the combination of HDC following by ABMT.

Materials and Methods

16pts. with high risk HD entered our trial (table I). Marrow involvement was excluded by 2 bone biopsies. HDC consisted in 2pts. of BCNU (700mg/mq), in 1p. of Cy (60mg/Kg x 2 days)+ TBI (10 Gy) and in 13 pts. of Cy (5g/mq) + VP-16 (400mg/mq) or VLB (15mg/mq) + BCNU (600mg/mq)(CVB protocol).
HDC was given 1 hour after BM harvesting. The BM suspension was kept at 4°C for 40-48 hours before reinfusion. Complete responders did not receive any further therapy after ABMT. Partial responders received a chemoradiotherapy for residual disease.

Results

Antitumoral responses are detailed in table II: 12/16pts. (75%) achieved a response and 10/16 (62,5%) a CR after HDC + ABMT.
Toxicity: extrahematological toxicity was mild consisting mainly in nausea lasting 24h in all patients and increase of liver enzimes and alkaline phosphatase. In one case was observed lung fibrosis. Profound aplasia (WBC 100/ , Platelets 20.000/ 1) occured in all patients, slightly longer in patients treated with wider chemo-radiotherapy protocols. One patient died of aplasia without hemopoietic reconstitution. The mean time to hematological recovery in the other 15 evaluable patients after BM reinfusion was WBC $1.0 \times 10^4/1 = 16$ days (range 9-31) and platelets $20 \times 10^9/1 = 16$ days (range 13-57).

Discussion

Using non frozen BM storage at 4°, we observed a fast hemopoietic reconstitution. Only in one case it was not observed reconstitution but in this case the study of thawed cells viability evaluated in vitro by a standard agar CFU-GM assay showed a low efficiency. The toxicity of the procedure is acceptable since only one case had lung fibrosis and in others liver enzimes and alkaline phosphatase increases returned within normal values 2-4 months after HDC. The response to HDC in our advanced resistant HD pts. has been impressive with 12/16 pts. (75%) having a significant response despite being truly resistant or relapsed to the most widely used combination chemotherapy (CCVPP or MOPP+ABVD+CEP+RT). At present, 7 pts. remain in CR 4 to 42 mo. after ABMT. The longest survivor, a case with bilateral lung HD, resistant to CcVPP+MOPP and RT, is in CR 42 mo. after HD BCNU. These preliminary data suggest that HDC and non frozen ABMT may be effective in resistant or relapsed HD. In the future, if these results will be confirmed in a larger series of patients, this approach might be of eligibility in poor prognosis HD earlier in the disease.

References

1)Bonadonna G., Santoro A.(1983): Update on malignant lymphomas, Bristol-Myers Company.
2)Carella A.M., et al.(1984): High-dose chemotherapy and non-frozen ABMT in resistant or relapsed malignant lymphomas. Cancer 54,2836-2839.
3)Carella A.M., et al.: Massive chemotherapy and non-frozen ABMT in advanced resistant Hodgkin's Disease. Eur.J.Cancer Clin.Oncol.(in press).
4)Spitzer G. et al. (1984): High dose chemotherapy with autologous bone marrow transplantation. Cancer 54,1216.
5)Tannir et al.(1983): High dose chemoradiotherapy and ABMT in patients with refractory lymphoma. Eur.J.Cancer Clin.Oncol.18,1091.

TABLE I

CLINICAL DETAILS OF ADVANCED HDpts TREATED BY HDC
AND NON-FROZEN ABMT

Cases	16
Age y.	26 (15-40)
Sex	10M, 6F
Histology (at diagnosis)	NS(8),MC(6),LD(1),EV(1)
Staging at harvesting	IIIB(1),IVA(2),IVB(13)
Response to Conventional chemot.:	
	CR 10
	NR 4
	PD 2
Mean Duration of 1th CR	10 mo.(range 1-64)
HDC:	2: BCNU(700mg/mq)
	1: Cy 60mg/Kgx2+TBI 10Gy
	13: CVB Protocol(Cy5g/mq +VP-16 400mg or VLB 15mg/mq + BCNU 600mg/mq)

NS: Nodular Sclerosis; MC: Mixed Cellularity; LD: Lymphoid Depletion; EV: Epitheloid Variety; CR: Complete Remission; NR: NO Response; PD: Progressive Disease

TABLE II

RESULTS OBTAINED BY HDC AND NON-FROZEN ABMT

Response to HDC:		
	CR	: 10/16(62,5%)
	PR	: 2
	CR+PR	: 12/16(75%)
	NR*	: 3
	PD*	: 1
Alive	10/16	
Alive in CR	7	
Mean CR duration (mo.):	19 (range 6-42)	
Died	6(1**CR, 2 NR, 1 Aplasia, 2 PR)	

* These pts. had received 4500 rads on the mediastinum and 2200 rads on both lungs before ABMT
** Cerebral Hemorrhage

Autologous BMT II
ABMT with Purged Bone Marrow

Exp. Hematol. (suppl. 17) 13:25 (1985)
© International Society for Experimental Hematology

Experimental Basis of the in vitro Treatment of Leukemic Bone Marrows with ASTA Z 7557

L. Douay, N. C. Gorin, J. P. Laporte, M. Lopez, and G. Duhamel

Laboratoire de Différenciation Cellulaire, CHU Saint-Antoine-CNTS Institut, Hôpital Saint-Antoine, Paris, France

In view of the in vitro treatment of leukemic bone marrows, we have previously shown that Cyclophosphamide derivatives such as ASTA Z 7557 may completely inhibit the in vitro proliferation of leukemic progenitors (CFU-L) but at the cost of simultaneous destruction of normal progenitor cells (CFU-GM, BFUe)(1). Initial studies of the behavior of treated marrows in long term marrow culture after incubation with doses of ASTA Z 7557 destroying 100% CFU-GM revealed that pre-CFU-GM are insensitive to ASTA at doses toxic on CFU-L, CFU-GM and BFUe (2). We report here our clinical experience with ASTA Z 7557 in order to treat the marrow of each individual patient with the highest possible dose of ASTA Z 7557 for maximum anti-leukemic activity, and yet spare enough normal stem cells for successful engraftment. Our experience on 32 bone marrow purging and 24 ABMT is presented. Establishment of the dose response curves for CFU-GM (n=37), BFUe (n=11) and myeloblastic CFU-L (n=10) demonstrated a wide range of sensitivity from patient to patient for all 3 progenitors, indicating that the optimal dose for in vitro treatment of the marrow should be adapted to each individual patient rather than constant. Whereas CFU-L, CFU-GM and BFUe grown in semi-solid cultures disclosed similar sensitivities to ASTA Z 7557, long term culture (LTC) studies (n=41) indicated a higher resistance of early progenitors with mean peak values of regenerating CFU-GM by day 14 of 165% (n=7), 56% (n=13) and 10% (n=8) respectively for marrow treated by moderate doses, high doses and very high doses of Asta Z, with mean values of residual CFU-GM of 40%, 4% and 0%, at time of initiation of LTC. Although marrows even totally deprived of residual CFU-GM did regenerate in LTC, our studies showed that the self renewal capacity of marrows for CFU-GM was related to the intensitivity of Asta Z treatment and in proportion to the surviving fraction of CFU-GM. In an effort to achieve a maximum tumor cell kill and yet spare a sufficient amount of normal stem cells to ensure consistent engraftment, we defined the optimal dose for marrow cleansing as the dose sparing 5 + 5%CFU-GM. This dose was established from a preincubation test (PIT) realized on a 10 ml marrow aspirate taken 15 days before marrow collection in each individual patient. In a series of 32 PIT leading to marrow cleansing procedure using doses of Asta Z ranging from 50 to 140 ug/2.10^7 buffy coat cells, the predictive value of the PIT was confirmed in 78% of the cases. Discrepancies which resulted in suboptimal marrow cleansing and unexpected high values for residual CFU-GM, were confined to our first manipulations and attributed mainly to variations in hematocrit values (4/7). For this reason, we attempted to incubate mononuclear cell suspension isolated over a Ficoll gradient (d:1,077) in view of avoiding the hematocrit parameter. In our hands, the dose response curves in these conditions were too steep to select appropriate doses of the drug to work with. We therefore elected to perform all our in vitro tests on buffy coat cells constantly adjusted to a final hematocrit of 5%. In these conditions the mean reproductibility between the PIT and the treatment of the whole collected marrow was 96+2.5%.

24 adult patients while in remission of AL were consolidated by Cyclophosphamide 60 mg/kg X 2 and total body irradiation at 10 Grays followed by ABMT with marrow cleansed by ASTA Z 7557 according to the specifications described above. All patients engrafted leukocytes (median day for recovery to 10^9/l = day 30). Delayed kinetics of recovery of platelets were observed in some ANLL patients. In the group of standard prognosis (13 patients), 11 patients have remained in CR or disease free with a median follow up of 12 months (12+ to 20+ months).

1) DOUAY L, GORIN NC, GEROTA I et al : Exp Hemat 1982, 10, 113-122

2) DOUAY L, GORIN NC, LOPEZ M et al : Exp Hemat 1984

Exp. Hematol. (suppl. 17) 13:26 (1985)
© International Society for Experimental Hematology

Autologous Bone Marrow Transplantation (ABMT) with Marrow Purged by ASTA Z 7557 as Consolidation Therapy for Acute Leukemia in Remission

J. P. Laporte, N. C. Gorin, L. Douay, M. Lopez, C. Salmon, A. Najman, and G. Duhamel

Hôpital Saint-Antoine, and Centre National de Transfusion Sanguine, Paris, France

24 adult patients (8 ALL, 16 ANLL) have been consolidated by Cyclophosphamide 60 mg/kg/day X 2 and TBI (10 Gy with lung shielding at 8 Gy) followed by ABMT with marrow purged by Asta Z 7557 while in complete or partial remission. No maintenance therapy was administered after ABMT. For each individual patient, the dose of Asta Z used for the in vitro incubation of the harvested marrow (15 - 140 microg/2.10^7 cells) has been calculated in pre-experiments in order to leave a surviving fraction of CFUc ranging from 0% to 10%. We had individualized two groups of patients :

1) Poor risk acute leukemia :
11 patients (Ph1 chromosome, secondary leukemia of breast cancer, partial remission, second or subsequent remission). The results are poor (6 deaths, 3 relapses (meningeal and medullary), 2 CR (3 months+, 4 months+)).

2) Standard risk (first complete remission) :
13 patients (5 ALL, 8 ANLL). 1 relapse at 14th month post-graft (ALL1), 1 death of liver veino-occlusive disease. The all 11 remain in complete remission, 2 at 20 months + after graft (median 13 months). The median of interval between CR and ABMT is 5 months.

We conclude :
1) The wide range of stem cells sensitivity to Asta Z justify the predetermination of the optimal dose of drug for each individual patient.
2) ABMT can successfully be done with pretreated marrow containing 5 + 5% CFUc.
3) Delayed kinetics of recovery of platelets are observed in ANLL.
4) ABMT in poor risk acute leukemia of adults is not associated with a high rate of long term unmaintained CR.
5) In standard risk A.L. in first CR, the procedure is safe with a high rate of persisting CR (11/13) and 5/13 CR ⟩17 months + post graft.
A long term follow-up is necessary to assess the value of this approach.

Exp. Hematol. (suppl. 17) 13:28–29 (1985)
© International Society for Experimental Hematology

In vitro Marrow Purging with Anti-DR Monoclonal Antibodies and Complement in High Dose Risk ALL

Preclinical Studies and Preliminary Clinical Experience

Dominique Maraninchi[5], Claude Mawas[1], Brynhild Mascret[5], Gérard Sebahoun[5], Jean-Albert Gastaut[5], Nicole Tubiana[5], Henri Perrimond[2], Joelle Scavennec[3], Gisèle Novakovitch[4], and Yves Carcassonne[5]

[1] Unité 119 INSERM, Marseille
[2] Service de Pédiatrie A, CHU Timone, Marseille
[3] Société Immunotech, Marseille
[4] Regional Blood Bank, Marseille
[5] Marrow Transplant Unit, Clinique des Maladies du Sang, Institut Paoli-Calmettes, Marseille, France

- Human DR antigens are histocompatibility antigens close to the Ia murine antigens. In mice, Ia is not expressed on CFU-S, but is present on more differenciated progenitors CFU-GM and BFU-E (1).
- DR is expressed to the membrane of most of the non T lymphoïd malignancies (2)- Anti DR Mo Ab could have large clinical indications to treat residual marrow leukemic contamination of such patients with the aim of autologous BMT.
- DR is expressed in man on GM-CFC, BFU-E and CFU-GEMM (3) suggesting that in vitro marrow treatment with anti DR monoclonal antibodies could affect haematological reconstitution after marrow transplantation.

The use of long term marrow culture provided the opportunity to evaluate indirectly human haematopoïetic stem cells by their ability to assure a long term production of differenciated precursors and progenitors (4).

We report here in vitro and in vivo data suggesting the lack of expression of DR antigens on human haematopoïetic stem-cells allowing their clinical use in marrow transplantation.

METHODS AND PATIENTS
Marrow samples were obtained from normal donors or patients with haematologic malignancies in Complete Remission at the time of marrow aspiratition prior to Bone Marrow Transplantation (BMT). Buffy coat cells were purified by centrifugation and diluted in alpha medium.

In vitro antibody treatment
Monoclonal antibodies (Mo Ab) were kindly provided by C. Mawas, M. Pieres (Centre Immunologie Marseille-Luminy) : B8.11, B8.12, B8.13,B8.15 are monomorphic anti DR Mo Ab, H140 is a murine anti Ia Mo Ab cross reacting with human DR locus (5). Marrow cells were incubated with each one and/or a pool of the Mo Ab at a final dilution of 1/500 at a cell concentration of 2×10^7 cells/ml. Incubation was done 1/2H at +4°C, then prescreened low-tox baby rabbit complement (Biogenzia) was added vol/vol 1/2H at +37°C. Cells were then washed twice. Residual cells were evaluated in comparison to complement treated marrow cells and seeded without cellularity adjustement. In vitro treatment of large volumes of marrow was done along the same general procedure, except that whole marrow was processed on Haemonetics V50 and that marrow was cryopreserved in plasma and DMSO prior final clinical use. In vitro haematopoïetic evaluation was done by GM-CFC assays in soft Agar with HPCM 15%. Long term marrow culture was done using the technic of S. Gartner et al (3).

PATIENTS
2 patients with poor prognosis DR positive Acute Lymphoïd Leukemias received autologous BMT from a cryopreserved marrow previously treated in vitro by the pool of anti DR Mo Ab and CT after a myelo-ablative conditionning regimen : Cyclo 60mg/kg x 2 - TBI 2.2 Gy x 5 and Melphalan 140 mg/m2 x 1- TBI 2.2 Gy x 5.

RESULTS
Marrow cultures - After marrow incubation with the anti DR pool of Mo Ab, 50% of marrow cells were DR positive using an indirect immunofluorescence assay and a morphologic control by immunogold (data not shown). DR expression on GM-CFC was heterogeneous in different experiments when evaluated with individual Mo Ab (Table I).

	B8.11	B8.12	B8.13	B8.15	H140
EXP 1	25%	41%	33%	–	100%
EXP 2	26%	12%	26%	16%	87%
EXP 3	2%	0%	2%	0%	33%

Table I – HETEROGENEITY OF EXPRESSION OF DR MOLECULES ON HEMATOPOIETIC PROGENITORS

Using the pool of 5 anti DR Mo Ab and CT, in 17 experiments, GM-CFC were reduced to 29 ± 6% (SEM) of the CT control. In 7 experiments, long term marrow cultures (Table II) showed that treatment with anti DR 1) didn't suppress in vitro developpement of adherent marrow micro-environnement 2)allowed long term production of GM-CFC and differenciated granulocytic precursors in an amount comparable to the complement control, up to 9 weeks of culture.

WEEKS	% CONTROL (CT)	n. Expts
0	29% ± 6	17
3	52% ± 13	7
5	68% ± 15	7
7	63% ± 19	7
9	51% ± 24	7

Table II : Production of GM-CFC in long term marrow cultures after treatment with anti DR Mo Ab pool and complement

Exp. Hematol. (suppl. 17) 13:27 (1985)
© International Society for Experimental Hematology

Long Term Effects of Autologous Bone Marrow Transplantation Performed in Children with Non-Hodgkin's Lymphoma of B-Cell Type

C. Baumgartner[1], E. A. Bleher[3], G. Brun del Re[2], U. Bucher[2], H. Frei[1], R. Greiner[3], A. Hirt[4], P. Imbach[1], Annette Lüthy[1], Angelika C. Stern[2], and H. P. Wagner[1, 4]

[1] Department of Pediatrics
[2] Central Hematology Laboratory
[3] Clinic for Radiotherapy, Inselspital, Bern
[4] Institute for Clinical and Experimental Cancer Research of the University, Bern, Switzerland

As the number of patients surviving after autologous bone marrow transplantation (ABMT) is increasing late effects of such procedures become a question of major concern. Our patients treated with ABMT for B-cell non-Hodgkin's lymphoma (B-NHL) have therefore been analysed for long-term toxicity.

17 pediatric patients with B-NHL (14 in first remission, 9 in Murphy stage III, 5 in stage IV and 3 in second remission) have undergone ABMT (1,2). The pretransplant regimen included vincristine 2 mg/m^2, adriamycin 60 mg/m^2, cyclophosphamide 45 mg/kg x4 and TBI 6 Gy single dose. Marrow decontamination with anti-Y 29/55 monoclonal antibody (3) and rabbit complement was performed in 7/17 patients.

One patient was lost due to acute toxicity and 7/17 succumbed to the tumor. 9/17 patients survive free of tumor for 13-67, median 36 months after ABMT. The age of the 9 survivors was at ABMT 4 10/12-15 9/12, median 9 4/12 years and in January 1985 7 4/12-20, median 10 8/12 years. All 9 survivors had ABMT in 1st remission (5/9 with marrow purging).

Five of 9 survivors are appearantly healthy and show normal physical and intellectual performance. Four of 9 survivors have specific problems probably or possibly related to the ABMT procedure: One of them (age, 10,5 years at ABMT, unpurged marrow, survival 67+ months) developed a papilloma of one ureter which was spontaneously expelled causing transient ureteral obstruction and hematuria (55 months after ABMT). Hematuria recurred several times without other evidence of a papilloma. The 2nd patient (age 7 years at ABMT, CNS disease, cranial irradiation 20 Gy, 23 doses of IT drugs, purged marrow, survival 39+ months) has a moderate psychoorganic syndrome. The 3rd patient (age 14 years at ABMT, CNS disease, cranial irradiation 24 Gy, 6 doses of IT drugs, purged marrow, survival 32+ months) has recovered from severe polyneuropathy and prolonged anorexia. He actually has bilateral cataract, retinopathy and severe caries. The 4th patient (age 9,5 years at ABMT, purged marrow, survival 13+ months) has persisting hepatopathy after venoocclusive disease resulting in multiple calcifications and decreased synthesis of blood clotting factors (slowly improving). The growth pattern was not significantly altered after ABMT except for a temporary decrease of body weight (fig. 1). Onset of puberty appears not to be altered after ABMT in the 3 patients beyond the age of 13 years. Susceptibility to infections was somewhat increased during the first year after ABMT. 4/9 patients had mild herpes zoster. No severe infections, however, were observed.

Long-term toxicity was observed more frequently in patients receiving purged marrow (3/5 patients) as compared to patients receiving untreated marrow (1/4 patients). In view of the heterogeneity of observed long-term sequelae, a specific toxic effect of the purging procedure appears to be unlikely.

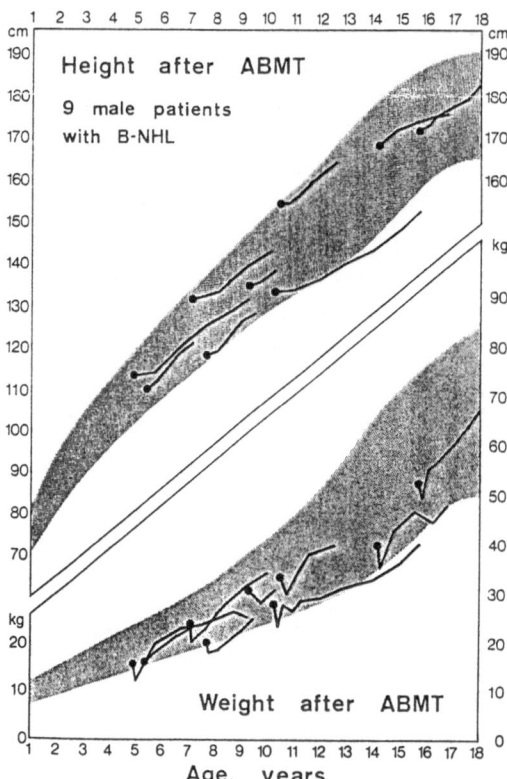

Fig. 1. Growth after ABMT. The shaded area indicates the normal range (3rd to 97th percentile).

References:
1. Baumgartner et al, Med Pediatr Oncol 12: 104-111, 1984
2. Baumgartner et al, Exp Hematol 11 (Suppl 14): 6, 1983
3. Forster et al, Cancer Res 42: 1927-1934, 1982

Clinical data on the 2 patients who received autologous BMT after anti DR + CT in vitro treatment and myelo-ablative conditionning regimens are detailed in Table III : both had full haematologic recovery and subsequent B cell reconstitution.

	PATIENT AU 72	PATIENT AU 79
AGE SEX	31 F	6 F
DIAGNOSIS	ALL 1st CR	ALL 2d CR
CONDITIONNING REGIMEN	Cy TBI 2.2 x 5	HDM-TBI 2.2 x 5
INFUSED NUCLEATED CELLS/Kg	0.6×10^8	2.1×10^8
INFUSED GM-CFC/Kg	2.5×10^4	8.1×10^4
GR £ <200/µl	14 DAYS	10 DAYS
GR £ <500/µl	15 DAYS	16 DAYS
Plts < 20 000/µl	24 DAYS	28 DAYS
Plts < 50 000/µl	41 DAYS	45 DAYS
BACTERIEMA	YES EARLY	YES EARLY
VIRAL INFECTION	HSV-HZV	HSV
FUNGAL INFECTION	YES EARLY	YES EARLY
B CELL RECONSTITUTION	YES	YES
Ig PRODUCTION	4 mths	3 mths
OUTCOME	ALIVE AND WELL 8.5 mths +	RELAPSE 5 mths ALIVE 6.5 mths +

Table III : Clinical data of autologous BMT patients after in vitro purge with anti DR + CT

DISCUSSION

- Our results confirm previous data showing that DR molecules are present on human haematopoïetic precursors and progenitors (5) (6). Results from long term marrow cultures suggest that more immature human stem-cells, closed to murine CFU-S, do not express sufficient DR molecules to be inhibited in a complement-mediated cell lysis. These results are in agreement with the recent reports of A. Keating and Al. (7).
- Furthermore, the clinical possibility to obtain a full hematologic reconstitution after TBI and autologous BMT treated in vitro with anti DR Mo Ab and CT suggests clearly that the level of expression of DR on human haematopoïetic stem cells is sufficiently low to authorize further haematopoïetic differenciation after DR depletion.
- These in vitro and in vivo results invite us to a wider use of anti DR Mo Ab in the aim to "purge" residual marrpw malignant cells in autologous BMT for non-T lymphoïd malignancies.

REFERENCES

(1) BASCH R.S., JANOSSY G, GREAVES M.F.
Murine pluripotential stem cells lack Ia antigen.
Nature 270 : 520, 1977

(2) NADLER L.M., RITZ J., GRIFFIN J.D. et al
Diagnosis and treatment of human leukemia and lymphoma utilizing monoclonal antibodies
Progress in Hematology 12 : 187-226, 1981

(3) FITCHEN J.H., LEFEVRE C., FERRONE S. et al
Expression of Ia like and HLA A-B antigens on human pluripotential haematopoïetic progenitor cells.
Blood 59 : 188, 1982

(4) GARTNER S., KAPLAN H.S.
Long term culture of human bone marrow cells
PNAS 77 : 4756,1980

(5) REBAI N., MALISSEN B., PIERES M. et al
Distinct HLA-DR epitopes and distinct families of HLA DR molecules defined by 15 either anti DR or allo anti Ia K cross reacting with human cells.
Eur. J. Immunology 1306, 1983

(6) FALKENBURG J.H.F., JANSEN J., V. der VAART-DUINKERKEN N. et al
Polymorphic and monomorphic HLA-DR determinants on human hematopoïetic progenitor cells.
Blood 63, 1125, 1984

(7) KEATING A., POWELL J., TAKAHOSI M. et al
The generation of human long term marrow cultures from marrow depleted of Ia (HLA-DR) positive cells
Blood 64 : 1159-1162, 1984

Total Body Irradiation

Exp. Hematol. (suppl. 17) 13:30 (1985)
© International Society for Experimental Hematology

Whole Body Irradiation Before Bone Marrow Transplantation
The "Kiel-Model" of Compensation

F. Brix[1], E. Dühmke[1], and N. Schmitz[2]

[1] Department of Radiology (Director Prof. Dr. H. Gremmel)
[2] II. Medical Department (Director Prof. Dr. H. Löffler) University of Kiel, D-2300 Kiel, Federal Republic of Germany

To avoid serious side effects from whole body irradiation before bone marrow transplantation, for example IP, a newly developed modality of irradiation has been established since 1983 by the Kiel Transplantation Center. 12 Gy are applicated within three days, two fractions of 2 Gy per day using an individually designed whole body compensator.

Compared to the poor dose distribution of a bilateral open field technique this sophisticated irradiation leads to a homogeneity within 3,5 % of the planned dose, delivered to any point in the midplane. Manufacturing of the compensator is based upon an adaquate number of CT-scans and considers the irregular body contour as well as the varying densities of different tissues.

Until now 2o patients (9ALL, 3AML, 4CML, 1megac.myel and 3SAA, 9 of them with high risc disease) have been irradiated and transplantated successfully. 13 of them are alive (day + 15 to + 524), six died early after transplantation (day + 11 to + 79), mostly because of severe aspergillosis due to immune deficiency, general sepsis, bacterial pneumonia and two because of IP. One died on day + 364 in relapse.

None of these survivors declared remarkable complains during or after irradiation. Only one patient endured GVHD grade I/II, five more times only grade I GVHD could be recognized. Neither clinical signs nore the radiographic follow up or the testified pulmonary function yielded any indications to restrictive pulmonary disease. Although the time of observation has been rather short, it seems very likely that the rate and degree of undesirable side effects, especially IP, can be reduced using this new irradiation technique.

Exp. Hematol. (suppl. 17) 13:31–32 (1985)
© International Society for Experimental Hematology

Low Early Mortality of Allogeneic Bone Marrow Transplantation by Use of Fractionated Total Body Irradiation, Cyclosporin-A, Long Lasting LAF-Isolation and Gut Decontamination

J. Burger and J. Gmür

Department of Internal Medicine, University Hospital, Zürich, Switzerland

In bone marrow transplantation the main reasons for treatment failure within the first months posttransplant were infection, interstitial pneumonia, GvHD and rejection (in SAA). A significant association with 6-month-mortality has been established for: 1) the use of high-dose-rate TBI, 2) the occurrence of moderate to severe GvHD, 3) more advanced disease, 4) patients of older age, 5) infection at the time of BMT and 6) high number of pre transplant transfusions and/or refractoriness to random platelets (1,2).

Patients (Table 1)

18 consecutive patients undergoing BMT between January 82 and December 84 (mean age 24 y, range 11-43 y) are presented: 6 AML (3 first, 1 second, 1 third remission, 1 second relapse); 3 ALL (2 second remission, 1 second relapse); 4 CGL (3 chronic phase, 1 blast crisis); 1 myelodysplasia and 4 severe aplastic anemia. Donors were in 16 an HLA-identical sibling, in one the HLA-identical mother and in one the HLA-A-different brother, all showing a reciprocal non-stimulatory MLC.

The patients were reviewed for the following poorly controlled risk-factors: Age (over 3o y); Disease status (blast crisis or relapse or AML $\geq$ 2.CR or ALL $\geq$ 3.CR); Infection at the time of BMT and (in SAA patients) refractoriness to random platelets. Two patients had no risk-factor, 5 patients one and 8 patients 2 or 3 risk-factors.

Transplantation protocol

Leukemia patients were conditioned according to standard protocols (3), SAA patients by a modified protocol using procarbazine, ALG and cyclophosphamide (4).

The following provisions were applied to reduce early mortality:

1) Radiation therapy:fractionated TBI with 6 x 2 Gy over 6 days, partial lung shielding (9.5 Gy absorbed lung dose), low dose-rate (2.7 cGy/min.).
2) Infection prophylaxis starting 2 weeks before and maintained for 5 weeks post BMT: Laminar-Air-Flow Isolation and complete gut decontamination (vancomycin, gentamycin, amphothericin, doses adapted to keep fecal germ-counts below 10^3/g).
3) GvHD prophylaxis: cyclosporine-A as continous infusion for at least 3 weeks, followed by oral medication in 2 daily doses for 4-9 months.
4) Interstitial pneumonia prophylaxis:Modality of radiation therapy (see 1); cyclosporine-A; CMV-negative transfusions; prophylactic CMV hyperimmun serum in CMV negative patients.

Results

Early mortality

Only 2/18 patients died within 6 month due to transplantation related complications. A 39 y old man (UPN 24) with refractory AML in second relapse died from GvHD on day +38, having preexisting non-A-non-B hepatitis. An 11 y old girl (UPN 21) died of renal failure under cyclosporin-A on day +64. This patient was back in Libya (scarse information after discharge). An additional patient died on day +171 of relapse of her AML M5 (FAB). The mean follow-up time of the whole group is 13.8 mts with one patient below 3 mts.

Table 1

UPN	Age	Disease, Status	aGvH	i Pn	Survival, mts
12	24	CGL, chronic phase	0	0	> 33, CR
26	16	CGL, chronic phase	0	0	> 5, CR
28	39	CGL, chronic phase	0	0	> 2, CR
17	43	CGL, blast crisis	I	0	+11, chron.GvH perf.ulcer
13	18	AML, 1st remission	0	0	> 31, CR
18	24	AML, 1st remission	I	0	> 18, CR
22	30	AML, 1st remission	I	0	+6, relapse
15	18	AML, 2nd remission	0	0	+11, relapse
14	32	AML, 3rd remission	I	0	> 28, CR
24	39	AML, 2nd relapse	IV	0	+1, aGvH
16	19	ALL, 2nd remission	I	0	+16, relapse
09	11	ALL, 2nd remission	0	0	+8, relapse
23	16	ALL, 2nd relapse	I	0	> 10, CR
25	24	Myelodysplasia	I	0	> 8, CR

UPN	Age	Dis.	refract./infected	Rej.	aGvH	i Pn	Survival, mts
11	12	SAA	yes/yes	no	0	0	> 36, well
20	19	SAA	yes/ no	no	0	0	> 14, well
21	13	SAA	yes/yes	no	?	0	+2, renal fail
27	26	SAA	yes/ no	no	0	0	> 3, well

refract./infected: refractory to random donor platelets or infected at the time of BMT. i Pn:interst.Pneumonia, Rej.: graft rejection. CR: complete remission.

Transplantation related complications

Only one patient had acute GvHD of more than grade I (UPN 24). No interstitial pneumonia occurred (with UPN 28) being still at risk at the time of this report).

In 15 patients 20 febrile episodes were observed. Ten of them were microbiologically documented: positive blood cultures for staphylococci (4) or corynebacterium (1); orofacial herpes simplex (5). Seven patients had clinically documented upper airway infections. Three patients had fever of unknown origin. No lifethreatening or lethal infection complications occurred.

Conclusion

This heterogenous group of 18 consecutive patients was treated according to a standardized BMT protocol aimed to reduce early posttransplant complications. In spite of the fact that 15 patients had at least one (8 of them 2-3) risk factors related to high early mortality (1,2), only two early death occurred. The low incidence of moderate or severe acute GvHD as well as the absence of interstitial pneumonia and lethal infections observed in this small patients group is presumed to be related to the rigorous isolation/decontamination conditions, the reduction of radiation toxicity and GvH prophylaxis with cyclosporin-A. These preventions may have an important impact on early outcome.

References

1. Bortin MM., Gale RP,. Kay HEM,. Rimm AA.: Bone marrow transplantation for acute myelogenous leukemia. Factors associated with early mortality. J.Am.Med.Ass. 249: 1166, 1983

2. Storb R., Prentice RL,. Thomas ED: Marrow transplantation for treatment of aplastic anemia: Analysis of factors associated with graft rejection. N.Engl.J.Med. 296: 61, 1977

3. Thomas ED,. Clift RA, Hersman J,. Sanders JE,. Stewart P,. Buckner CD,. Fefer A,. Guffin R,. Smith JW,. Storb R.: Marrow transplantation for acute nonlymphocytic leukemia in first remission using fractionated or single-dose irradiation. Int.J.Rad.Onc.Biol.Phys. 8: 817, 1982

4. Gmür J., Frick PG., von Felten A.: Successful allogeneic bone marrow transplantation with the same donor after graft rejection: application of a modified conditioning regimen. Blut 39: 47, 1979

Exp. Hematol. (suppl. 17) 13:33 (1985)
© International Society for Experimental Hematology

Evaluation of Cyclophosphamide and Different TBI Regimens (Single Dose or Fractionnated) in Allogeneic Marrow Transplantation for Hematologic Malignancies

D. Maraninchi[1], B. Mascret[1], J. L. Lagrange[1], J. P. Guillet[1], J. A. Gastaut[1], G. Sebahoun[1], H. Perrimond[2], J. Camerlo[1], and Y. Carcassonne[1]

[1] Marrow Transplant Unit, Clinique des Maladies du Sang, Institut Paoli-Calmettes, 232 Boulevard Sainte Marguerite, F-13273 Marseille, Cedex
[2] Service de Pédiatrie, CHU Timone, Marseille, France

The combination of Cyclophosphamide and 10 Gy total body irradiation has been the most widely used as a preparation to bone marrow transplantation. The limits of this regimen were both the occurence of lethal interstitial pneumonia–variable between teams and patients situations–and relapse, specially in patients grafted beyond the 1st RC. Several studies showed that lethal interstitial pneumonia was less frequent using fractionnated regimens (1) (2) and that the higher total doses allowed by these regimens could decrease the risks of relapse. We report here our experience in 48 patients receiving single dose or fractionnated TBI in the aim to define the most adequate regimen for patients with standard or high neoplasic risks at the time of BMT.

PATIENTS AND METHODS

PATIENTS

48 patients are evaluated : 10 had Acute Myeloïd Leukemia, 22 Acute Lymphoïd Leukemia, 9 Chronic Myeloïd Leukemia (CML) and 7 malignant Lymphomas. Median age was 18 years ranging 6–35 years with 27 males and 21 females.

At the time of bone marrow transplantation (BMT) 13 patients were in relapse, 1 patient in 3d Complete Remission (CR), 7 patients in 2d CR, 37 patients in 1st CR or 1st chronic phase of CML.

Patients were divided in two groups according to their status at the time of BMT : patients in 1st or 2d CR and 1st chronic phase of CML were defined with "standard neoplasic risk" ; patients in other situations were defined with "high neoplasic risk".

METHODS

- All patients were conditionned by Cyclophosphamide 60mg/kgx2 followed by TBI in different regimens. Each regimen was initialy experimented in "high risk" patients ; after 14 consecutive patients in the 3 first TBI regimens, all patients with "standard risk" received TBI 2.2 Gyx5 and all "high risk" patients received TBI 2.4 Gy x5 until the end of the study.

- TBI was done with a Linear Accelerator Saturne (18 MV) with a low radiation rate (< 5cGy/mi.). All patients had Lung Shielding at a total Lung dose of less than 8 Gy. Fractionnated regimens were done with one fraction each day of 5 successive days. Patients were managed in LAF rooms and had GVH prophylaxis by MTX or Cyclosporin.

RESULTS

In the first 5 patients, who received TBI 10 Gy in one dose, 3 died from pneumonia, 2 are alive and well (one with high risk-one with standard risk). In the following 4 patients prepared with TBI 2 Gy x 5, one with high risk-relapsed, 3 are alive and well. Over the 29 patients who received TBI 2.2 Gy x 5, only one-with

standard risk-relapsed and only two died from pneumonia, 21 are alive and well. In the 10 patients with high risk receiving TBI 2.4 Gy x 5, 6 relapsed and no patient is still alive in remission.

TBI REGIMEN	10 Gy x 1	2 Gy x 5	2.2 Gy x 5	2.4 Gy x 5
N pts (High Risk)	5 (1)	4 (1)	29 (2)	10 (10)
LETHAL PNEUMONIA	3 (60 %)	0	2 (7 %)	0
RELAPSE	0	1	1	6
ALIVE AND WELL	2 (40 %)	3 (75 %)	21 (75 %)	0 (0 %)
MED. FOLLOW-UP	37 mths +	33 mths +	14 mths +	–

Table I – Outcome in the different TBI regimens

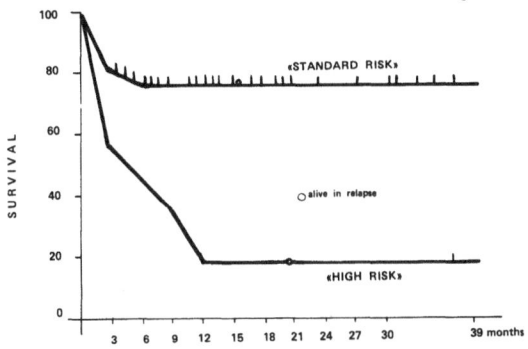

Fig. n°1 – Survival according to the neoplasic risk

DISCUSSION

Fractionnated TBI regimens reduced the incidence of lethal pneumonia (2/43) compared to TBI in single dose (3/5). The rate of relapse is low in standard risk patients (1/34) but remains high in "high risk" patients (7/14), even receiving TBI 2.4 Gy x 5.

Giving a 75% plateau of survival, the regimen Cy + TBI 2.2 Gy x 5 seems suitable for standard risk patients. The use of higher doses of TBI didn't improve the results in high risk patients with a 18% survival. New approaches of leukemia ablative regimens might be developped for high risk patients.

REFERENCES

(1) THOMAS E.D. : The role of marrow transplantation in the eradication of malignant diseases. Am. Cancer Soc. 49 : 1963, 1982

(2) GOOLDEN AWG, GOLDMAN JM, KAM KC et al : Fractionation of whole body irradiation before bone marrow transplantation for patients with leukemia Br. J. Radiol. 56 : 245, 1983

Exp. Hematol. (suppl. 17) 13:34 (1985)
© International Society for Experimental Hematology

Low Dose Total Body Irradiation in Allogeneic Bone Marrow Transplantation for Hematological Malignancy: Incidence of Interstitial Pneumonitis and Relapse after Longterm Follow-Up

F. Charpentier[1], J. P. Vernant[1], J. Dutreix[3], C. Cordonnier[1], M. Rodet[2], M. Kuentz[1], P. Bierling[2], N. Duedari[2], P. Mannoni[2], B. Dreyfus[1], and H. Rochant[1]

[1] BMT Unit [2] Blood Center, Hôpital Henri Mondor 51, ave du Maréchal de Lattre de Tassigny, F-94000 Creteil
[3] Institut Gustave Roussy, F-94800 Villejuif, France

Between September 78 and May 81, 13 adults (mean age 27± 7 years) with acute myeloid leukemia (AML) in 1st remission (n=11) or chronic myeloid leukemia (CML) in 2nd chronic phase, were given donor buffy coat cells, Cyclophosphamide (60 mg/kgx2), and low dose total body irradiation (TBI) as conditioning regimen for allogeneic bone marrow transplantation (BMT) from an HLA identical sibling donor.
Methotrexate was given for graft versus host disease prophylaxis, according to the Seattle scheme (1).
TBI was performed with a 5.5 MV Xrays beam in a horizontal direction. The distance between source and patient midline was 4 m. The reference dose at the abdominal midplane was 8 grays. The lungs were shielded at 4 grays. The dose rate on the patient midline during irradiation was about 10 cGy min -1 but the average dose rate was reduced to 4 to 5 cGy min -1.
BMT was performed within 4 months of complete remission for patients with acute leukemia (mean 91 ± 16 days).
The incidence of interstitial pneumonitis (iPn) was low, in spite of systematic prophylactic leukocyte transfusion during aplasia (2) : only one case occured, 4 months after BMT, resolutive, and CMV antibody levels raised (1/20 to 1/160) in the following month.
Five patients died : 1 veno occlusive disease (CML), 1 acute GVHD (AML), 1 thrombotic microangiopathy (AML) 1 fulminant measles (AML) and 1 relapse (AML). The incidence of relapses remained low with 2 cases (15 %):

1 AML5 (3) at 4 months, and 1 AML 5 at 40 months (still alive 20 months later). 7 patients are living in persistent remission (54 to 72 months after BMT) with a Karnofsky performance score of 100 %. The disease free survival rate is 53,8 % with a "plateau" obtained at 40 months.
Therefore low dose irradiation, used in a attempt to decrease iPn rates, doesn't appear to be responsible for a high incidence of relapses when transplantation is performed early after remission is achieved in patients with acute myeloid leukemia.

REFERENCES :

1 - THOMAS ED, BUCKNER CD, et all.
One hundred patients with acute leukemia treated by chemotherapy, total body irradiation, and allogeneic marrow transplantation.
Blood, 49 : 511, 1977.

2 - WINSTON DJ et all.
CMV infections associated with leukocyte transfusion.
Ann. of Intern. Med. 93 : 671, 1980.

3 - BENNETT JM, CATOVSKY D, DANIEL MT et all.
Proposals for the classification of acute leukemias.
B.J. of Haematology, 33 : 451, 1976.

Exp. Hematol. (suppl. 17) 13:35 (1985)
© International Society for Experimental Hematology

Attempt for a Complete Protocol of TBI

W. Kallinger[1], G. Alth[2], G. Müller[2], W. Hinterberger[3], H. Kolbabek[2], M. Danzer[1], W. Schmidmeier[4], J. Klumaier[5], and H. Koren[2]

[1] Phys.-techn. Prüfanstalt für Radiologie und Elektromedizin, KH Lainz, Wolkersbergenstraße 1, A-1130 Wien
[2] Sonderabteilung für Strahlentherapie, KH Lainz, Wolkersbergenstraße 1, A-1130 Wien
[3] I. Medizinische Universitätsklinik, AKH, Lazarettgasse 14, A-1090 Wien
[4] St. Anna Kinderspital, Kinderspitalgasse 6, A-1090 Wien
[5] Zentralröntgeninstitut, KH Lainz, Wolkersbergenstraße 1, A-1130 Wien, Austria

As the dose inside tissue is strongly dependent on the density of the desired object, every patient is scanned in 8 planes on the CT. In the following the calculation of lung dose is done by a treatment planning system using an inhomogeneity correction. The dose inside the lung is calculated pixel by pixel for every patient undergoing TBI. It can be shown that the resulting dose distribution will always lead to differences inside the lung of the order of 0.5-1 Gy. However these differences exist only in small areas, the edges of the lung. The mean lung dose, defined as the average over the lung area, is the most representative number and is calculated individually. It can be seen that the dose values and the dose differences inside the lung vary strongly. The reason for this is, that the relation between lung area and lung body area within the CT-slice is varying strongly from patient to patient. Therefore the shielding of the lung is calculated individually for every patient and the resulting dose is reduced below 8 Gy. Similarly the dose distribution and shielding is calculated for neck and head. After the 8th patient the doserate was lowered from 12-20 down to 4cGy/min on the body surface during radiation on. Additionally with the reduction of doserate the total absorbed dose in the abdomen midplane was not considered a criterion of radiation anymore. We believe, the abdomen dose should result from the average of the dose on 4 points on the surface in the lung plane with 10.5 Gy. A planning technique measuring these 4 points with TLD´s without calculating the correct lung size is missing the enormous differences in lung dose.

CONCLUSION: As is shown above the authors claim, that dose planning for TBI must be done individually as there may be unknown dose inside the lungs due to the big variations of the area of the lung. It is necessary to find the range of dose which is needed for the irradiation of the lung without exceeding a maximum of 8 Gy in certain areas, keeping the risk at a minimum. In order to find these limits - as the statistics from one institute will be to small - the protocols of the IBMR should be changed and extended to the following.

Point 30 B: Dose rate at body surface (during radiation on) frontal field ..... cGy/min

backside field ..... cGy/min

lateral field left ..... cGy/min

lateral field right ..... cGy/min

Point 30 D: total dose in .. fractions within ... days

1. Midplane dose head ..... Gy

   Maximum dose head ..... Gy

2. Midplane dose neck ..... Gy

   Maximum dose neck ..... Gy

3. Midplane dose lungs ..... Gy

   Maximum dose lungs ..... Gy

   Minimum dose lungs ..... Gy

   Mean dose lungs ..... Gy

4. Midplane dose abdomen ..... Gy

   Maximum dose abdomen ..... Gy

5. Dose to the ribs ..... Gy

6. Treatment planning done

   yes   no

7. Treatment planning done on CT-basis

   yes   no

8. Lung shielding constructed individually

   yes   no

9. Dose checked during irradiation

   yes   no

10. Accuracy of dose dertermination

    in free air ..... %

    inside the patient ..... %

Exp. Hematol. (suppl. 17) 13:36 (1985)
© International Society for Experimental Hematology

Allogeneic Bone Marrow Transplantation for Leukemias and Hematologic Malignancies in Bologna

G. Bandini[1], P. Ricci[1], M. Baccarani[1], L. Gugliotta[1], M. Gobbi[1], G. Visani[1], M. R. Motta[1], C. Guardigli[1], S. Rizzi[1], A. Zaccaria[1], G. Sermasi[2], A. Ferri[3], E. Emiliani[4], and S. Tura[1]

[1] Institute of Hematology "L.&A. Seràgnoli" University of Bologna and St. Orsola Hospital, Bologna
[2] Blood Transfusion Centre, St. Orsola Hospital, Bologna
[3] Department of Medical Physics, St. Orsola Hospital, Bologna
[4] Institute of Radiotherapy, St. Orsola Hospital, Bologna, Italy

Since Feb. '83 to Dec. '84 we performed 30 allogeneic bone marrow transplants (BTM) in hematologic malignancies. All the patients (pts) were HLA identical, MLR negative with the donor sibling. Conditioning followed the Seattle protocol; TBI was given from a single Co^{60} source at a low (3-5 rads/min) dose rate. Pts with Chronic Granulocytic Leukemia (CGL) were additionally given Daunomycin 1.5 mg/kg on day – 5; those with CGL in transformation also received Cytosine Arabinoside 200 mg/M^2/day in continuous infusion in 4 days. The pt with myeloma was given also melphalan, 5 mg/kg in 5 days. GVHD prophylaxis was attempted with Cyclosporin-A, given i.v. from day – 1 to + 5, then p.o. for 4 months, if GVHD was absent; doses were gradually decreased after day 50. Details of the patients and results are shown in the table. All pts with CGL are in hematological and cytogenetic remission. The major problems of our BMT programme are a high relapse rate in acute myeloid leukemia and a high frequency of chronic GVHD in CGL.

Table - Analysis performed at January 15, 1985.

U.P.N. age/sex	diagnosis	months from diagnosis	acute GVHD	chronic GVHD	outcome	survival (days)	Karnofsky score
1. 31/F	M_4 (1st CR)	5	1, skin	No	Relapse	269	0
3. 24/F	M_4 (1st CR)	5	1, skin	No	Relapse	208	0
4. 13/M	M_5 (1st CR)	6	0	Minor	Relpase	620 +	40
7. 24/M	M_3 (1st CR)	10	4, skin, gut, liver	–	GVHD, infection	46	0
22. 14/M	M_2 (1st CR)	9	1, skin	Minor	Well	224 +	100
23. 24/F	M_3 (1st CR)	5	2, skin	No	Well	133 +	80
30. 19/F	M_4 (1st CR)	5	0	–	Well	42 +	100
31. 39/M	Sec.ry leukemia*	8	0	–	Well	35 +	90
2. 17/M	L_2 (1st CR)	4	3, skin	Mild	Chronic GVHD	670 +	90
5. 28/M	L_2 (2nd CR)	24	2, skin	Moderate	CNS relapse	460	0
6. 21/M	LB Lymphoma	3	0	No	Well	590 +	100
8. 17/F	L_2 (2nd CR)	7	0	No	Well	480 +	100
28. 17/M	L_2 (2nd rel)	14	2, skin	–	Well	63 +	100
15. 36/F	Myeloma	22	2, skin	Minor	Well	357 +	90
9. 28/F	CGL ch. ph.	24	0	Minor	Well	470 +	100
10. 31/F	CGL acc. ph.	24	2, skin	Moderate	Chronic GVHD	450 +	90
11. 29/F	CGL ch. ph.	42	1, skin	Moderate	Chronic GVHD	440 +	80
12. 37/M	CGL ch. ph.	140	0	Moderate	Tuberculosis	345	0
13. 42/M	CGL ch. ph.	26	0	Severe	Chronic GVHD	410 +	70
14. 40/F	CGL ch. ph.	9	0	Minor	Well	367 +	90
16. 31/M	CGL ch. ph.	7	0	Mild	Bacterial pneumonia	184	0
17. 25/M	CGL bl. ph.	15	3, skin	Severe	Chronic GVHD	308 +	70
18. 33/M	CGL acc. ph.	19	1, skin	Severe	Chronic GVHD	293 +	40
19. 46/M	CGL ch. ph.	13	3, skin, liver, gut	–	GVHD, infection	67	0
20. 28/M	CGL ch. ph.	7	3, skin	Minor	Well	251 +	100
21. 13/F	CGL ch. ph.	5	3, skin	No	Well	238 +	100
24. 19/M	CGL ch. ph.	18	1, skin	No	Well	125 +	100
25. 28/M	CGL ch. ph.	51	2, skin, gut, liver	–	GVHD, pneumonia	54	0
27. 32/F	CGL ch. ph.	13	0	–	Well	90 +	90
29. 35/M	CGL ch. ph.	23	3, skin, gut, liver	–	GVHD, Encephalopathy	55 +	20

* Primary disease Hodgkin's lymphoma.

Work supported by Italian C.N.R., Oncology Finalized Projects No. 84.00834.44 and 84.00432.44.

Exp. Hematol. (suppl. 17) 13:37 (1985)
© International Society for Experimental Hematology

Allogeneic Bone Marrow Transplantation for Thalassemia Major by Busulphan – Cytoxan Protocol and Cyclosporin – Acyclovir Prophylaxis

G. Torlontano, P. Di Bartolomeo, G. Di Girolamo, D. Natale, G. Bonanni, L. Velluto, M. Maldini, F. Barboni, E. Beltrandi, and A. Iacone

Cattedra di Ematologia e Divisioni di Ematologia e di Anestesia, Chieti-Pescara, Laboratorio Analisi Ospedale Malpighi, Bologna, Italy

Although much progress is being achieved in transfusi_ on therapy and iron chelating treatment, homozygous thalassemia patients have a bad quality and limited expectancy of life with conservative therapy. They u_ sually dye by the second or the third decade because of myocardium and liver iron overload. Allogeneic bone marrow transplantation (BMT) has been demonstrated to be an efficacious form of therapy for patients with congenital bone marrow disorders. Essential to propo_ se such form of therapy is to reduce at most the risk taken during the procedure. To this purpose, we have selected for BMT young thalassemic patients under 8 yr of age, little transfused, without parenchimal damage and with an HLA-identical and MLC-nonreactive sibling to serve as marrow donor.

Between May 1983 and October 1984, 5 patients (4 with beta-thalassemia major and 1 with double heterozygosis beta-thalassemia-hemoglobin Lepore), ranged in age from 2 to 7 yr, underwent BMT using their HLA-identi_ cal and MLC-nonreactive beta-thalassemia heterozygous siblings as marrow donors. They had received between 15 and 45 transfusions before BMT. The preparative re_ gimen consisted of busulphan (3-3.25 mg/Kg day for 4 consecutive days) and cyclophosphamide (50 mg/Kg/day for 4 consecutive days). Patients were nursed in "re_ verse isolation" rooms and received acyclovir orally as prophylaxis against herpetic virus infections. Cy_ closporin A was given to prevent graft-versus-host di_ sease (GvHD). The dose of nucleated cells infused was always above 5 x10^8/Kg body weight. One patient (uni_ que patient number, UPN, 28) dye on day +12 with func_ tioning graft because venocclusive disease of the li_ ver, staphylococcus aureus septicemia and pneumonia. The remaining 4 patients achieved complete hematologi_ cal chimerism, as proved by cytogenetic examinations and red cell markers. In all cases analysis of both beta/alfa globin chain synthesis ratio and hemoglobin electrophoretic pattern from bone marrow and periphe_ ral blood samples after BMT documented a picture con_ siting with thalassemia trait. In 1 patient (UPN 23) progressive autologous reconstitution occurred 6 months after grafting, as proved by gradual decrease of beta/alfa globin chain synthesis ratio and increase of fetal hemoglobin level (above 25 %). At 12 mo post BMT this patient shows a mixed chimerism and poor re

quirement of blood transfusions. The remaining 3 pati_ ents are living, well and hematologically normal wi_ thout GvHD between 6 and 20 mo after BMT. Fetal hemo_ globin levels are less than 2 %. The following table summarizes data of transplanted patients.

				BETA/ALFA GLOBIN RATIO				
	SEX/			Before	After BMT			OUTCOME
UPN	AGE	TR.	GvHD	BMT	3 mo	6 mo	10 mo	(1/20/85)
16	F/2	15	I	0.18	0.38	0.41	0.42	+ 611
23	F/2	16	NO	0	0.48	0.30	0.15	+ 393
26	M/7	45	I	0	0.43	0.42	0.43	+ 304
28	M/4	42	/	0.12	/	/	/	12
32	F/2	23	I	0	0.49	0.49		+ 173

(TR. : transfusions before BMT)

These results, as well as those of others (1-4), indi_ cate that BMT is fesible in patients with congenital bone marrow disorders as thalassemia major. For the future, two main objectives must be followed, i.e. a careful selection of patients to be transplanted and the choice of the optimal antihematopoietic preparati_ ve regimen.

References :
1) Thomas ED, Buckner CD, Sanders E, et al. Lancet 1982, ii, 227.
2) Lucarelli G, Polchi P, Izzi T, et al. Exp Hematol 1984, 12 (Suppl 15), 95.
3) Ioshi R, Barrett AJ, Ingram L, et al. Exp Hematol 1984, 12 (Suppl 15), 97.
4) Di Bartolomeo P, Di Girolamo G, Natale D, et al. XX Congr ISH, Buenos Aires, September 1-7, 1984.

Supported by M.P.I., Grant 40 %, 1982 and 1983.

Exp. Hematol. (suppl. 17) 13:38 (1985)
© International Society for Experimental Hematology

Allogeneic Bone Marrow Transplantation (BMT) for Chronic Myelogeneous Leukemia (CML) in Chronic Phase (CP)

G. Papa [1], W. Arcese [1], G. Arcangeli [2], F. R. Mauro [1], A. Bianchi [1], A. Guerra [2], G. Isacchi [1], T. Gallerano [1], M. Venditti [3], D. Diverio [1], G. Adorno [1], M. Purpura [4], L. Quintiliani [4], A. Filippini [5], and F. Mandelli [1]

[1] Institute of Hematology, University "La Sapienza", Rome
[2] Medical Institute of Scientific Research (I.M.R.S.), Rome
[3] Chair of Semeiotica Medica III, University "La Sapienza", Rome
[4] Laboratory of Histocompatibility, Centro Nazionale Trasfusione Sangue
[5] Chair of Surgical Clinic V, University "La Sapienza", Rome, Italy

INTRODUCTION

Allogeneic BMT seems to be a promising therapeutic modality for patients with CML. An actuarial 3-years disease-free survival of 60-70% can be achieved in patients grafted during CP of the disease (1, 2, 3). The results of BMT in accelerated phase and blastic phase of CML are poorer then in CP; the major problems are due to transplant -related complications (2) or to increased frequency of recurrent leukemia (3). This report summarizes the experience with allogeneic BMT performed during CP of CML at the Institute of Hematology of the University of Rome.

PATIENTS AND METHODS

Between August 1983 and December 1984, 11 Ph^1 positive CML patients, 10 in first and 1 in second CP, received allogeneic BMT from HLA identical siblings. The age range was 17 to 43 years (median 30 yrs); disease duration of CML at time of BMT ranged from 8 to 123 months (median 32 mo). All patients were previously-treated with hydroxyurea and/or busulfan. No patient was splenectomized. One patient underwent allogeneic BMT during second CP obtained by intensive chemotherapy (BAVC regimen) and infusion of cryopreserved peripheral stem cells (4). The conditioning regimen consisted of Cyclophosphamide (120 mg/kg b.w.) and 10.20 GY TBI at six doses of 1.7 GY each and administered in three daily fractions over two days. The nucleated cell dose of bone marrow infused ranged from 1.03 to 3.7 x 10^8 /kg b.w. of the recipient with a median cell dose of 2.1 x 10^8/kg b.w. The first patient received i.v. Methotrexate (MTX) for prevention of GVHD. The other 10 patients received Cyclosporine-A (CSA) i.v. and orally. Three patients received, in addition to CSA, donor marrow in vitro incubated with a monoclonal rat anti-human lymphocyte antibody (CAMPATH-1) and autologous complement to obtain T-cell depletion. Reverse barrier isolation, gut decontamination with sterile food and non absorbable antibiotics, oral Acyclovir, high dose i.v. Sandoglobulins and oral Cotrimoxazole were employed for prophylaxis against infections.

RESULTS (Table)

Survival. Ten of 11 patients survive at follow-up periods ranging from 42 to 383 days with a Karnofsky score of 90-100% The actuarial survival at one year for all 11 patients is 90%. No hematological or cytogenetic relapse has been observed.

Toxicity and mortality. Acute-GVHD occurred in 6 out 11 evaluable patients (54.5%). Of these 3 had grade I, 2 grade II and 1 grade III A-GVHD. Two out of the 9 patients at risk showed some evidence of chronic GVHD. Neither acute nor chronic GVHD were observed among the 3 patients who received T-depleted marrow and CSA. Infections post BMT were as follows: septicemia (3); pneumonia (1); CMV-related interstitial pneumonitis (I.P.) (1). Other major non infective

complications included an hemolytic crisis in Rh incompatible graft, a CSA related bilateral deltoid paralysis with electromiographic proven peripheral polyneuropathy and an early post-transplant pulmonary oedema syndrome (P.O.S.), which resolved without complications. The patient on MTX prophylaxis died on day +111 for CMV-related interstitial pneumonitis.

PTS	GVHD		COMPLICATIONS	SURVIVAL	KARNOFSKY
	A	C		days	%
1*	III	L	sepsis, CMV-I.P.	died, 111	–
2	0	–	deltoid paralysis	+ 383	100
3	I	–	convulsions	+ 347	100
4	II	S	hemolysis, pneumonia hypertension	+ 314	100
5	I	–	nephrotoxicity	+ 252	100
6	0	–	nephrotoxicity	+ 233	100
7**	0	–	P.O.S., hypertension	+ 195	100
8	II	–	sepsis	+ 138	100
9	I	–	sepsis, CVC abscess	+ 104	90
10**	0	–	–	+ 69	100
11**	0	–	–	+ 42	100

*MTX to prevent A-GVHD.   **In addition to CSA, patients received donor BM in vitro treated by CAMPATH-1.

CONCLUSIONS

The small series and the short follow-up of our patients cannot bring to any conclusions as to incidence of leukemic relapse. However some considerations about the outcome of the early post-transplant period may be drawn. Mucositis, severe A-GVHD and CMV-related I.P. appeared only in the patient on MTX prophylaxis. It is noteworthy that among CSA patients aged more than 25 yrs, A-GVHD was observed in all 4 patients (age: 25,31,33,36 yrs) treated with CSA alone and in none out of 3 patients (age: 33,36,43) given CSA in association with CAMPATH-1 treated donor BM. The administration of CSA was associated to a number of side effects that were common: nausea, vomiting, nephrotoxicity and hypertension; unusual: bilateral deltoid paralysis with peripheral polyneuropathy; debated: P.O.S.

REFERENCES

1) Champlin R.E. and Gale R.P.: Cancer Treat. Rep. 68:145-161,1984
2) Goldman J.M. et al.: Exp. Hematol. 12 (suppl.15): 34-35,1984
3) Speck B. et al.: The Lancet, i: 665-668,1984
4) Papa G. et al.: New Trends in Experimental Hematology, eds. C. Peschle and C. Rizzoli, Serono Symposia Review 7:346-348,1984

Exp. Hematol. (suppl. 17) 13:40 (1985)
© International Society for Experimental Hematology

Bone Marrow Transplantation Versus Chemotherapy alone for Acute Nonlymphoblastic Leukemia

A. Marmont, A. Bacigalupo, M. T. Van Lint, F. Frassoni, and A. Carella

Department of Haematology, Ospedale San Martino, Genova, Italy

The question whether allogeneic bone marrow transplantation (BMT) carries greater advantage for patients with ANLL as compared to chemotherapy (CT) alone has been and is still debated intensively (1,2). The issue has been further complicated by recent results with autologous BMT (3). In this contribution a retrospective analysis from our clinical experience is presented.

Materials and Methods.

From December, 1978 to July, 1984, 37 patients aged 3-44 with ANLL were brought into CR by means of the "7 and 3" CT regimen, with consolidation of the C type (4). Nineteen patients with HLA-histocompatible siblings were transplanted, 18 in first and 1 in second CR. Three were conditioned according to the original Seattle protocol (CY 120 - TBI 10 Gy in single dose), and 17 with fractionated TBI (3.33 Gy x 3; 5). Other 18 patients with no HLA-histocompatible siblings were treated with CT alone (4). Overall and disease-free survival at 2 years (DFS) were as following:

	Overall survival	DFS
BMT	70%	64%
CT	21%	13%

Both in the raw data and in the survival curves

BMT vs CHEMO in 1st rem. ANLL

survival for both groups was calculated starting from the achievement of CR. BMT was performed frome 1 to 12 months after remission.

DISCUSSION

Measuring overall survival and DFS from the onset of CR was considered a necessary adjustment to obtain a better evaluation (2). Although it must be pointed out that there was only 1 patient in the FAB M4-M5 cathegory for the BMT group, as contrasted with 10 patients for the CT group, the main points of this study are (a) the DFS plateau for the BMT group, which is still holding, and (b) the highly significant difference from the CT curve. Admittedly, more efficient CT protocols are now employed (6), and a new approach is advocated (7,8), so that we are limited with data that are not especially mature. In addition, we agree with Begg et al. as to the necessity of placing the issue in proper perspective. Large scale, prospective, biologically randomized studies are clearly indicated, but it must be also realized that the introduction of new drugs and/or new manipulations is susceptible of changing both our approach and our management of ANLL.

References

1. Gale,R.P.,Champlin,R.E.-In Gale R.P.(ed) "Recent Advances in Bone Marrow Transplantation"; Liss,N.Y.,1983.
2. Begg,C.B. et al - J.Clin.Oncol.2:369-378,1984.
3. Burnett,A.K. et al - Lancet 2:1068-1070,1984.
4. Rai, K.R. et al - Blood 58:1203-1212,1981.
5. Vitale, V. et al. - Brit.J.Haematol. 55:547-554,1983.
6. Carella,A.M. et al.-Leukemia Res.,in the press.
7. Santer,Chr.et al.-Lancet 1:379-382,1984.
8. Champlin, R.et al.-Lancet 1:894-895,1984.

Exp. Hematol. (suppl. 17) 13:39 (1985)
© International Society for Experimental Hematology

Allogeneic BMT for Chronic Myelocytic Leukaemia (CML): Some Ph+ Bone Marrow Cells May Resist Cyclophosphamide and TBI Conditioning but are Gradually Deleted during Donor-Type Haemopoietic Reconstitution

W. Hinterberger[1], W. Schmidmeier[2], A. Hajek-Rosenmayr[3], P. Höcker[4], B. Volc-Platzer[5], G. Grabner[6], W. Kallinger[7], G. Alth[7], H. Kolbabek[7], A. Laszkowicz, W. Mauritz[9], W. Graninger[10], H. Gadner[2], K. Lechner[1], M. Fischer[1], G. Stingl[5], I. Schwarzinger[1], I. Druml[1], and E. Deutsch[1]

[1] First Department of Medicine, University of Vienna
[2] St. Anna's Children Hospital, Vienna
[3] Institute for Blood Group Serology, Vienne (National Blood Group Reference Laboratory, WHO and National Tissue Typing Reference Laboratory, Council of Europe)
[4] Blood Transfusion Service, University of Vienna
[5] First Department of Dermatology, University of Vienna
[6] Second Department of Ophtalmology, University of Vienna
[7] Department of Radiotherapy, Community Hospital Lainz-Vienna
[8] Second Department of Surgery, University of Vienna
[9] Department of Anesthesiology, University of Vienna
[10] Department of Chemotherapy, University of Vienna, Austria

Introduction: The conditioning regimen for BMT in CML, consisting of Cyclophosphamide and TBI, is supposed to permit eradication of Ph+ haemopoiesis. Cells from successfully grafted patients have a donor-karyotype and re-appearance of Ph+ cells is considered as a reliable sign of relapse. Our own observation, however, illustrates that persistence of Ph+ cells after the conditioning must not necessarily reflect resisten leukaemia or early relapse.

Patients: 10 consecutive patients, allografted from their HLA-matched siblings, are described: 7 patients were in chronic phase. 3 patients were in "accelerated" phase, as judged on Busulfan-unresponsive anemia and thrombocytopenia (Nr 3), an evolving new clone (Nr 7) or an increase of blasts in blood and marrow (Nr 9). Pat. Nr 4 was admitted in Tdt+ lymphoid blast crisis (Table 1).

Patient Nr	Age, Sex	Duration (Months)	Phase of Disease	Treatment before BMT	Donor Age
1	25, m	11	Chronic	Busulfan	23, m
2	28, m	10	Chronic	Busulfan	38, m
3	32, m	8	Accel.	Busulfan	25, m
4	29, f	36	Blastic	Busul., VCR, PRED	16, f
5	38, f	14	Chronic	Busulfan	34, m
6	33, f	42	Chronic	Busulfan	25, f
7	32, m	16	Accel.	Busulfan	37, f
8	34, f	48	Chronic	Busulfan	25, m
9	14, f	87	Accel.	Busulfan, M-Bromol	10, m
10	32, m	8	Chronic	Busulfan	36, m
	X=32	X=15			X=25

Bone Marrow Transplantation Procedure: Conditioning included Cyclophosphamide (2 x 60 mg/kg, days -5, -4) and 1000 rad TBI, delivered from a Co^{60} source at 7-17 rad/min (Nr 1-3) or 3-4 rad/min (Nr 4-10). Lungs were shielded to 800 rad. MTX was given as CNS prophylaxis on days -6 and -3, and was later given as GVH-D prophylaxis until day 100 (Seattle scheme). No patient was splenectomized or had received splenic irradiation.

Clinical Results: 3 patients died, 7 patients are alive 129-506 days post graft. Patients 1 and 3 died from CMV-pneumonitis (autopsy-proven). Patient 2 died from veno-occlusive liver disease. One patient (Nr 7) developed grade IV GVH-D of the gut, but recovered after treatment with Prednisolone, ATG and Cyclosporine-A. 3 patients developed chronic GVH-D of liver and skin (Nr 6, 7, 10), all of them responded favorably to Azathioprin/Prednisolone.

Haemopoietic Reconstitution: Prompt engraftment was documented in all patients. All survivors have normal blood counts at present. Serially performed cytogenetics (G-banding technique) revealed the presence of Ph+ mitoses 30 to 60 days in the bone marrow of 3 of 8 evaluable patients. Beyond 100 days, however, Ph+ metaphases were only demonstrable in patient 6 (day 120 after BMT). This patient is still in complete clinical and haematological remission. A recent cytogenetic analysis failed from technical reasons (Table 2).

Table 2

Patient Nr	Cytogenetics before BMT	Cytogenetics after BMT 30-60 Days	>100 Days	Survival (Days)	Karnovsky Score
1	46 XY, Ph+	46 XY, Ph-	---	100	0 %
2	46 XY, Ph+	---	---	47	0 %
3	46 XY, Ph+	---	---	43	0 %
4	n.e., Tdt+	46 XX, 5% Ph+	46 XX, Ph-	> 506	100 %
5	46 XX, Ph+	46 XY, Ph-	46 XY, Ph-	>422	90 %
6	46 XX, Ph+	46 XX, 27 % Ph+	46 XX, 17 % Ph+	>414	90 %
7	46 XY, Ph+, 5q-	46 XX, 11 % Ph+	46 XX, Ph-	>319	90 %
8	46 XX, Ph+	46 XY, Ph-	46 XY, Ph-	>305	100 %
9	46 XX, Ph+	46 XY, Ph-	46 XY, Ph-	>187	100 %
10	46 XY, Ph+	46 XY, Ph-	46 XY, Ph-	>129	90 %

(10.11.1985)

Discussion: Our results confirm previous experience documenting the possibility of eradicating Ph+ haemopoiesis after intensive chemo-radiotherapy. After patients 3, our irradiation protocol was changed to a lower dose rate in order to minimize the risk of pneumonitis. Our concern was then a possibly increased risk of leukaemic relapse. Indeed, the detection of Ph+ cells in 3 of 8 evaluable patients 30 to 60 days after BMT seemed to justify our concerns. However, Ph+ cells were no longer demonstrable in subsequent investigations in 2 of 3 patients. None of the surviving patients has so far shown any sign of clinical and haematological relapse. Thus, the persistence of chemo-radioresistant Ph+ cells obviously requires other considerations than late reappearance of Ph+ cells, which is, by common clinical experience, a sign of haematological relapse. We have no clues about the nature of cells carrying the Ph+ karyotype immediately after BMT. Chemo-radioresistance of some lymphoid cells of Ph+ karyotype, being devoid of haemopoietic repopulation capacity, could suitable explain this phenomenon. A longer follow up period is clearly needed to clarify the significance of such chemo-radio resistant Ph+ cells in the early period after BMT.

Exp. Hematol. (suppl. 17) 13:41 (1985)
© International Society for Experimental Hematology

Bone Marrow Transplantation Versus Chemotherapy for Patients under 15 Years of Age in 2nd Remission Acute Lymphoblastic Leukaemia (ALL)

F. Frassoni, A. Bacigalupo, M. T. Van Lint, M. Congiu, A. Carella, M. Martinengo, G. Dini, A. Comelli, L. Massimo, and A. Marmont

Department of Haematology, Ospedale San Martino, Genova, and
Istituto G. Gaslini, Genova, Italy

Recently the European Bone marrow Transplant Group (EBMT) has reported a significantly different relapse rate for ALL, according whether in first or subsequent remission (1). However, as far as ALL in children is concerned, the choice of BMT in 1st remission remains on open question since more than 50% of patients can be cured with chemotherapy (CT)(2). However, once relapse has occured, the mean survival of patients does not excedes 8 months. Therefore BMT in children with ALL in 2nd remission represent a crucial task.
Patients.31 patients under 15 years of age with ALL in 2nd remission were either transplanted with their HLA identical sibs(14 pts.) or were treated with standard CT (17 pts.)(3).
Transplant procedures. All patients received cyclophosfamide 60 mg/kg. on day -7,-6,. Ten pts. were give 330 rads of TBI for 3 consecutive days and 4 received 200x2 rads for 3 consecutive days according to a protocol activated in Nov. 1983 because a low relapse rate with this procedure had been reported (4) .TBI was delivered at 4-6 rads/minute.Lung were shielded in order to receive 20% less of the total dose. The care of the patients during transplantation has been described(5). 2/14 patients received methotrexate(MTX) or Cyclosporin A(CyA)for GvHD prophilaxis.Chemotherapy.The treatment of childhood ALL and the maitenance therapy has been described(3).Survival of the patients was calculated using Kaplan-Meier method.
Status of the patients.1)BMT group:1st relapse occurred for 6 patients in therapy, for 4 patient off therapy, and 4 patients were borderline (within 1-2 months after stop therapy).2)chemotherapy group:1st relapse occurred in therapy in 11 patients ,off therapy in 4 patients and 2 patients were borderline.
RESULTS AND DISCUSSION.
Engrafment was seen in all patients.Acute graft versus host disease: grade O-I ,II,III-IV GvHD was observed in 4,6,4 pts. respectively.Chronic graft versus host disease was seen in 6 pts.
Grafted patients:two pts. died of acute GvHD .Relapse occurred in 5 pts.(5/12) at 3,6,6,11,12

months after BMT.These patients had relapse in therapy or were borderline patients. No relapse was observed in patients who had experienced 1st relapse off therapy with a follou-up at 12-41 months after BMT.One of these patients had 1st relapse only in the CNS again relapsed in CNS 6 months post-BMT; he was reinduced and he is still in CR 29 months after BMT.Interstitial Pneumonitis(IP) has not been observed using either two TBI regimens.Chemotherapy patients. 14/17 had a 2nd relapse 1-24 months after 2nd CR. All of them were reinduced and 5/14 achieved a further remission, but none of them survived more than 11 months.2/17 patient are still in 2nd CR with a follow-up of 21,24 months.The actuarial survival at 30 months is 47% for the grafted patients and 0% for the petients non-grafted; the disease free survival at 24 months is 50% for the grafted patients and 14% for the chemotherapy group. This study is in keeping with the data of the literature(1) indicating a sizable relapse rate in pts. with ALL grafted in 2nd remission. In addition it poits out that relapses occur with higher frequency in pts.who had 1st relapse in therapy. However, 8/14 pts. are currently in CR 11 to 41 months .after BMT, whereas only 2/17 non grafted pts. are still in 2nd CR.(P 0.02). Interestingly, 3 patients relapsed after BMT had a sex mismatched graft:they were successfully reinduced, and the remission marrow was found to be 100% of donor origin. However, these pts. experienced complete remission for no more than two years.

References
1)Zwaan F.E. et al. Brit.J.Haematol. 58,33,1984;
2)Riehm H. et al Am.J.Pediatr. Hematol Oncol 2,299,1980.
3)Dini G.et al.Haematologica 68,202,1983.
4)Dinsmore R. et al. Blood 62,381,1983.
5)Marmont A. et al.Haematologica 68,351,1983.
This work was supported by CNR Progetto Finalizzato 82.00349.96-83.00870.96, and A.I.R.C. Milano, 1983.

Exp. Hematol. (suppl. 17) 13:42–43 (1985)
© International Society for Experimental Hematology

Autologous Bone Marrow Transplantation (ABMT) for Acute Leukemias (AL) in Remission

A. M. Carella[1], G. Santini[1], F. Frassoni[1], V. Rizzoli[2], A. Porcellini[3], M. Martinengo[1], A. Congiu[1], D. Giordano[1], S. Nati[1], and A. M. Marmont[1]

[1] Division of Haematology, Ospedale San Martino, Genova
[2] Department of Haematology, Parma
[3] Division of Haematology, Pesaro, Italy

It has been reported that ABMT may be successful in patients with AL treated in first CR (Gorin for the European ABMT group). Recently, Burnett also reported a high success rate in first CR ANLL using non-frozen ABMT. We are now reporting our experience in eleven (11) pts. with ANLL and ALL receving ABMT in CR.

Patients and Methods

Four pts. (2 ALL, 2 ANLL) were in their first CR. The duration of CR ranged from 1 to 32 mo. (median, 11 mo.). Five pts. (3 ALL, 2 ANLL) were in their second CR: these pts had experienced their first relapse 8,10,34 mo. (ALL) and 3 mo. (ANLL) after achieving a first CR. The second CR were observed in ALL pts. by VM-26 + Cytarabine and by Idarubicin (demetoxydaunorubicin) for ANLL pts. Two pts. (1 ALL- 1 ANLL) received ABMT while were in third CR. The relevant clinical data of patients is outlined in table I. According to the FAB classification there were in ALL group 5 L2 non B non T, 1 L3 SIg+ and 1 L2 E Ros+ (all pts had high risk characteristics at the diagnosis) and, for ANLL, 2 M1, 1 M2 and 1 M4 (the M2 patient had q8- q21+ traslocation). Except four ALL pts., that received high-dose BCNU (800mg/MQ) and non-frozen ABMT, the others received Cy 60mg/Kgx2 and after a rest day, TBI 10 Gy (ANLL pts.) or fractionated TBI (4 Gy for 3 d.) in ALL pts. A median of 0.94x10 (range 0.57-1.8x10) nucleated BM cells/Kg body weight were reinfused. The median CFU-GM recovery was 1.0x10 /Kg (range 0.4x1.6x10). Peripheral blood neutrophils and platelets attained level 500/mmc and 20.000/mmc at a median of 17 (range 15-29) and 29 (range 16-56 days) following marrow reinfusion.

Results

4/11 (2 ALL in 2nd CR, 2 ANLL in 1st CR) are surviving 11 mo. after ABMT, with a median survival from diagnosis of 22 mo. (range 16-48 mo.)(Table II). The others experienced early relapse or died for BMT procedure.

Conclusions

These preliminary results point out: 1) absence of early relapse in ALL pts. treated with BM "purged" fractionated TBI and conventional chemotherapy with CNS prophylaxis after ABMT; 2) promising results in ANLL treated with ABMT in first CR; 3) a very low incidence of extrahematological toxicity.

TABLE I
CLINICAL DATA OF PATIENTS ON ADMISSION

Number of pts.	11
Age y.	22(range, 16-46)
Sex	M7, F4
N.courses to enter 1st CR	ALL : 1
	ANLL : 2
N.days to enter 1st CR (median)	ALL : 20(16-42)
	ANLL : 30(28-64)
N.mo. CR/ABMT(1st CR only)	ALL : 8(6-14)
	ANLL : 5(2-8)
Survival after ABMT (mo.median)	ALL : 7mo.(2-18)
	ANLL : 6mo.(1-11)
N. pts. alive and well (January, 1985)	ALL :2(9mo.after ABMT)
	ANLL :2(11mo.after ABMT

TABLE II
AUTOLOGOUS BMT IN REMISSION AL

	Age/sex		Diagnosis	Disease status	BM storage	BM Treat. by ASTA-Z	Maintenance post ABMT	Survival pre (mo.)	post (mo.)	Outcome
B.L.	18	M	ALL/L3*	3th CR	4°C	-	-	12	6	Died(relapse)
P.E.	20	F	ALL/L2*	1st CR	4°C	-	-	11	7	Died(relapse)
M.V.	18	M	ALL/L2*	2nd CR	4°C	-	-	12	7	Died(relapse)
S.D.	24	M	ALL/L2*	1st CR	4°C	-	-	10	18	Died(relapse)
M.M.	38	M	ALL/L2T	3th CR	4°C	-	-	17	3	Died(relapse)
D.MA.	22	M	ALL/L2*	2nd CR	FROZEN	yes	yes***	40	10	Alive CR10mo.
P.M.	16	M	ALL/L2**	2nd CR	FROZEN	yes	yes***	16	10	Alive CR10mo.
B.M.	36	F	ANLL/M2	1st CR	FROZEN	-	-	11	11	Alive CR11mo.
S.M.	19	F	ANLL/M4	1st CR	FROZEN	yes	yes****	7	11	Alive CR11mo.
M.L.	46	M	ANLL/M1	2nd CR	FROZEN	-	-	11	-	Died cardiac failure)
C.B.	22	F	ANLL/M1	2nd CR	FROZEN	-	-	9	-	Died (gram negative sepsis

* non B, non T; ** Common

*** VCR+prednisolone x 4 wks followed by 6MP 50mg/mq daily + MTX 15mg/mq every ten days. Both pts. were treated with this scheme day +60 from ABMT for 6mo.

**** Idarubicin p.o 80mg/mq every two wks for 4 wks day +80 from ABMT.

Exp. Hematol. (suppl. 17) 13:44–45 (1985)
© International Society for Experimental Hematology

In vitro Purging with ASTA-Z of Autologous Bone Marrow Transplantation (ABMT) in Acute Leukemia and Lymphoma

Vittorio Rizzoli[1], Lina Mangoni[1], Gino Degliantoni[1], Cecilia Caramatti[1], Daniele Costi[1], Rodolfo Maramotti[3], Michele Carella[2], Gino Santini[2], and Alberto Marmont[2]

[1] Cattedra di Ematologia, Università di Parma
[2] Divisione di Ematologia, Ospedale di Genova
[3] Servizio di Anestesia e Rianimazione, Ospedale di Parma, Italy

INTRODUCTION

Bone marrow transplantation (BMT) is the best therapeutic strategy for acute leukemia. The goal of this method is to completely destroy the residual tumor cells and replace leukemic marrow with normal hemopoietic cells. The allogeneic BMT is the method of choice but it is possible in a small number of the patients because of the difficult to have an HLA identical donor.

Autologous bone marrow transplantation (ABMT) is now adays a tool by which it is possible to treat patients laking histocompatible donor. For this method the patient's own hematopoietic stem cells are harvested during partial or complete remission cryopreserved in liquid nitrogen then reinfused following treatment with intensive chemo-radiotherapy.(1,2,3,).

The limit of ABMT,however,is the possibility that the malignant cells present in the remission marrow determine the relapse of disease. To minimize the chance of bone marrow contamination with tumor cells, in vitro techniques have been developed to deplete malignant cells from bone marrow suspension, sparing the normal stem cells compartment before the reinfusion; at present, physical, pharmacological and immunological methods have been proposed to in vitro bone marrow "purging"(4,5).

In this brief report we analyze the results obtained with ABMT in leukemia and lymphoma after in vitro purging with Maphosphamide(ASTA Z) a new derivative of cyclophosphamide, wich is demonstrated an in vitro active drug able to destroy malignant cells, sparing normal stem cell compartment.(6).

MATERIALS AND METHODS

Patients. Patients wuth acute lymphatic leukemia (ALL),acute non lymphoid leukemia(ANLL) Hodgkin's disease(HD) and non Hodgkin lymphoma(NHL) are included in the study.The criteria of patient selection are:age <40 years, absence of significant liver, renal and heart disfunctions,poor prognosis, evidence of remission marrow(number of blasts<5%).The details of patients are summarized in table I. As conditioning regimen patients received high doses of chemotherapy plus total body irradiation(TBI) at single dose,except patients whose are treated by chemotherapy alone.

Bone marrow collection. Bone marrow is collected after at least three weeks from the end of chemotherapy, by multiple aspiration from posterior iliac crests,under general anestesia. The amount of bone marrow collect must be enough to obtain 4×10^8 cells/kg of patients body weight.

Bone marrow purging. To purifie bone marrow from the malignant cells, we used ASTA Z at a final concentration of 100 µg/ml . ASTA Z is a stabilized metabolite of 4-hydroperoxy-cyclophosphamide(4HC), the cytotoxic efficacy of wich on malignant cells corresponds to the activity of 4HC..The suspension is incubated 30 minute at 37°C in water bath, cooled to 4°C for 5 minutes, centrifuged then resuspended at a final concentration of 4×10^7 /ml for the cryopreservation.

Before and afer in vitro purging, samples of bone marrow cells are kept for the evaluation of in vitro colony growth.

Bone marrow transplant. Prior to reinfusion the cells are tawed by a rapid immersion in water bath at 37°C. The viability of cells is evaluated by trypan blue dye test exclusion and reinfused into patients immediatly after the end of conditioning regimen. The cells are reinjected at doses ranging from 0.9 to 2×10^8 cells/kg body weight.The engraftment is documented by the evaluation of hematologic recovery. None of the patients received chemotherapy after ABMT.

Supportive care. All patients are hospitalized in laminar air ventilated room.During the period of post transplant aplasia, patients are supported with platelets and paked red blood cells transfusions. A broad spectrum of antibiotic and antimicotyc drugs is administered until the patients are fever free and the total leucocyte count rises above $1,000/mm^3$ with absolute granulocyte number over $500/mm^3$.

Tab.I Clinical data of patients treated with ABMT in vitro purged with ASTA Z(100 µg/ml).

N. of cases	age	diagn.	remiss. before ABMT	regimen	remission after ABMT
4	15-34	ALL	1st CR[a]	Cy-TBI[b]	32+,12+,5+ 0.3, G.I. haemorrage
2	15-17	ALL	2nd CR	Cy-TBI	21+relapse 8+
1	49	ANLL	1st CR	Bu[c]Cy	7+
1	32	ANLL	2nd CR	Bu-Cy	0.5 sepsis and renal failure
6	17-30	NHL	3 PR, 3 CR	BAVC[d]	18+,9+,6+, 3+,11+ re-lapse,0.3 G.I.hemorrage
1	21	HD	PR	Cy-TBI	6+

[a] Complete Remission
[b] Cyclophosphamide 50 mg/kg 4 days
[c] Busulfan 4 mg/kg 4 days
[d] BCNU 200mg/m^2d.4,ARA-C and VP16 1200 mg/m^2q12h dd -5-2, Cycloph. 180 mg/kg.q24h dd -5-2

RESULTS

The survival time of the patients are shown in Fig. 1 and Fig.2.

The post transplant clinical course of the patients is characterized by severe cytopenia,fever,infections and alopecia,in all cases. Two patients with pregressed gastric or peptic ulcer had moderate hemorragic symptoms of the G.I. tract.

In eight cases oral mucositis of variable duration and severity occurred. Three patients had liver disfunction and moderate renal toxicity.

The hematologic recovery was evaluated by the daily count of total leucocytes, granulocytes, platelets. The nadir of bone marrow aplasia occurred within 3-6 days after the end of conditioning regimen;the hematologic recovery occurred at 14 th -18 th day.

At the time of discharge all patient were in good clinical conditions. Neither consolidation nor manteinance therapy was given after ABMT.

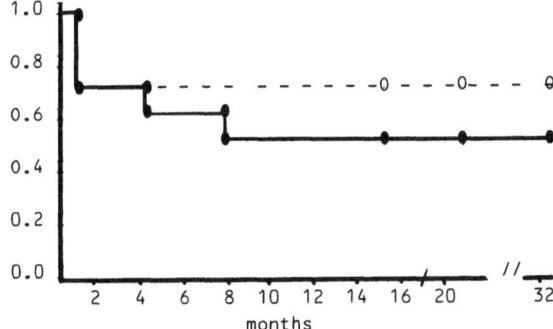

Fig.1. Survival time of ALL and ANLL patients treated with purged ABMT.
O- - Ooverall survival,●——●disease free survival

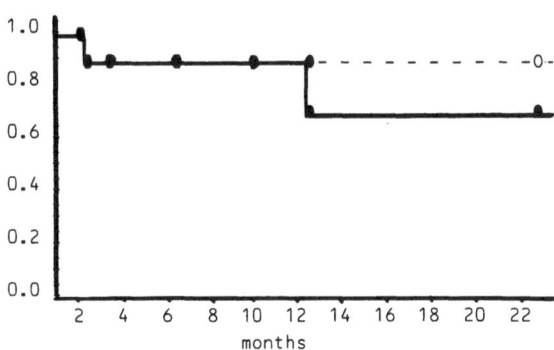

Fig. 2. Survival time of lymphoma patients treated with purged ABMT
O- - -Ooverall survival,●——●disease free survival

DISCUSSION

The evaluation of the survival time of treated patients shows that 6 of 8 patients with leukemia and 6 of 7 patients with lymphoma are surviving for 5 to 32 and 3 to 18 months respectivelly after ABMT.;10 of them are in complete remission.Our previous data (6) on the effect of in vitro treatment of bone marrow with ASTA Z demonstrated that the in vivo hematologic recovery is delayed when compared with the data obtained in patients transplanted with ABMT without pharmacological purging; in all cases however,we never observed any complication related with the treatment of bone marrow cells with the drug.Thus the in vitro cleansing of bone marrow with the method described does not affect the clinical course of the post transplant period.

It remains to be seen whether the ASTA Z is able to completely destroy the residual tumor cells in the remission marrow and if this treatment can be equally made in 1st or 2nd remission.

REFERENCES

1. Abrams RA., Levine A.S., Deisseroth AB.(1981)The use of intensive antineoplastic therapy in association with hematopoietic reconstitution. Medical Complications in Cancer Patients.Raven Press New York 292.

2. Gale R.P.(1980) Advances in the treatment of acute myelogenous leukemia. N. Engl. J. Med. 300:1189.

3. Gorin N.C., David R., Stachowlach J. (1981) : High dose chemotherapy and autologous bone marrow transplantation in acute leukemias, malignant lymphomas and solid tumors. A study of 23 patients. Eur.J.of Cancer 17:557.

4. Rizzoli V., Caramatti C.,Mangoni L.,(1983) : The effect of 4 HC and VP16 213 on leukemic and normal myeloid progenitor cells. Exp.Hemat., 11 suppl.14: 9.

5. Ritz J., Schlossman S.F.(1982) Utilization of monoclonal antibodies in the treatment of leukemia and lymphoma.Blood 59, 1:1

6. Rizzoli V., Mangoni L., Caramatti C., Degliantoni G., Costi D. (1983): The in vitro bone marrow purging in autologous bone marrow transplantation. Haematologica, 68:51

This investigation was supported by grant 84.00767.44 from the CNR,Rome, Italy.

Exp. Hematol. (suppl. 17) 13:46 (1985)
© International Society for Experimental Hematology

Autologous Bone Marrow Transplantation in Children Acute Lymphoblastic Leukemia

E. Plouvier, P. Herve, A. Noir, M. Flesch, J. Y. Cahn, E. Racadot, P. Henon, P. Lutz, A. Boilletot, C. Behar, and M. Munzer

Bone Marrow Transplantation Unit, Pediatric Clinics, Hôpital Saint-Jacques, F-25000 Besançon, France

Autologous bone marrow transplantation (A.B.M.T.) following intensive therapy represents a new approach to the treatment of children with acute lymphoblastic leukemia (A.L.L.) in complete remission (C.R.) (1,2). This study presents the results and toxicity observed in twelve children with A.L.L., treated with intensive therapy and A.B.M.T.

PATIENTS AND METHODS

They were two girls and ten boys and their age ranged from 3 to 15 years with a mean of 8 years. One girl, with B-ALL (L3), was autografted in first C.R. Eleven children were autografted in second C.R. : 8 had L1 lymphoblasts, and 3 had L2 lymphoblasts (F.A.B. classification).

Four children had bone marrow harvested during the first C.R., because they had "poor prognosis" A.L.L. (B phenotype, lymphoblasts 100 x 10^9/L at diagnosis, ...). The median time between C.R. and harvesting was 12 months.

Eight children had bone marrow harvested during the second C.R., with a median time of 10 months between second C.R. and harvesting.

Seven bone marrows were treated ex-vivo with metabolite of cyclophosphamide (ASTA-Z) (3) and four bone marrows with anti-CALLA monoclonal antibodies and rabbit complement. Before ex-vivo treatment, the marrow cells were washed and concentrated with an IBM-2991 cell washer, and mononuclear cells were isolated by means of discontinuous "Ficoll-Hypaque" density gradients.

In the girl with B-ALL, the conditioning regimen was the "modified" B.A.C.T. : BCNU : 200 mg/m^2 on days 1, 2, 3 ; aracytine : 200 mg/m^2 on days 2, 3, 4, 5 ; cyclophosphamide : 1600 mg/m^2 on days 2, 3, 4, 5 and 6-thioguanine : 200 mg/m^2 on days 2, 3, 4, 5.

Eleven children were conditioned with total body irradiation (T.B.I.) followed by cyclophosphamide (60 mg/kg/day x 2). T.B.I. was administered in on single dose (10 grays) for one patient, and was fractionated for ten chilren (12 to 13,2 grays).

Autologous bone marrow was infused 48 hours after the last dose of chemotherapy.

Children received oral non-absorbable antibiotics for total gut decontamination, and Ketoconazole for fungal infection prophylaxis.

No child received maintenance therapy after A.B.M.T.

RESULTS

Sustained engraftment occured in all children. Peripheral blood neutrophils attained a level 0,5 x 10^9/L at a median of 32 days (range 18-58), and platelet recovery to a level 50 x 10^9/L was reached at a median of 37 days (range 22-115).

The intensive therapy was well tolerated, and no death was observed for the first three months postgraft. Two cases of bacterial septicemia (Staphylococcus epidermidis, Branhamella catarrhalis) were documented, and one severe pulmonary infection was observed.

Four children developed localized herpes zoster infection at months 3, 6, 6, 8 post-transplantation but all resolved quickly. One boy presents one moderate and unilateral cataract which began 15 months after A.B.M.T.

At the present time, the results of this study are the following :
- one girl, with B-ALL, relapsed 8 months after A.B.M.T. and died three months after relapse,
- one boy died 112 days post-graft, following cerebral hemorrhage (platelets 10 x 10^9/L),
- two boys relapsed 8 and 9 months after graft,
- in fact, eight children remained in second C.R., without any maintenance therapy, from 7 to 47 months after A.B.M.T., and the median survival time was 18 months.

DISCUSSION

In spite of the short follow-up for some children, the low incidence of relapse appears to be encouraging in this study and five children remained in second C.R. more than 12 months after graft.

A.B.M.T. with ex-vivo treated bone marrow is proven to be an attractive alternative to children who lack HLA identical donors, in the management of ALL in second remission.

A French protocol is being put into practice to compare autologous transplant with treated marrow versus allogenic transplantation in childhood ALL in second C.R.

REFERENCES

1 - SALLAN SE, BAST RD, LIPTON JM et al. : 'Autologous bone marrow transplantation in C ALLA positive acute lymphoblastic leukemia". In "Minimal residual disease in acute leukemia". Lowenberg B, Hagenbeck A, eds Boston/The Haye/Dordsecht/Lancaster/Martinus Nijhoff 1984, 255-264.

2 - RAMSAY W, LEBIEN TW, NESBIT M et al. : "Autologous bone marrow transplantation for acute lymphoblastic leukemia following marrow treatment BA1, BA2, BA3 and rabbit complement". Blood (in press).

3 - HERVE P, CAHN JY, PLOUVIER E et al. : "Autologous bone marrow transplantation for acute leukemia using transplant purified with a metabolite of oxazaphosphorines (ASTA-Z) : first clinical results". Invest New Drugs 1984, 2, 245-252.

Exp. Hematol. (suppl. 17) 13:47 (1985)
© International Society for Experimental Hematology

Autologous Bone Marrow Transplantation (ABMT) for Patients with Chronic Granulocytic Leukemia (CGL) in Blastic Phase (BP)

G. Meloni, A. Pulsoni, P. De Fabritiis, F. Malagnino, E. Montefusco, G. Papa, A. Sandrelli, F. Simone, and F. Mandelli

Institute of Hematology, Department of Human Biopathology, University of Rome, Italy

Autologous hemopoietic stem cell infusion after high dose chemo/radiotherapy performed in BP of CGL is able to reinduce II CP in 90% of patients; however the median survival does not last more than 6 months. This report concerns 5 patients with Ph1 positive CGL in BP treated with BAVC regimen followed by hemopoietic stem cells reinfusion. An intensification program of cyclic chemotherapy has been applied after ABMT with the aim to prolong the survival of these patients. Since 1980 the majority of CGL patients seen at the Institute of Hematology of Rome were subjected to collection and cryopreservation of hemopoietic stem cells from bone marrow (BM) or peripheral blood (PB). Details of the methods have been described elsewhere (1,2). Of the 5 patients presented in this report 4 received stem cells collected from PB and 1 from BM. Four patients were males, median age was 39 years (range 29-41). Therapy during CP consisted of hydroxyurea; no splenectomy had been performed in any patient. Type of transformation was myeloid in 4 cases and mixed in one. BAVC conditioning regimen consisted of BCNU 800 mg/mq day 1; AMSA 150 mg/mq/day on days 2-4; VP-16 150 mg/mq/day days 2-4; CA 300 mg/mq/day c.i. days 2-4. Stem cells were reinfused 24 hours after last dose chemotherapy with a median of 11×10^8 (range 3-21) nucleated cells/kg body weight. After complete hematological reconstitution (25-30 days) from autologous infusion an intensification program of cyclic chemotherapy was begun consisting of 3 courses of L-VAMP (VCR 1.5 mg/mq i.v. hour 0, MTX 200mg/mq c.i. hours 1-3, CA 500 mg/mq c.i. hours 3-7, ASNASI 5000 U/mq i.m. hour 24, PDN 40 mg/mq/day days 1-5); 3 courses of DAT (DNR 60 mg/mq i.v. day 1, CA 60 to 150 mg/mq/8 hours s.c. days 1-5, 6-TG 70 mg/mq/8 hours p.o. days 1-5) and 3 courses of HiDAC (CA 1 g/mq/12 hours c.i. in 3 hours on hour 0,12; ASNASI 6000 U/mq i.v. on hour 18). RESULTS All patients obtained II CP; 1 patient died on day 10 after BM engraftment from cerebral hemorrhage. Recovery of PMN>500/µl occurred on day 8 through 19 and PLTs>50000/µl on day 10 through 22. One patient had an HLA compatible donor and underwent allogeneic BM transplantation during II CP, 3 months after ABMT. He is now alive and well at 6 months in complete hematological and cytogenetic remission. In other 3 patients the BP relapsed after 3,5.3,8 months, with a survival of 7.5+,9.6,9.6 months after ABMT, respectively. One patient developed an extramedullary relapse presenting as mediastinal T-cell lymphoblastic lymphoma 8 months after ABMT. Cytogenetic analyses, performed on the tumour mass and on pleural effusion, revealed the presence of complex numerical and structural chromosome abnormalities, including a duplicate or triplicate Ph1 chromosome. The patient died after 1.5 month for rapid progression of disease with BM still in CP.

Pt.	I CP months	ABMT result	Subsequent treatment	II CP months	Survival months
1	24	II CP	–	0.1	0.3
2	28	II CP	chemoth.	8	9.6
3	50	II CP	chemoth.	5.3	9.6
4	37	II CP	BMT	3	9.3+
5	40	II CP	chemoth.	3	7.5+

Four patients had BM cytogenetic investigations both at diagnosis of BP and during the II CP. Two patients at BP displayed chromosome abnormalities additional to the Ph1, which were not seen at II CP. The patient who presented the extramedullary relapse showed at II CP a reduction of Ph1+ cells from 90% to 20%.
DISCUSSION ABMT in patients with CGL in BP allows high proportion of return to the CP, invariably followed after 3-8 months by a new BP which is always fatal (3,4). Patients with HLA identical donor but in which transformation occurs before allogeneic BMT may be autografted and then transplanted in II CP. Preliminary good results were obtained in fact in patients reverted to the CP with intensive chemotherapy and transplanted at that time. The role of a post-ABMT intensive polychemotherapy program is still undefined and needs to be evaluated in more extended trials although in our experience it seems of little value in prolonging II CP duration.

REFERENCES
1) G. Meloni et al. Leukemia Res., in press.
2) G. Meloni et al. Proc. 8 Corso Naz. Agg. Emat. 1982
3) R.E. Champlin et al. Cancer Treat. Rep. 68,1:145,1984
4) A. Haines et al., submitted for publication.

Exp. Hematol. (suppl. 17) 13:48 (1985)
© International Society for Experimental Hematology

Intensive Cytotoxic Therapy Followed by Autologous Bone Marrow Transplantation in Haematological Malignancies
A Report of 25 Patients

L. F. Verdonck, A. W. Dekker, M. L. van Kempen, K. Punt, and G. C. de Gast

University Hospital Utrecht, The Netherlands

INTRODUCTION

We report our experience with intensive cytotoxic therapy followed by autologous bone marrow transplantation (ABMT) in 25 patients with a non-Hodgkin lymphoma of high grade malignancy (NHL), refractory Hodgkin's disease (HD) and acute leukaemia (AL).

MATERIALS AND METHODS

Patients:

The median age of the patients was 27 years (range 15-53) and male-female ratio 2.1:1. Fifteen patients had a (non-localised) NHL, of whom thirteen with bulky disease (> 10 cm) and one with bone marrow involvement at presentation. All patients received multiple courses of combination chemotherapy before the ABMT procedure. Thirteen received CNS prophylaxis. At the time of ABMT four patients had a drug-resistant NHL, five were in partial remission (PR) and six were in complete remission (CR)(five in 1st CR and one in 2nd CR). Two patients had a (refractory) HD and had received extensive treatment with combination chemotherapy and radiotherapy and were non-responsive to any (conventional) treatment at the time of ABMT. Eight patients had an AL; four an acute non-lymphocytic leukaemia (ANLL), three a (bad risk) acute lymphocytic leukaemia (ALL) and one an acute undifferentiated leukaemia (AUL). They received remission-induction and consolidation treatment and all received CNS prophylaxis.

Bone marrow procurement

Bone marrow aspiration and cryopreservation occurred after confirmation of no tumour involvement of the bone marrow. Bone marrow aspiration in patients with an AL occurred in 1st CR. The bone marrow of one patient with a T-ALL was purged in vitro with an immunotoxin (WTI-Ricin A).

Cytoreductive treatment

Patients with a NHL and an AL received cyclophosphamide (120 mg/kg) and total body irradiation (800 rad) and patients with HD received cyclophosphamide (6 g/m^2) and etoposide (1,2 g/m^2). None received post-transplant cytoreductive treatment.

RESULTS

NHL: Three out of four patients with a drug-resistant NHL achieved a CR but all relapsed within 6 months. Five out of five patients with a NHL in PR achieved a CR but two relapsed 3 and 5 months after ABMT and one died in aplastic phase because of sepsis, two are in CR 4+ and 33+ months after ABMT. Three out of six patients with a NHL in CR are in CR 18+, 19+ and 36+ months after ABMT, two relapsed 8 (transplanted in 2nd CR) and 11 months after ABMT and one died 7 months after ABMT because of an ANLL without recurrence of his T cell NHL.

HD: Two out of two patients with a therapy-resistant HD achieved a CR but one relapsed 2 months after ABMT and the other died of therapy-related toxicity.

AL: Three patients with an ANLL were treated in 1st CR and two are in CR 17+ and 18+ months after ABMT, one relapsed 7 months after ABMT. One patient with an ANLL was treated in 2nd CR and relapsed 3 months after ABMT.

Two patients with a poor risk ALL were treated in 1st CR and both relapsed 3 and 6 months after ABMT (the one with in vitro purging of the BM with an immunotoxin relapsed after 6 months). One patient with a poor risk ALL was treated in 2nd CR and relapsed 2 months after ABMT. One patient with an AUL was treated in 1st CR and is in CR 4+ months after ABMT.

Toxicity of the ABMT procedure was acceptable with three therapy-related deaths (all patients with end-stage disease and poor clinical condition).

CONCLUSIONS

These preliminary results indicate that intensive cytoreductive treatment followed by ABMT may improve disease-free survival in patients with a NHL in CR (and PR?) and ANLL in 1st CR. No conclusions can be drawn for patients with a poor risk ALL in 1st CR. For patients with a HD this treatment may be of value in an earlier phase of their disease.

Exp. Hematol. (suppl. 17) 13:49 (1985)
© International Society for Experimental Hematology

Autologous Non-Frozen Bone Marrow Transplantation
Report of 16 Cases

G. Santini[1], A. M. Carella[1], A. M. Congiu[1], F. Frassoni[1], M. Martinengo[1], S. Nati[1], D. Giordano[1], V. Rizzoli[2], A. Porcellini[3], and A. M. Marmont[1]

[1] Division of Haematology, Ospedale San Martino, Genova
[2] Institute of Haematology, Parma
[3] Division of Haematology, Pesaro, Italy

5Pts. with non-Hodgkin lymphoma (NHL) and 11Pts. with solid tumor (mediam age 44 years, range 12-63) were treated with high dose chemotherapy ± TBI and autologous non-frozen bone marrow transplantation (ABMT). In all cases bone marrow was harvested in general anesthesia, kept at 4°C for 36-48 hours, and then reinfused.

Conditioning regimens: 1) BCNU 600-1000mg/m, median 730mg/m (7 glioblastoma, 2NHL); 2) BCNU 600mg/m +VP-16-213 600mg/m (4 lung cancer); 3) BCNU 600mg/m +CTX 5g/m +VP-16-213 400mg/m (2 NHL); 4) CTX 120mg/Kg + TBI 10Gy (1 NHL).

NHL: 5 Pts.; 2 in 1st complete remission (CR), 1 in 2nd CR, 1 in 1st relapse, 1 in 2nd relapse. All patients with high-grade malignancy NHL (3 lymphoblastic, 2 centroblastic); 3 out 5 are now in CR at 35 (1st relapse), 8 and 43 (both in 1st CR) months post-ABMT. Of the two remaining: one is alive in relapse at 17 months (2nd CR), while the second died in relapse at 18 months (2nd relapse).

GLIOBLASTOMA: 7 Pts. (5 in 1st CR, 2 in 2nd CR) all after surgery and total brain irradiation (40Gy). One patient, in 2nd CR, is currently in persistent CR 47 months post-ABMT and 55 months from diagnosis. The other 6 Pts. died in relapse 10,11,13,14,15,16 months after ABMT and 14,15,16,17,18,26 months from diagnosis respectively.

LUNG CANCER: 4 Pts. A) 1 adenocarcinoma and 1 epidermoidal carcinoma were treated with ABMT as first regimen: a partial response was obtained in one case (died for infection), but the disease progressed in both of them; B) 2 small cell carcinoma in 1st CR: 1 is in CR 14 months after ABMT and the second died in relapse 5 months after ABMT. Total number of infused nucleated marrow cells was $1.2 \pm 0.5 \times 10$ /Kg (± SD), with a recovery from the original aspirate of 72±27%. Total number of infused CFU-GM was $3.3 \pm 1.6 \bar{x} 10$ /Kg, with a recovery of 84±19%. Hemopoietic recovery was prompt after ABMT: patients had median granulocyte level 500/mm on day + 14 (range 0-20), and median platelet count 20.000/mm on day + 19 (range 0-33).

In conclusion these data indicate that ABMT using non-frozen marrow is feasible and associated with low toxicity. The ABMT is effective in prolonging survival in glioblastoma after surgery and total brain irradiation. A possible role of the ABMT in high-grade malignancy NHL is suggested althought more data are required. Little effect was seen in lung tumors.

HIGH-DOSE CHEMOTHERAPY ± TBI AND AUTOLOGOUS NON-FROZEN BONE MARROW TRANSPLANTATION

Pathology	Cases	Patient status	Treatment	Anti-tumor effectiveness	Overall survival	Comments
Glioblastoma	7	RC	BCNU	1Pt. in persistent CR 47mo.+	1Pt./60mo.+	3 cases of mild lung fibrosis
Lung Tumors	4	RC 2; initial diagnosis 2	BCNU+VP-16	1Pt. in persistent CR 14mo.+	1Pt./25mo.+	1 case died of infection
NHL						
Centroblastic	1	1st RC	BCNU	persistent CR 43 mo.+	46 mo.+	ABMT after 3 CHOP
Lymphoblastic	1	1st relapse	"	CR 35 mo.+	43 mo.+	mediastinal involvement
Centroblastic	1	2nd relapse	BCNU+CTX+ VP - 16	partial remission	67mo.	died for progression disease 18mo. after ABMT
Lymphoblastic	1	2nd RC	"	relapse 10mo. after ABMT	38 mo.+	leukaemic relapse
Lymphoblastic	1	1st RC	CTX+TBI	persistent CR 8 mo.+	18 mo.+	-

Exp. Hematol. (suppl. 17) 13:50 (1985)
© International Society for Experimental Hematology

Circulating Stem Cells in Patients with Akute Leukaemia in Remission

K. Geißler, W. Hinterberger, P. Bettelheim, P. Höcker, M. Fischer, and K. Lechner

1st Department of Medicine, Division of Haematology and Blood Coag., University of Vienna and Blood Transfusion Service, Vienna, Austria

FIG.1

Introduction: The results of allogeneic bone marrow transplantation in patients with acute leukaemia (AL) in complete remission (CR) suggest, that supralethal chemo-radiotherapy is capable of eradicating leukaemia. However, graft versus host disease and the lack of HLA-compatible donors in more than 50% of patients remain the mature problems of this procedure. These limitations have led to interest in using autologous stem cells for rescue after supralethal chemo-radiotherapy. In order to examine peripheral blood from AL-patients in remission as a possible source of stem cells for autografting, we determined the number of circulating granulocyte/macrophage committed progenitor cells (CFU-GM), erythroid committed progenitor cells (BFU-E) and pluripotent progenitor cells (CFU-MIX) in 13 patients with acute myeloid leukaemia (AML) and 10 patients with acute lymphocytic leukaemia (ALL) during and after maintenance chemotherapy.

Patients: AML-patients received weekly thioguanine (100 mg/m², d 1 to 5) and cytosine-arabinoside (100 mg/m², d 6) or cycles of daunoblastine (45/m², d 1), vincristine (1 mg/m², d 1) and cytosine arabinoside (100 mg/m², twice daily, d 1 to 5) at intervals of 6 weeks. ALL-patients received 6-mercaptopurine (50 mg/m², daily), methotrexate (5 mg/kg, twice weekly), and 14 d cycles of vincristine (1 mg/m², d 1,7,14) and prednisolone (2 mg/kg, d 1 to 14) at intervals of 7 weeks.

Methods: CFU-GM were assayed by the method of Pike and Robinson. BFU-E and CFU-MIX were cultured using a modification of the clonal assay described by Fauser & Messner. No investigations were performed during infectious episodes, during leukopenia (<2000/μl) or when violations of the treatment protocol were detected.

Results: Fig 1 shows the stem cell numbers in the PB of patients with AL during and after maintenance chemotherapy. Results are expressed as median values of all investigations performed in the same patient. Shaded areas represent values for normal peripheral blood. In 8 AML-patients on maintenance chemotherapy circulating CFU-GM were significantly (p < 0.01) decreased compared with normal subjects. 5 AML-patients being off chemotherapy had likewise reduced CFU-GM (p<0.05),

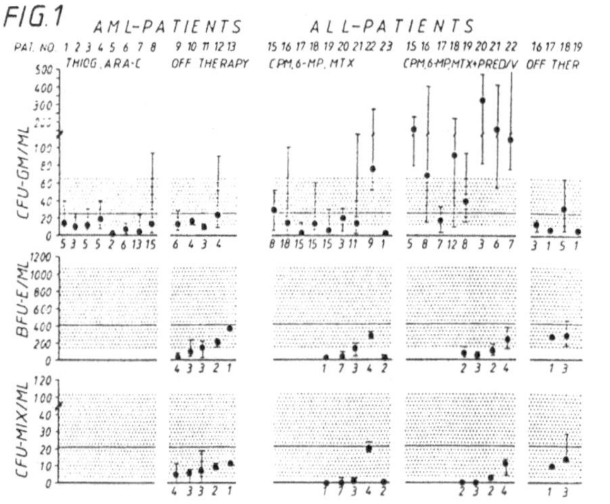

BFU-E (p < 0.05) and CFU-MIX (p < 0.05), respectively. In 9 ALL-patients on maintenance chemotherapy numbers of circulating CFU-GM, BFU-E and CFU-MIX were decreased (p< 0.01). Cycles of vincristine and prednisolone caused a tenfold expansion of circulating CFU-GM, whereas no increment of BFU-E and CFU-MIX could be observed. In 2 ALL-patients being off chemotherapy, all stem cell classes were found to be in the range of normal controls.

Conclusions: If the CFU-MIX content is considered to be an indicator of the reconstitutive capacity, periperhal blood from patients with AML and ALL during and after chemotherapy is a poor source of stem cells for autografting. Taken the number of CFU-GM as a measure of the reconstitutive capacity peripheral blood of pred/vcr treated patients would contain more cells being able to restore haemopoiesis after supralethal therapy. The discrepancy between the numbers of CFU-GM and CFU-MIX in pred/vcr treated patients indicates that one has to be very cautious in predicting the reconstitutive capacity by means of CFU-GM determinations only.

References:
Dicke KA et al (1979) Lancet,i, 514-517
Fauser AA & Messner HA (1978) Blood 52 1243-1248
Hinterberger W et al(1984)Scan J Haematol,33,244-251
Pike BL & Robinson WA (1979) J Cell Physiol,76,77-84
Thomas ED et al (1975) N Engl J med 292, 832-843

Supported by Grant 4100 of the "Fonds zu Förderung der Wissenschaftlichen Forschung in Österreich" and by the "Kommission für Leukämieforschung und Knochenmarktransplantation" of the Austrian Academy of Sciences

Exp. Hematol. (suppl. 17) 13:51 (1985)
© International Society for Experimental Hematology

Bone Marrow (BM) Processing and Cryopreservation for Autologous Bone Marrow Transplantation (ABMT)

J. García, R. Ayats, P. Madoz, P. Sardà, C. Pastoret, L. Vila, E. Martínez, and M. L. Rutllant

Unitat de Recerca Biomèdica, Servei d'Hematologia, Banc de Sang, Hospital de la Santa Creu i Sant Pau, Barcelona, Spain

INTRODUCTION

Successful chemo-radiotherapy followed by autologous bone marrow infusion is nowadays a widespread treatment applied to an increasing number of malignancies.

While its therapeutic objective is quite clear in the treatment of solid tumours and lymphomes, where bone marrow is free of disease, the rational use of this kind of treatment in leukemia is doubtful.

We report our experience in bone marrow harvesting, fractionation, concentration by density sedimentation and cryopreservation, in order to perform autologous bone marrow infusion. We also describe our experience in monitoring the complete process by CFU-GM cultures using different sources of CSA.

PATIENTS AND METHODS

BM harvesting and cryopreservation, in order to perform ABMT, were done in 14 patients (3 Hodgkin diseases, 2 CGL in CP, 3 ANLL in first complete remision and 6 non Hodgkin lymphomes).

Harvesting was done by multiple punctures in iliac crests (1). BM concentration was performed by means of IBM-2991 blood cell processor (2, 3). BM mononuclear cell (MNC) cryopreservation, using DMSO at final concentration of 10%, was carried out in an automatic freezer (Cryoson-BV6) at 1º C/min. rate (4).

Throughout BM process we have performed viability controls by Blue Trypan exclusion and CFU-GM cultures using Pike & Robinson thecnique (5).Human placental conditioned medium (HPCM) was used as a source of colony stimulation activity (CSA). Moreover, feeder layer (FL) and FL plus α-thyoglicerol were employed in thawed material.

REFERENCES

1.- Thomas et al. Blood, 36, 507. 1970.
2.- Gilmore et al. Brit. J. Haematol. 50, 619. 1982.
3.- Hervé et al. Rev. Fr. Transf. XXVI, 2. 1983.
4.- Hervé et al. In "Bone Marrow transplantation in Europe". Touraine Ed. Excerpta Medica, Amsterdam, p. 80. 1979.
5.- Pike & Robinson. J. Cell Physiol. 76, 77. 1970.
6.- Schlunk et al. Cryobiology, 18, 111. 1981.
7.- Aglietta et al. Cryobiology, 21, 486. 1984.

RESULTS

Table 1. B. M. CONCENTRATION RESULTS (IBM-2991)

- Volume reduction	= 85%
- Reduction of RBC contamination	= > 99%
- Reduction of platelets contam.	= 55%
- Mononuclear cells recovery	= 172%
- CFU-GM recovery	= 127%

Table 2. CFU-GM CULTURES THROUGHOUT B.M. PROCESS

PN	BASAL	FRESH BM	IBM Fr.	+DMSO	THAWED HPCH	THAWED F-L
1	25	148	70	110	NG	NG
2	42	205	165	100	75	80
3	160	37	60	54	36	41
4	21	107	75	55	88	94
5	21	37	43	14	32	54
6	220	249	105	143	224	190
7	97	105	160	124	52	95
8	67	45	37	35	7	26
9	44	107	60	57	30	169
10	182	90	81	145	68	190
11	200	25	19	11	80	50
12	76	128	90	132	1	115
13	17	16	3	1	26	ND
14	54	102	55	58	108	96
MEAN	87±72	100±68	73±46	74±50	63±57*	100±56*
% RECOVERY	100	79±40	73±43	88±81	112±54	

NG = No Growth.   ND = Not done.   (•) p > 0,1
Results in number of CFU-GM/10^5 MNC seeded.
Addition of α-TG in a concentration of 10^{-4} to 10^{-5} M sometimes corrects the low stimulation observed with HPCM.

DISCUSSION

In agreement with other authors (2, 3), in our experience BM fractionation by blood cell processor (IBM-2991, using Ficoll-Metrizoate) is a feasible method which yields a high degree of purification of Mononuclear cells (MNC).Problems derived from hemolysis and cell clumping are thus avoided. The fact that cryopreservator introduction and removal does not alter CFU-GM recovery confirms the lack of toxicity of DMSO at low temperatures during a short period of time and a tolerable osmotical cell behaviour.

In addition our standard freezing program seems to be acceptable in terms of CFU-GM recovery either from bags or samples.

In thawed material we agree with others (6, 7) about the importance of the source of CSA used. HPCM does not seem to be the best one. In our results FL is, statistically, a better CSA in 6 out of 12 cases studied.

Exp. Hematol. (suppl. 17) 13:52 (1985)
© International Society for Experimental Hematology

Buffy Coat Collection and Incubation with a Cytotoxic Compound (ASTA Z 7557) in Patients with Previously Untreated Chronic Granulocytic Leukemia (CGL)

P. Höcker[1], W. Hinterberger[2], K. Geissler[2], O. Haas[3], W. Schidmeier[3], K. Gerhartl[1], and K. Lechner[2]

[1] Blood Transfusion Service
[2] 1st Department of Medicine
[3] Division of Haematology and Haemostaseologie, University of Vienna and St. Anna Children Hospital, Vienna, Austria

Introduction: Conventional treatment with cytostatics and/or irradiation can barely prolong survival in patients with CML. Allogeneic BMT has frequently led to Philadelphia (Ph)-negative haemopoiesis with the option of long term survival. For patients lacking suitable bone marrow donors, collecting of enough autologous buffy coat cells and subsequent autografting in blast crisis is another approach (1). In a recent report, a rather unexplainable finding was described: Following autografting with unpurged bone marrow in a patient with Ph[+] CML, a transient Ph[-] haemopoiesis in vivo was restored (2). This observation was confirmed (3) in patients who were autografted with unpurged blood-derived buffy coat cells.
For patients with AML, purging of remission bone marrow with a Cyclophosphamide derivative, ASTA Z 7557 has widely been used. This compound, to our best knowledge, has not been used for CML patients. This initial report describes our preclinical experience in treating Ph[+] buffy coat cells in vitro with ASTA Z 7557.
Patients and Methods: 3 newly diagnosed patients with Ph[+] CML underwent leucapheresis with an AMINCO cell separator. The number of myeloid progenitor cells (CFU-GM) per ml blood and per ml buffy coat suspension are shown in Table 1:

Pat.	CFU-GM/ml (peripheral blood)	CFU-GM/ml (buffy-coat)
1	2965	31783
2	1835	24998
3	778	7211

Each buffy coat was subsequently divided in 2 portions: One portion was enriched with $Me_2SO(4)$ and cryopreserved. The other portion was FICOLL-separated and the cell concentration was adjusted to 2.10^7 cells/ml. After a 30 min incubation with ASTA Z 7557 at 100ug/ml final concentration (5,6) cells were washed twice, enriched with Me_2SO, and cryopreserved. Prior and at the end of the cryopreservation CFU-GM cultures and Cytogenetics (G-banding technique) were performed.

Results and Discussion: The preparation for freezing, which included preincubation with ASTA Z 7557, washing and subsequent enrichment with Me_2SO eliminated detectable CFU-GM in the samples of patients 1 and 2. Sample 3 still contained measurable CFU-GM (Table 2).

Pat.	CFU-GM/ml (+ ASTA Z) (+ Me_2SO_4)		CFU-GM/ml (without ASTA Z) (+ Me_2SO_4)		duration of Storage (days)
	pre	post	pre	post	(Freezing+Storage)
1	0.0	333.0	14549	20493	77
2	0.0	0.0	4829	1130	16
3	181.0	317.6	3089	2904	113

After freezing and storage in liquid nitrogen, however, CFU-GM were detectable in the samples of patients 1 and 3. Without preincubation with ASTA Z 7557, a wide range of recovery of freezing was seen. Cytogenetic analysis demonstrated persistence of Ph[+] metaphases in the sample of patient 1. In samples 2 and 3 no suitable metaphases were harvested.
Thus, our observation demonstrates that ASTA Z 7557 does not preferentially eradicate Ph[+] cells. The persistence of normal stem cells in CML is controversial. To define the usefulness of ASTA Z 7557 for bone marrow purging, selected patients having coexisting normal stem cells should be studied. For patients having only Ph[+] leukaemic cells, however, our very limited experience seems to argue against the use of ASTA Z 7557 in purging unseparated patient buffy coat cells.

References:
1. Goldman et al., Brit.J.Haematol.45:223-231 (1980)
2. Gorin et al. Europ.J.Cancer Clin Onc.:20:1-9 (1984)
3. Reiffers et al. Brit.J.Haematol.55:382-383 (1983)
4. Hagenbeck et al. Invest.New Drugs 2:237-243 (1984)
5. Herve et al. Exper.Haematol 12 (Suppl 14),133-134 (1984)
6. Körbling et al. Blut 48:189-199 (1984)

Exp. Hematol. (suppl. 17) 13:53 (1985)
© International Society for Experimental Hematology

Purging of Bone Marrow with the B-Lymphocyte Specific Monoclonal Antibody Y29/55 and Complement: Exclusion of Antigenic Modulation †

Angelika C. Stern [1], C. Baumgartner [2], G. P. Brun del Re [1], H. K. Forster [3], A. Hirt [4], A. Morell [4], H. P. Wagner [2, 4], and U. Bucher [1]

[1] Central Hematology Laboratory and
[2] Department of Pediatrics, University Hospitals, Inselspital, CH-3010 Berne
[3] Pharma Research, Hoffmann-La Roche, CH-4002 Basel
[4] Institute for Clinical and Experimental Cancer Research, University of Berne, Tiefenauspital, CH-3004 Berne, Switzerland

Introduction. The murine monoclonal antibody (mAB) anti-Y 29/55 (IgG2A) reacts with malignant B-lymphocytes obtained from patients with chronic lymphocytic leukemia (CLL) or non-Hodgkin's-lymphoma (NHL) (1). We have used this antibody for in vitro complement (C') induced elimination of lymphoma cells in human bone marrow (b.m.) prior to autologous b.m. transplantation (2). Certain mAB are known to induce antigenic modulation. This could interfere with optimal C'-mediated cell lysis (3). Optimal incubation conditions have been defined with CLL-cells:
Cell concentration: $\leqslant 20 \times 10^6$ cells/ml, mAB concentration: 50-250 µg/ml, concentration of C': 25%, time of incubation: 15' for mAB alone and 90' together with C' at 20°C. — This study was performed to evaluate possible antigenic modulation induced by anti-Y 29/55.

Materials and methods. CLL-cells (5×10^6 or 20×10^6 cells/ml) or Daudi-cells (2×10^6 cells/ml) were preincubated with anit-Y 29/55 (100 µg/ml) for 30', 2 h or 24 h at 4°C, 20°C or 37°C. The cells were washed twice and tested for the presence of antigen or antigen-antibody complexes on the cell surface. — Assessment was done by either determining susceptibility to C'-mediated cell lysis or by indirect immunofluorescence. Adult rabbit serum prepared in our own laboratory was used as C' source.

Results:

Fig. 1

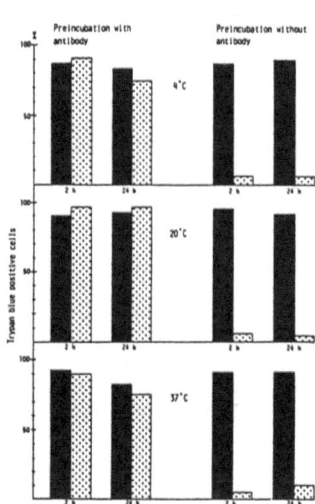

Legend to Fig. 1: It shows the C'-mediated lysis of CLL-cells (20×10^6/ml) after preincubation with 100 µg/ml anti-Y 29/55 (left panel) or without mAB (right panel) for 2 h or 24 h at 4°C, 20°C or 37°C. Cell lysis was assessed by dye exclusion (Trypan blue) after a second incubation (90', 20°C) with 50 µg mAB and C' or with C' alone.

Fig. 2

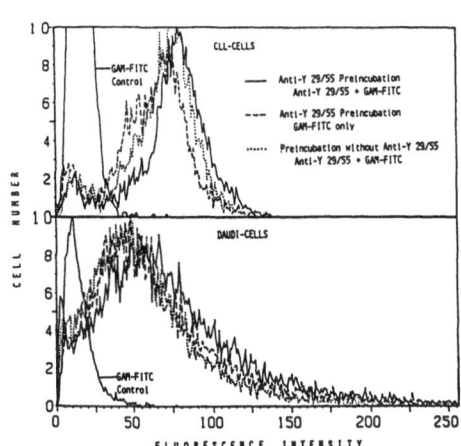

Legend to Fig. 2: 5×10^6 CLL-cells/ml or 2×10^6 Daudi-cells were preincubated with or without 100 µg/ml anti-Y 29/55 for 24 h at 37°C. The cells were washed twice and then stained for indirect immunofluorescence analysis with either 10 µg mAB and goat anti mouse FITC (GAM-FITC) or GAM-FITC alone. — The intensity of immunofluorescence was measured by cytofluorograph (10^4 cells/sample).

Conclusions. Only minor differences were found between mAB pretreated and untreated cells, proving stability of antigen and antigen-antibody complexes on the cell surface. Thus the mAB anti-Y 29/55 does not induce significant antigenic modulation. This shows that anti-Y 29/55 positive tumor cells can be effectively removed by C'-mediated lysis.

References
1. Forster H.K. et al.: Cancer Res. 42:1927, 1982.
2. Baumgartner C. et al.: Exp. Hematol. 12:404, 1984.
3. Ritz J. et al.: Blood 59(1):1, 1982.

† Supported by the Swiss National Foundation for Scientific Research.

Exp. Hematol. (suppl. 17) 13:54 (1985)
© International Society for Experimental Hematology

Purging of Bone Marrow with the Monoclonal Anti Calla Antibodies VIL-A1, VIB-E3 and VIB-C5 as a Prerequisite for Autologous Bone Marrow Transplantation

G. P. Brun del Re[1], Angelika C. Stern[1], C. Baumgartner[2], W. Knapp[3], A. Hirt[4], A. Morell[4], U. Bucher[1], and H. P. Wagner[2, 4]

[1] Central Hematology Laboratory and
[2] Department of Pediatrics, University Hospitals, Inselspital, CH-3010 Berne, Switzerland
[3] Institute of Immunology, University of Vienna, A-1090 Vienna, Austria
[4] Institute for Clinical and Experimental Cancer Research, University of Berne, Tiefenauspital, CH-3004 Berne, Switzerland

Adult patients with common acute lymphoblastic leuk-emia (cALL) have a poor prognosis despite an improve-ment of conventional chemotherapy. In patients lack-ing a suitable HLA identical donor of bone marrow (b.m.), intensive chemo- and radiotherapy and trans-plantation of in vitro purged autologous b.m. could be an alternative to induce long term remissions. We have therefore tested the in vitro cytotoxicity of the monoclonal anti CALLA antibodies (mAB) VIL-A1, VIB-C5 and VIB-E3 together with complement (C').

Materials and methods

Antibodies: VIL-A1, VIB-C5 and VIB-E3 are murine mAB of IgM-class which lyse CALLA positive cells in the presence of rabbit C', VIB-C5 also with human C' (1). VIB-C5 and VIB-E3 do react with myeloid cells and B cells too. The mAB-concentration in the ascitic fluid varied between 1-5 mg/ml.
As C' source we used fresh serum of young rabbits, prepared in our own laboratory.
Cells: The influence of the in vitro treatment on CFU-c was tested with b.m. cells of healthy donors. VIL-A1 positive tumor cells were obtained from pa-tients with cALL (b.m. or peripheral blood).
Conditions for the in vitro treatment: Separated mono-nuclear cells (20x10⁶/ml albumin solution) were pre-incubated with mAB (0.00005-500 µg/ml). After 15 min 25 % rabbit C' was added and left at room temperature for 90 min. The cells were then washed twice and re-suspended in Hank's solution.
Cell lysis was assessed by dye-exclusion (trypan blue). Additionally a mixture of bisbenzimide labelled nor-mal b.m. cells and VIL-A1 positive tumor cells was treated in vitro with either VIL-A1, VIB-C5 or VIB-E3 and C'. Remaining viable (ethidiumbromide negative) leukemic cells were identified by indirect immuno-fluorescence (VIL-A1, VIB-C5 or VIB-E3 plus GAM-FITC).

Patient: A 42 years old female with cALL was treated with chemotherapy according to the high risk protocoll 33/83 of the Swiss Group for Clinical Cancer Research (SAKK). Relapse occurred 10.5 months after diagnosis. After 2 cycles with DNR, VP-16, VCR and PRD the b.m. was collected, treated in vitro with VIL-A1 and C' and cryopreserved. At the moment of collection the b.m. contained about 5 % of blasts. The autologous b.m. was reinfused after a regimen with Cytoxan 60 mg/kgx2 and TBI 6x200 cGy.

†Supported by the Swiss National Foundation for Scientific Research.

Results

CFU-c content in normal b.m. was not affected by in vitro treatment with VIL-A1 and C'   . The same result was obtained with VIB-C5 and VIB-E3 (not shown here). The loss of CFU-c by additional freezing and thawing was not more than 25 %.
Maximal lysis of CALLA-positive cells was achieved at a mAB-concentration above 0.05 µg/ml and a C' concen-tration of 20 % or more. With each mAB a plateau was already reached after 30 min of incubation (Fig. 1). After treatment of the mixture of b.m. and tumor cells with either VIL-A1, VIB-C5 or VIB-E3 and C' no more viable VIL-A1 positive cells could be detected. But after purging with VIL-A1 and C' 1-2 % of viable VIB-C5 or VIB-E3 positive tumor cells were still present.

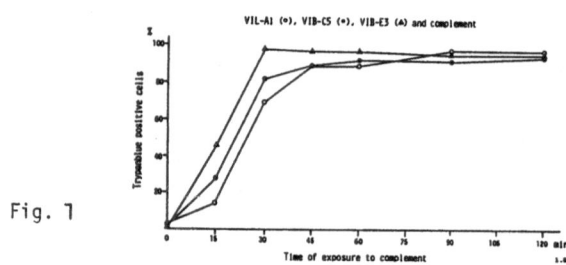

Fig. 1

The patient described showed after massive chemothera-py, TBI and transplantation of VIL-A1 purged marrow (0.33x10⁵ CFU-c/kg) rapid hematological reconstitu-tion (0.5x10⁹/ℓ neutrophils day 21, 50x10⁹/ℓ platelets day 18). Discharged from hospital on day 21. Septi-caemia with Strept. viridans responded promptly to pe-nicillin. A therapy resistent relapse occurred on day 60.

Conclusions

Our results demonstrate that in vitro purging of auto-logous b.m. with VIL-A1, VIB-C5, VIB-E3 and C' does not interfere with the regeneration capacity of hemo-poietic stem cells in vitro. The same applies for VIL-A1 in ABMT. These mAB induce rapid and virtually com-plete C'-mediated lysis of reactive leukemic cells by combination of the three anti CALLA mAB.

Reference

1. Knapp et al.: Cancer Detect Prev 6:281-86 (1983).

Exp. Hematol. (suppl. 17) 13:55 (1985)
© International Society for Experimental Hematology

Treatment of Disseminated Malignant Histocytosis in First Remission with Intensive Chemotherapy and Cryopreserved Autologous Bone Marrow

W. Kaulfersch[1], C. H. Urban[1], I. Slavc[1], , G. Maurer[1], I. Teubel[2], and P. Höcker[3]

[1] Department of Pediatrics, University of Graz
[2] Blood Transfusion Service, Department of Surgery, University of Graz
[3] Blood Transfusion Service, Allgemeines Krankenhaus Wien, Vienna, Austria

Introduction: Malignant Histiocytosis (MH) is a non hereditary rapidly fatal disease characterized by a neoplastic proliferation of atypical histiocytes, predominantly within lymphoid and haematopoeitic organs. Median duration of survival is two years after Adriamycin-based chemotherapy (CHOP) with complete remission rates from 57 % to 92 % (1). Despite early responsiveness of MH to chemotherapy the disease is still frequently relapsing at the end or shortly after therapy. On the contrary Phillips et al.(2) report a disease free survival rate of 56+ months in a patient with MH who has been treated with cyclophosphamide,total body irradiation (TBI) and autologous bone marrow transplantation (ABMT).

Case report: Our patient, a 17 year old boy, had a 2 months history of recurrent fever, weight loss and painful swelling of his right inguinal lymphnodes. Ultrasonography and computed tomography revealed extensive intra- and retroperitoneal nodal involvement. A preliminary diagnosis of B-cell Non-Hodgkins' Lymphoma (NHL) was based on the histomorphological and histochemical examination of the lymphnodes. Liver, spleen and bone marrow were not involved. Polychemotherapy according to the Austrian protocol for NHL (B-plan) was started and complete remission (CR) was achieved after 3 weeks.

Diagnosis had to be revised on immunhistochemical criteria (Lymphknotenregister der Deutschen Gesellschaft für Pathologie,Kiel) to MH. Chemotherapy was stopped on day 45. Bone marrow morphologically free of tumor cells was collected from the patient and stored in liquid nitrogen. BACT chemotherapy (Fig.1) was utilized as preparative regimen prior to ABMT.

Leucocytes were $4,3x10^9$/l on day 9,reticulocytes 10%o on day 18, and thrombocytes $51x10^9$/l on day 28 after ABMT. The posttransplant course was uneventful and the patient is in good condition and free of disease for now 10+ months since ABMT.

	Day						
	1	2	3	4	5	6	7
BCNU 200 mg/m^2	•						
Cytosine arabinoside 200 mg/m^2		•	•	•	•		
Cyclophosphamide 1600 mg/m^2		•	•	•	•		
6-thioguanine 200 mg/m^2		•	•	•	•		
Cryopreserved bone marrow							•

Fig.1: BACT Chemotherapy and day of ABMT

Discussion: MH still is a highly malignant disease with a poor prognosis. Recently clinical studies exploring the use of high-dose therapies with predominantly bone marrow toxicity supported by ABMT have proven a high response rate and an increase in survival rates in patients with responsive tumors, but who have a low cure rate (3). These strategies are best applied early in the clinical course before extensive damage from chemotherapy can accumulate.

Among other tumors with low cure rates and a poor prognosis, the one case reported by Phillips et al. and our own one may tentatively suggest that high-dose tumor ablative therapy and ABMT might be an alternative approach in the treatment of disseminated MH.

References:

1) Tseng A et al. The treatment of Malignant Histiocytosis. Blood,64, 48-53,1984.
2) Phillips GL et al. Treatment of resistant malignant lymphoma with cyclophosphamide, total body irradiation, and transplantation of cryopreserved autologous marrow. N Engl J Med, 310, 1557-61,1984.
3) Spitzer G et al. High-dose chemotherapy with autologous bone marrow transplantation. Cancer, 54, 1216-25,1984.

Aplastic Anemia I

Treatment

Exp. Hematol. (suppl. 17) 13:56–57 (1985)
© International Society for Experimental Hematology

Treatment of Severe Aplastic Anemia in Europe 1970–1983
A Report of the EBMT SAA Working Party

A. Bacigalupo, F. Di Giorgio, M. Congiu, M. T. Van Lint, F. Frassoni, M. G. Daga, L. Gogioso, and A. M. Marmont

Divisione Ematologia, Ospedale San Martino, Istituto Scientifico Tumori, Genova, Italy

List of Centers contributing patients to the EBMT study (according to number of patients).
Hôpital Saint Louis, E. Gluckman Paris; Kantonspital, B. Speck Basel; Hammersmith Hospital, C. Gordon Smith London; Ospedale San Martino, A. Marmont Genova; Postgraduate School of Haematology, A. Granena Barcelona; University Hospital I.P., F. Zwaan Leiden; University Hospital Dept of Pediatrics, J. Vossen Leiden; Westminster Hospital, J. Barrett London; Huddinge Hospital, G. Gahrton Huddinge; University Hospital, W. Hinterberger Vienna; Klinik Innere Medizin, H. Heimpel, Ulm; University Hospital J. Gmur Zurich; Medizinische Universitaetsklinik, P. Ostendorff Tubigen; Cliniques Universitaires Saint Luc, A. Ferrant Bruxelles; Ospedale Civile, G. Torlontano Pescara; The Finsen Institute, P. Ernst, Copenhagen; Hôpital E. Herriot, J. Touraine Lione; Ospedale Civile, G. Lucarelli Pesaro; Hotel Dieu, J. James Paris; Center Hospitalier Regional de Nancy, P. Bordigoni Nancy Cedex; Cattedra Ematologia Università, W. Arcese Roma; Hôpital Nice Nice; Hopital Bellevue, F. Freicon St. Etienne; University Hospital, A. Toivanen Turku; Academisch ziekenhuis, G. Tricot Leuven; Charing Cross Hospital, G.D. Pegrum, London; The Royal Infirmary, A. Parker Edindurgh; Ospedale Civile, G. Carotenuto S. Giovanni Rotondo; Clinica Pediatrica, M. Lo Curto Palermo; Cattedra di Ematologia Università, V. Silingardi Modena; Royal Free Hospital, H. Prentice London;

778 patients with severe aplastic anemia (SAA), were treated with immunosuppression (IS) or bone marrow transplantation (BMT) between january 1.1970 and december 31.1983.

707 patients were evaluable (alive more than 1 year or dead). The overall survival is 49% at 11 years .The longest survivor has been followed for 4090 days from BMT.

IMMUNOSUPPRESSION. 310 patients were treated with IS and evaluable. The overall survival is 60% at 1 year (201 patients at risk), 50% at 4 years (57 patients at risk), 48% at 9 years (1 patient at risk). Survival was not influenced by the year of treatment : 49% for patients treated between 1976

and 1980 and 48% for patients treated between 1981 and 1983. As to the IS protocol horse ALG (HALG) alone , rabbit ALG (RALG), HALG in combination with prednisolone at high or low doses, or HALG followed by haploidentical bone marrow infusion all produced survivals ranging from 38% (HALG+BM) to 66% (HALG+low dose steroids). The effect of age on survival was as follows: 161 patients over 20 showed a 51% survival compared to 43% for 149 patients under 20 years of age.

143 patients died of consequences of marrow failure : 49% of infections, 34% of hemorrhage and 17% of other causes. 80% of all deaths occurred within 1 year from treatment; however patients continued to be at risk of death for 6 years.

IS : 310 patients
EBMT SAA Working Party 1985

BONE MARROW TRANSPLANTATION. 397 patients were treated with BMT.

Donor. 9 patients received a syngeneic BMT, 367 received a BMT from an HLA identical sibling, and 21 from donors other than HLA identical siblings. The survival was 88% for twins, 49% for HLA identical sibs, and 39% for other donors. This last figure is certainly encouraging

Year of BMT. The survival was 30% for patients grafted in 1970-1975 , 41% for patients grafted in 1976-1980 and 63% for patients grafted in

1981-1983.

Sex and age. There was no effect of sex on survival. Unexpectedly patients under 20 years or over 20 years showed identical survival (50%).

Conditioning Regimen. Given the significant differences of survival according to the year of treatment, different conditioning regimens were compared for patients grafted between 1980 and 1983.

The survival was 33% for 6 patients prepared with cytoxan (CY)+ total lymphoid irradiation (TLI), 40% for 10 patients prepared with CY+ TBI, 61% for 75 patients prepared with CY alone, 64% for 31 patients prepared with CY+ buffy coat, and 70% for 43 patients conditioned with CY+ toraco abdominal irradiation.

Previous treatment. There was no difference between patients grafted without previous IS treatment, and patients grafted after failing one course of IS.

Graft versus host disease. 49%, 20%, 23% had grade 0-I, II, III-IV acute GvHD. The information was not available in 8% of patients. Patients with grade 0-II GvHD showed a 73% survival compared to 37% survival for patients with grade III-IV GvHD.

There was no difference in the incidence and mortality of GvHD for 79 patients given methotrexate (MTX) or 92 patients given cyclosporin A (CyA) between 1980 and 1983. The figures are as follows for MTX and CyA respectively: 45%,42% grade 0-I, 29%, 30% grade II, 20%,26% grade III-IV and 14%,13% lethal GvHD.

The survival was 71% for CyA patients and 55% for MTX patients. It is interesting to note that the lower mortality in CyA treated patients as compared to MTX treated patients is not due to a decreased mortality of GvHD nor of rejection (14% and 5% respectively in both groups), but mainly to a decreased number of deaths related to infections.

GvHD represented 22% ,38% and 41% of all causes of death for patients grafted in 1970-75, 1976-80 and 1981-83 respectively.

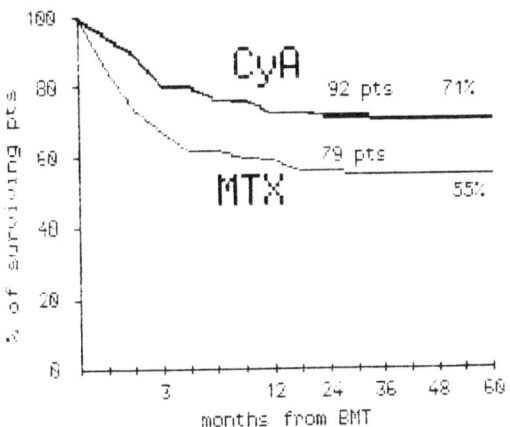

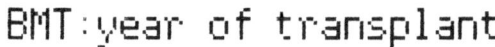

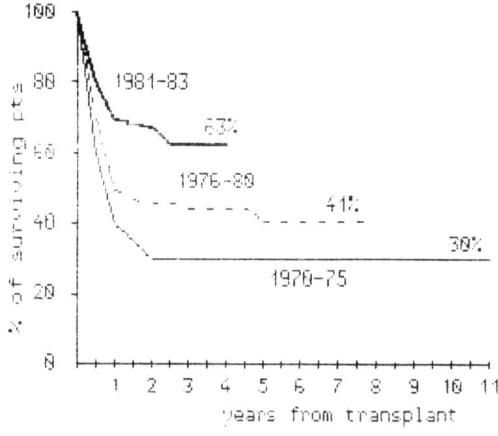

Rejection.61%,16% and 15% of deaths were caused by rejection respectively in 1970-75, 1976-80 and 1981-83. 28 patients, excluding syngeneic graft recipient, received a second transplant after rejecting their first graft : the survival was 17%; one patient is alive and well 3000 days post-BMT. The mortality of rejection varied according to the conditioning regimen: it was 13% for CY, 14% for CY+BC, 5% for CY+TBI, 0% for CY+TLI and 0% for CY+TAI. Therefore the addition of irradiation reduced the occurrence of graft rejection but was associated with an increse of overall mortality in patients receiving TBI or TLI (61% and 66%):this was not the case for patients receiving CY+TAI (30%).

Interstitial pneumonia. 13% and 4% respectively of deaths were caused by IP in 1976-80 and 1981-83.

CONCLUSIONS. This preliminary analysis follows two previous reports of the EBMT SAA Working Party (1,2). It points out to a lack of improvement for IS therapy in the past 10 years, with a cure rate close to 50%. On the contrary a significant improvement is seen for BMT: a survival of 30% and 40% respectively in the early and mid seventies, and over 60% in the early eighties. Improvement is probably associated with a number of factors associated with the transplant procedures,among which cyclosporin A seems to be of great relevance. Rejection and interstitial pneumonia are currently rare complications.

References
1)E. Gluckman, A.J. Barrett, W. Arcese, A. Devergie, P. Degoulet (1981): Bone Marrow Transplantation in Severe Aplastic Anaemia: a survey of the European Group for Bone Marrow Transplantation (EGEBMT). Br.J.Haematol. 49:165-173.
2)E. Gluckman, A. Devergie, A. Poros, P. Degoulet (1982): Results of immunosuppression in 170 cases of severe aplastic anemia: Report of the European Group of Bone Marrow Transplantation (EGBMT). Br.J.Haematol. 51:541-550.
This work was supported by A.I.R.C.,Milano 1983 and by the E.B.M.T.

Exp. Hematol. (suppl. 17) 13:58–60 (1985)

Therapy of Severe Aplastic Anemia

R. Storb and K. Doney

For the Seattle Bone Marrow Transplant Team, Seattle, Washington, USA

An earlier study of the International Aplastic Anemia Study Group had shown that newly-diagnosed patients with severe aplastic anemia treated by supportive therapy with or without oral or intravenous androgens had a survival of approximately 20% at 5 years, with most of the deaths occurring within the first 6 months of diagnosis (1). Most surviving patients had spontaneous hematologic recovery sufficient to live without the need for transfusions, while some still required continued transfusions. A subsequent study by the study group confirmed the grim prognosis of patients with aplastic anemia undergoing supportive therapy (2).

The Seattle team began using Upjohn horse antihuman thymocyte globulin (ATG) in 1978, in a dose of 40 mg/kg on each of four successive days, to treat 19 patients with severe aplastic anemia (3). Now, seven years after treatment, seven of the 19 patients (37%) are alive; all are transfusion-independent (3). Two of the seven survivors recovered their hematological function spontaneously more than 1 year after ATG treatment. A subsequent study involving 54 patients treated with ATG at a dose of 16 mg/kg on each of 10 successive days, followed by androgens, showed that HLA haploidentical marrow infusion had no effect on the incidence of response or survival. Projected survival at 40 months was 60% for the group not receiving marrow, and 48% for the group receiving mismatched marrow. Twenty of the surviving patients in both groups had complete or partial hematologic responses, and the remaining 15 survivors had either minimal improvement or no response (4). A subsequent prospective randomized trial was undertaken to compare the efficacy of murine anti-human T cell monoclonal antibody to that of ATG. One of 12 patients who received monoclonal antibody therapy had a partial response, while 11 failed to respond, compared to four of 13 patients receiving ATG who had complete or partial responses. Currently, seven of 12 patients given monoclonal antibody are surviving at 15-25 months, compared to 10 of 13 patients given ATG (5,6). It is possible that the survival curves in the last two trials will continue to decline, in view of the fact that some patients continue to be transfusion-dependent.

An interesting finding was the significant association between clinical recovery after ATG therapy and the presence in the circulating blood of a population of small mononuclear cells phenotypically associated with the erythroid lineage (7). Perhaps the availability of reliable prognostic in vitro tests will allow separating those patients who

might benefit from immunosuppressive therapy from those who would benefit from marrow transplantation.

Eight patients with severe aplastic anemia, including one radiation accident, were given syngeneic transplants, and they are surviving 3-22 years (8,9). Five of these grafts were successful without preceding immunosuppression. In one, the graft was successful only after conditioning with cyclophosphamide (CY), and in two grafts, failed despite CY. Recovery was seen in one of these two after additional ATG and in the other after conditioning with CY and total body irradiation (TBI) in preparation for a third graft, suggesting that some cases of aplastic anemia may involve mechanisms other than stem cell failure.

Ninety-three multiply-transfused patients were conditioned with CY, and then given marrow infusions from HLA-identical siblings (10,11). Forty-five percent of the 93 patients are surviving between 3.75 and 13.75 years after grafting. Graft rejection was a major problem, with an incidence of 36%. Analysis of the clinical data and experiments in canine DLA-identical littermate marrow graft recipients suggested that rejection was due to sensitization through multiple blood transfusions (12,13).

Forty-three previously untransfused patients were given HLA-identical marrow grafts following CY, and more than 80% are surviving between 2.5 and 12.25 years (14). Graft failure was the exception among the untransfused patients, supporting the notion that rejection is the result of transfusion-induced sensitization.

An attempt at abrogating rejection in HLA-identical sibling marrow transplants for aplastic anemia using a combination of CY and TBI in 20 patients was effective (11). However, the treatment was accompanied by an increased incidence of acute GVHD and multiple infectious complications with a resulting poor survival. This regimen was abandoned in early 1976.

Based on the observation that a large marrow cell dose resulted in a decreased rejection rate in multiply-transfused patients and the observation in experimental animals of the presence of circulating hemopoietic stem cells, a subsequent group of 65 multiply-transfused patients were given CY, marrow and buffy-coat cell infusions from HLA-identical siblings (10,15). 70% of these are surviving between 2.75 and 9.25 after grafting; 13% died from rejection.

Acute and chronic GVHD have been major problems despite methotrexate prophylaxis (16,17). Therefore, a subsequent group of 46 patients with HLA-identical sibling marrow donors was given CY, marrow and buffy-coat cell infusions. Patients were then randomized to receive either methotrexate or a combination of cyclosporine and methotrexate post-grafting. While the incidence of acute GVHD was significantly lessened in the cyclosporine/ methotrexate group, it is too early to assess the impact of this treatment on chronic GVHD and survival (unpublished observations). It is of interest that only two of these 46 patients rejected their grafts. Actuarial survival at two years is 80%.

Eighteen transplants were carried out using family members who genotypically shared one HLA haplotype, and phenotypically were matched for one or more HLA antigens on the other haplotype (11). Most of these transplants have been carried out following conditioning with CY. The majority failed because of graft rejection. Currently only four patients are alive, one two months, and three between 1 and 7 years after transplantation. More effective conditioning regimens are needed in this incompatible situation.

Nine Seattle patients had Fanconi anemia and were given HLA-identical sibling grafts following CY or (in one case with preleukemia) CY and TBI, and five are long-term survivors, with survival ranging from 2-1/4 to more than 1-1/2 years (18). Four patients had paroxysmal nocturnal hemoglobinuria-associated aplastic anemia, and all are surviving between 15 and 55 months after transplantation (19). Fourteen patients had hepatitis-associated aplastic anemia and 11 are surviving between one and 12 years (20). Ten patients referred as aplastic anemia were found to have preleukemia based on marrow histology and the finding of clonal cytogenetic abnormalities (21). Three of the 10 were prepared for HLA-identical sibling marrow transplantation by CY alone, and the abnormal cell clone either persisted or reemerged within six months of transplantation. All three patients died with leukemia. The other seven patients were treated with CY plus TBI before transplantation, and six of these seven are alive and well without evidence of disease from 19 to 37 months after transplantation. Results suggest that CY alone is incapable of eradicating the abnormal clone, and that CY combined with TBI is more effective.

Based on our current data, we believe that marrow transplantation is the treatment of choice for patients below the age of 40 years who have an HLA-identical sibling (22). For patients between the ages of 40 and 50, the results of marrow transplantation are not as good, largely because of increasing problems with GVHD. In these patients, ATG should first be tried before considering marrow transplantation.

REFERENCES

1. Camitta BM, Thomas ED, Nathan DG, et al. A prospective study of androgens and bone marrow transplantation for treatment of severe aplastic anemia. Blood 53: 504-514, 1979.

2. Camitta B, O'Reilly RJ, Sensenbrenner L, et al. Anti-thoracic duct lymphocyte globulin therapy of severe aplastic anemia. Blood 62: 883-888, 1983.

3. Doney KC, Weiden PL, Buckner CD, et al. Treatment of severe aplastic anemia using antithymocyte globulin with or without an infusion of HLA haploidentical marrow. Exp Hematol 9: 829-834, 1981.

4. Doney K, Dahlberg SJ, Monroe D, et al. Therapy of severe aplastic anemia with anti-human thymocyte globulin and androgens: The effect of HLA-haploidentical marrow infusion. Blood 63: 342-348, 1984.

5. Doney KC, Torok-Storb B, Dahlberg S, et al. Immunosuppressive therapy of severe aplastic anemia. In: Aplastic Anemia: Stem Cell Biology and Advances in Treatment. Young NS, Levine AS, Humphries RK, (eds). New York: Alan R. Liss, Inc., 1984, pp 259-270.

6. Doney K, Martin P, Storb R, et al. A randomized trial of antihuman thymocyte globulin versus murine monoclonal anti-human T-cell antibodies as immunosuppressive therapy for aplastic anemia. Exp Hematol, in press.

7. Torok-Storb B, Doney K, Sale G, et al. Aplastic Anemia: Subsets of patients identified by flow microfluorimetry. N Engl J Med, in press.

8. Appelbaum FR, Fefer A, Cheever MA, et al. Treatment of aplastic anemia by bone marrow transplantation in identical twins. Blood 55: 1033-1039, 1980.

9. Appelbaum FR, Cheever MA, Fefer A, et al. Recurrence of aplastic anemia following cyclophosphamide and syngeneic bone marrow transplantation - evidence for two mechanisms of graft failure. Blood, in press.

10. Storb R, Thomas ED, Buckner CD, et al. Marrow transplantation for aplastic anemia. Semin Hematol 21: 27-35, 1984.

11. Storb R, Thomas ED, Appelbaum FR, et al. Marrow transplantation for severe aplastic anemia: The Seattle experience. In: Aplastic Anemia: Stem Cell Biology and Advances in Treatment. Young NS, Levine AS, Humphries RK, (eds). New York: Alan R. Liss, Inc., 1984, pp 297-313.

12. Storb R, Prentice RL, Thomas ED, et al. Factors associated with graft rejection after HLA-identical marrow transplantation for aplastic anaemia. Brit J Haematol 55: 573-585, 1983.

13. Storb R, Weiden PL, Deeg HJ, et al. Rejection of marrow from DLA-identical canine littermates given transfusions before grafting: Antigens involved are expressed on leukocytes and skin epithelial cells but not on platelets and red blood cells. Blood 54: 477-484, 1979.

14. Storb R, Thomas ED, Buckner CD, et al. Marrow transplantation in thirty "untransfused" patients with severe aplastic anemia. Ann Intern Med 92: 30-36, 1980.

15. Storb R, Doney KC, Thomas ED, et al. Marrow transplantation with or without donor buffy coat cells for 65 transfused aplastic anemia patients. Blood 59: 236-246, 1982.

16. Storb R, Prentice RL, Buckner CD, et al. Graft-versus-host disease and survival in patients with aplastic anemia treated by marrow grafts from HLA-identical siblings. Beneficial effect of a protective environment. N Engl J Med 308: 302-307, 1983.

60

17. Storb R, Prentice RL, Sullivan KM, et al. Predictive factors in chronic graft-versus-host disease in patients with aplastic anemia treated by marrow transplantation from HLA-identical siblings. Ann Intern Med 98: 461-466, 1983.

18. Deeg HJ, Storb R, Thomas ED, et al. Fanconi's anemia treated by allogeneic marrow transplantation. Blood 61: 954-959, 1983.

19. Szer J, Deeg HJ, Witherspoon RP, et al. Long-term survival after marrow transplantation for paroxysmal nocturnal hemoglobinuria with aplastic anemia. Ann Intern Med 101: 193-195, 1984.

20. Witherspoon RP, Storb R, Shulman H, et al. Marrow transplantation in hepatitis-associated aplastic anemia. Am J Hematol 17: 269-278, 1984.

21. Appelbaum FR, Storb R, Ramberg RE, et al. Allogeneic marrow transplantation in the treatment of preleukemia. Ann Intern Med 100: 689-693, 1984.

22. Thomas ED, Storb R. Acquired severe aplastic anemia: Progress and perplexity. Blood 64: 325-328, 1984.

Supported in part by grants CA 30924, CA 18221, CA 15704, and CA 18029 awarded by the National Cancer Institute, DHHS, and by the Upjohn Co., Kalamazoo, Michigan.

Exp. Hematol. (suppl. 17) 13:61 (1985)
© International Society for Experimental Hematology

Immunosuppressive Therapy (IT) of Severe Aplastic Anemia (SAA) with ATG, Prednisolone (PRED) and Cyclosporin A (CSA)

W. Heit, D. Bunjes, N. Frickhofen, A. Ragavachar, and H. Heimpel

Department of Internal Medicine III, University of Ulm, D-7900 Ulm, Federal Republic of Germany

IT in SAA with ALG/ATG + Pred is the therapy of choise in patients not elegible for allogeneic bone marrow transplantation. The overall response rates reported in the literature are promising but revealed a great deal of variability in different groups (40-60%) (1). Our own experience with equine ALG or rabbit ATG + Pred in 20 consecutively treated cases with SAA was unsatisfactory. 3/5 patients exposed to equine ALG (Lymphoser) and 1/15 cases treated with rabbit ATG (Fresenius Corp.) achieved a partial response (PR) after 3 months (total PR: 4/20 or 20%). Thus, a new protocol was introduced in February 1984 including CSA, ATG and Pred (CAP-Protocol) (Table 1). The rationale of the CAP-protocol is to achieve a cytoreductive effect with ATG and Pred which is to be maintained by the inhibitory effect of CSA on T-cell proliferation (2). Nine consecutive patients with SAA had been treated by October 1984 and the response rates after 2 months are summarized in Table 2. 2/9 early deaths due to bacterial and fungal infection occurred within 4 weeks of treatment without evidence of hemopoietic recovery, 7/9 cases are alive and tolerated the protocol without difficulties. One patient was exposed to CSA and Pred alone because of hypersensitivity to ATGAM (Upjohn Corp.) and achieved complete response (CR). There is suggestive evidence from two patients that the quality of their PR is CSA-dependent. So far, our preliminary experience with CAP indicates that cyclosporin A is an effective component of our immunosuppressive regimen for the treatment of SAA.

TABLE I: IT-REGIMEN IN SAA WITH CSA, ATG and Pred. (CAP)

CYCLOSPORINE A: THERAPEUTICAL BLOOD LEVEL: 400-800 ng/ml[+]

D 1	:	2 x 5 mg/kg i.v
D 2 - 8	:	3 - 5 mg/kg i.v.
D 9 - 84	:	2 x 2 - 6 mg/kg p.o.[++]

PREDNISOLONE:

D 1 - 8	:	5 mg/kg i.v.
D 9 - 15	:	1 mg/kg i.v.
D16 - 28	:	0,5 mg/kg p.o., dose reduction and stop.

ATG (ATGAM):

D 2 - 8	:	20 mg/kg (4 mg/kg/h)

+ blood level control: D1-15: daily, D16-84: 2 x - 1 x /week

++ after D85: therapeutical Level: 200-400 ng/ml, stop by mos 6

Table II. IT IN SAA WITH CAP

CR/PR	:	5 / 9[+]	(56%)
MR	:	2 / 9	
early death[++]	:	2 / 9	

[+] 1/9: No ATG CR after CSA and Prednisolone

[++] day 23 and 25

REFERENCE

1. Aplastic Anemia
   NS. Young, ES Levine,
   R.K Humphries (Eds.)
   Prog. Clin. Biol. Res. Vol 148
   A.R. Liss, N.Y. 1984

Exp. Hematol. (suppl. 17) 13:62 (1985)
© International Society for Experimental Hematology

Cyclosporin (CSP) for Therapy of Severe Aplastic Anemia (SAA) and Pure Red Cell Aplasia (PRCA)

L. Debusscher, R. Paridaens, J. Otten, M. Malarme, and P. Stryckmans

Institut J. Bordet and Hôpital Saint-Pierre, Brussels, Belgium

The following experimental and clinical observations prompted us to test the efficacy of Csp (a) the prevention of CFU-GM suppressor T cells by in vitro preincubation with Csp of SAA T cells (1) (b) a reduced occurrence of allograft failure by the use of Csp as anti-gvh prophylaxis (2), (c) the immune pathogenesis repeatedly demonstrated in PRCA and (d) a recent report illustrating the need for alternatives to classical treatments (3).

We treated by Csp, administered orally, twice daily, 5 patients with SAA unsuitable for bone marrow grafting and 2 patients with primary type PRCA, previously untreated by immunosuppression.

Both PRCA patients, aged 67 and 82 years, who had required respectively 36 and 66 units of packed red cells during their 8 and 13 months evolution showed a rise in their reticulocytosis 20 and 10 days after Csp initiation. In PRCA 67, the complete response obtained with low atoxic doses of Csp (4mg/kg/day) lasted during the 140 days of Csp administration and for 4 months after its withdrawal. A second complete remission, obtained after Csp resumption, is still ongoing. In PRCA 82, low daily doses (5 mg/kg/day) are given since 100 days resulting in a good partial remission (Hb levels at 10 g/dl).

The 5 SAA patients aged from 14 to 80 years. Their diagnosis (according to the criteria of the International Aplastic Anemia Study Group) had been made since 20-24-43-137-380 days at start of Csp.

In SAA 80, the drug was stopped after 67 days for total uneffectiveness. In SAA 64, an incipient increase of granulocytes was noticeable on day 37 when Csp had to be interrupted for severe but rapidly reversible renal failure. In SAA 14, the partial remission obtained is only possibly related to drug administration.

In SAA 62, an excellent partial remission is clearly related to Csp. After a 13 months evolution, her granulocytes were acceptable (mean 1,480/mm3) but her clinical status was quite critical with severe diffuse bleedings due to extreme thrombocytopenia unresponsive to massive platelet transfusions, despite several previous therapeutic attempts (prednisolone, high dose prednisolone, antithymocyte globulins). Fourteen days after start of Csp, given at 6 to 10 mg/kg/day, a rise in platelets counts became evident, reaching 65,000/mm3 on day 47. The patient has been in excellent condition without any need for transfusion, with platelets around 35,000 and Hb levels at 11 g/dl, during the 494 days of Csp treatment which resulted in rather low (100ng/ml)

through plasma levels due to diphantoïn administration. Seventy days after Csp interruption she relapsed, requiring a RBC transfusion. Presently, after resumption of the drug, a second response becomes evident.

In SAA 20, Csp was started as first treatment 24 days after diagnosis. A response was noticeable at day 30. The completely normalized blood parameters obtained after 5 months deteriorated when Csp doses were reduced and reimproved to normal with drug reincrease.

In the two PRCA, the low effective Csp doses, resulting in trough plasma levels around 100 ng/ml did not cause any significant toxicity. Higher Csp levels (± 500 ng/ml) needed to be optimal in SAA, led to severe toxicity in 2 cases (1 gingival hypertrophy and 1 renal failure). Both problems were rapidly reversible after drug withdrawal. In the other cases, tremor, hirsutism, paresthesia, weight gain, hyperuremia and hyperbilirubinemia were transient and acceptable.

In conclusion : Csp as a single agent is effective in SAA (2/5) and PRCA (2/2). There seems to be no cross-resistance with prednisolone and antithymocyte globulins. SAA requires apparently higher doses than PRCA. Tolerance is mostly fair, even in elderly patients. Maintenance treatment appears warranted.

References

1. Podesta M., Bacigalupo A., Frassoni F., Raffo M., Piaggio G., Repetto M., Van Lint M., Marmont A. : Generation of CFU-C suppressor T cells. VI. Effects of Cyclosporin A. Acta haematol. 1983; 70 : 163-169
2. Hows JM., Palmer S., Gordon-Smith EC. : Use of cyclosporin A in allogeneic bone marrow transplantation for severe aplastic anemia. Transplantation 1982; 33 : 382-386.
3. Clark DA., Dessypris EN., Krantz SB. : Studies on pure red cell aplasia. XI. Results of immunosuppressive treatment of 37 patients. Blood 1984; 63 : 277-286.

Exp. Hematol. (suppl. 17) 13:63 (1985)
© International Society for Experimental Hematology

Bone Marrow Transplantation in Thalassemia Major

Paola Polchi, Maria Galimberti, Teodosio Izzi, Claudio Giardini, Emanuele Angelucci, Patrizia Politi, and Guido Lucarelli

Diviso of Hematology, Pesaro, Italy

Bone marrow transplantation in patients with thalassemia major has been successfully performed for last 3 years.

In our center 30 patients less then 8 y o underwent transplant from an HLA-identical donor after preparation with Busulfan 14-16 mg/kg in 4 days and Cytoxan 200 mg/kg in 4 days.

Patients were in very different clinical conditions pre-transplant as far as concerning hepatomegaly, syderosis, skeleton deformities, hepatitis, number of transfusion, correct chelation therapy.

Four of these patients were untransfused at transplant time, others had received 4-80 RBC transfusions (median 25).

Twentysix (87%) patients are surviving 2-25 months: 4 are alive with thalassemia and 22 are cured.

Four patients (13%) died of transplant related complications at +7,+28,+38,+50 days after transplant: 1 of ARDS,1 of Pneumocystis Carinii pneumonia, 1 of VOD, 1 of ac.GVHD and P.I.

Rejection of graft has been observed in 6 of these patients (20%).

Two of six did not reconstitute marrow and died aplastic at +28,+38 days.

Four others had prompt graft documented within 11 and 18 days by bone marrow cells kariotype and Hb-chain synthesis; subsequentely their thalassemic marrow replaced the graft within 32-46 days from transplant.

Acute GVHD (grade II-IV) affected overall six patients and was cause of death in one. Chronic GVHD with a Karnofsky score less then 80% affects only 1 of these patients.

It appears from our observations that a young thalassemic patient with a suitable HLA-identical donor can be cured by bone marrow transplantation with low risk of transplant related complications.

References:
1-THOMAS E.D.,BUCKNER C.D. et al.: Lancet 227:29,1982.
2-LUCARELLI G.,IZZI T.,POLCHI P. et al.: Exp. Hematol.11.,Suppl.13,1983.
3-LUCARELLI G.,POLCHI P.,IZZI T. et al.: Exp. Hematol.12:676, 1984

Exp. Hematol. (suppl. 17) 13:64–65 (1985)
© International Society for Experimental Hematology

Aplastic Anemia: A Disease of "Seed" and "Soil"

C. Nissen, A. Gratwohl, A. Würsch, and B. Speck

Department of Research and Department of Internal Medicine, Kantonsspital Basel, Switzerland

INTRODUCTION

Aplastic anemia (AA) can be cured by BMT, indicating that the primary defect is intrinsic to the "seed". Hemopoiesis in AA can also recover after immunosuppression, suggesting that the "soil" is the primary site of disease.

We have found abnormalities of hemopoietic precursor cells in AA patients in vitro, from which we have concluded that the "seed" is abnormally sensitive to changes occurring in the "soil" (1).
We are now reporting results of extended experiments.

PATIENTS AND METHODS

Bone marrow from patients with aplastic anemia (AA) at different stages of disease - including patients in complete autologous hemopoietic remission -, from patients with paroxysmal noctural hemoglobinuria (PNH), from patients with recovering bone marrow function after chemotherapy induced aplasia, and from normal controls was cultured in methylcellulose for detection of CFU-C and BFU-E directly, and after a 1 hr preincubation in liquid medium at the following conditions:

1) Neutral medium
2) 66 % complement in isotonic medium (0.16 M NaCl)
3) 5 % complement in isosmolar sucrose medium (i.e. at low ionic strength)

Serum from adult rabbits, baby rabbits and fresh autologous human serum were used as source of complement. After thorough washing, cells were incubated in methylcellulose at the same concentrations as untreated cells.

RESULTS AND DISCUSSION

1) Preincubation in neutral medium

Untreated marrow from patients with AA, even in apparent complete hematological remission, and from patients with PNH grew poorly, as expected. Liquid preincubation in neutral medium unexpectedly increased growth from CFU-C and BFU-E up to tenfold, whereas growth from normal marrow was not significantly changed. The reason for this improvement of plating efficiency after liquid preincubation is not known. Since this procedure is routinely used for removal of cell bound antibodies, it is conceivable that AA and PNH-precursors are liberated from inhibitory antibody by liquid preincubation.

2) Effect of 66 % complement in isotonic medium

1/3 batches of adult rabbit serum strongly reduced colony formation in patients with AA and PNH, but not in normals, nor in patients recovering bone marrow function after BMT or chemotherapy induced aplasia. Toxicity of adult rabbit complement was completely abrogated by selective blockage of the antibody-dependent "classical" complement pathway, and by absorbtion of the serum with human buffy coat, indicating that heterophilic rabbit-anti-human antibodies were responsible for precursor cell toxicity of rabbit serum. None of 3 batches of baby rabbit complement nor autologous serum inhibited colony formation by normal and aplastic precursors in isotonic medium.

3) Effect of 5 % complement in isosmolar sucrose

Reduction of ionic strength increases susceptibility to complement mediated cell damage. This is the basis of the

"sucrose test", which is routinely adopted for detection of RBC sensitivity to complement in PNH. Complement sensitivity is not restricted to mature blood cells in PNH. Bone marrow precursors, including colony forming cells of the myeloid and erythroid line, are reduced by a preincubation in sucrose with 5 % fresh human serum (2).
We found that the sucrose test on hemopoietic precursor cells is also positive in patients who have AA, but no PNH. Nontoxic baby rabbit serum or fresh human serum can be used as a source of complement. Colony forming capacity was reduced to approximately 50 % in all of 13 patients tested, only 1 of them had clinical PNH, 3 had a weakly positive sucrose test but no hemolysis. 9/13 were in complete hemopoietic recovery.

Preliminary results indicate that the IgG fraction (97 % pure) from a patient with relapsing aplastic anemia and a positive sucrose test, potentiates complement mediated damage to precursor cells in patients with AA and PNH. In addition, this fraction lyses PNH RBC, but not normal erythrocytes, in the presence of complement.

It is of concern that this precursor cell abnormality persists even in apparent complete hemopoietic recovery after immunosuppression. These patients are probably not "cured" inspite of normal bone marrow cellularity and peripheral blood counts. They remain at risk of relapse or development of PNH. In contrast, patients with a stable hemopoietic graft after BMT for AA have no such abnormalities. Thus, BMT is likely to "cure" AA, at the cost of high treatment related mortality, whereas immunosuppression is likely to induce autologous hemopoietic recovery without life threatening complications, but with a questionable long term outcome.

CONCLUSIONS

AA is a PNH-like disease with sensitivity of precursor cells to complement, i.e. an intrinsic disease of the "seed". However, the presence of complement sensitive precursors is compatible with normal hemopoietic function. Additional changes in the "soil" are obviously required for manifestation of the disease. We propose and will further study the possibility that an immunoglobulin to which normal cells are resistant, is involved in complement mediated lyses of precursor cells in PNH and AA.

References
1. C. Nissen et al
   Exp. Hematol Vol 12 No 6 1984, p. 472

2. Dessypris et al
   N Engl. J Med. 309: 690 - 693, 83

Exp. Hematol. (suppl. 17) 13:66–67 (1985)
© International Society for Experimental Hematology

Failure of Identical Twin Bone Marrow to Restore Haemopoiesis in 2 Patients with Severe Aplastic Anemia (SAA) without Immunosuppressive (IS) Conditioning

Failure to Detect in vitro Inhibition of Normal Donor CFU-GM by Patient Mononuclear Blood Cells (MNC) and Bone Marrow Cells (BMC), but Impaired Capacity of Patient MNC to Generate Colony Stimulating Factor (CSF)

W. Hinterberger, K. Geissler, M. Fischer, E. Kabrna, and P. Höcker

1st Department of Medicine, Blood Transfusion Service, University of Vienna, Lazarettgasse 14, A-1090 Wien, Austria

Introduction: The role of mononuclear cells (MNC) in the regulation of aplastic haemopoiesis is poorly understood. Evidence for an important role of T-lymphocytes in SAA is strengthened by a frequent clinical response after treatment with Anti-T-cellglobulin. The occurrence of SAA in patients who are fortunate enough to have an identical twin bone marrow donor can provide insight into "immune"-mediated aplasia, as half of these patients ultimately require pretreatment with Cyclophosphamide to obtain haemopoietic recovery. We had the rare opportunity to study mononuclear leucocytes and bone marrow cells from 2 patients with SAA who ultimately required Cyclophosphamide to recover following twin bone marrow grafting. In coculture studies performed with donor cells, major or minor histocompatibility differences as a cause of colony growth alteration could be excluded (1).

Patients and Methods: The clinical course of patients A and B is depicted in Table 1:

	Pair A-A	Pair B-B
1. Conditioning	0	0
1. Marrow Infusion Cell Number	Day 0 4.7×10^8/kg	Day 0 2.5×10^8/kg
	no Take	no Take
2. Conditioning	Cy 200 mg/kg	Cy 200 mg/kg
2. Marrow Infusion Cell Number	Day 78 2.7×10^8/kg	Day 133 3.5×10^8/Kg
	Nomalization	Norsalization
Survival	⟩ 620 days	⟩ 285 days

Prior to the 1. bone marrow infusion both patients were pretransfused. The stimulation index in both pairs was 1.02 and 1.06, respectively. On day 60 after the 1. bone marrow infusion, patient A had a cellular bone marrow. There was, however, no sign of improvement of blood cell counts. Donor buffy coat cells, given in order to provide "accessory" cells on 4 consecutive days, failed to improve haemopoiesis. The bone marrow of patient B remained hypocellular throughout. After Cyclophosphamide and the 2. bone marrow infusion, the clinical course of both patients was uneventful. They have normal blood counts and their Karnovsky score at present is 100%.

Coculture Studies: Myeloid progenitor cells (CFU-GM) were assayed as described (2). Bone marrow and peripheral blood cell samples were separated on FICOLL-HYPAQUE (spec. weight 1.077, 40 min, 400 g) and washed twice in RPMI 1640 culture medium. For the enumaration of myeloid stem cells, test cells were incubated in 0.8% methylcellulose (Methocel*, Dow Chemicals) at 10^5 cells/ml.

Assay for Patient's MNC derived Colony Inhibiting and Stimulating Activity: 10^6 patient derived MNC were suspended in feeder layers consisting of 1 ml Agar (0.5%)-McCoy medium, enriched with 20% fetal calf serum. Additional experiments included coculture of 10^6 donor MNC with $2 \cdot 10^5$ patient MNC. Such feeder layers were covered with 1 ml upper layer containing 10^5 FICOLL-separated syngeneic donor bone marrow cells. Duplicate cultures were incubated at 37°C in 5% CO_2, in full humidity. Aggregates with 40 cells were scored as colonies.

Results:

Assay for Bone Marrow Cell derived Colony Inhibitory Activity (Pair A): Bone marrow cells from the donor and the patient were mixed at 1:1 giving a cell number of 10^5 cells/ml culture medium. Each culture was activated with 10^6 donor derived MNC, suspended in 1 ml feeder layers: In this experiment, the measured number of colonies was virtually identical with the expected number (Figure 1). Thus, patient derived bone marrow cells in this experiment failed to disclose inhibition of normal syngeneic bone marrow cells.

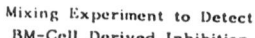

Mixing Experiment to Detect
BM-Cell Derived Inhibition

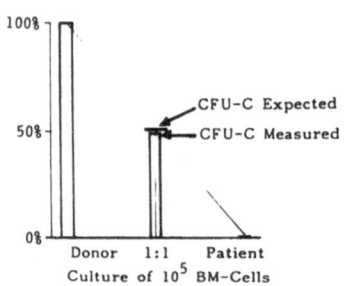

Supported by Grant 4100 of the "Fonds zu Förderung der Wissenschaftlichen Forschung in Österreich" and by the "Kommission für Leukämieforschung und Knochenmarktransplantation" of the Austrian Academy of Sciences

Assay for Patient's MNC derived Colony Stimulatory or Inhibitory Activity : The number of colonies obtained upon stimulation with 10^6 donor's MNC was scored as 100%. Autostimulation (Culture without cells in feeder layers) revealed 12% and 4% colony growth, respectively. Addition of 2.10^5 patient's MNC to donor's MNC was not inhibitory (104% and 105%, respectively). Patient's MNC generated much less Colony stimulating Activity than MNC from the donors (37% and 24%, respectively). To exclude a lower proportion of monocytes in the MNC fraction as a possible cause of diminished CSF release (2% and 7%, respectively), the proportion of monocytes was increased to 15%: No increase of CSF release was observed. These experiments thus failed to demonstrate inhibition of patient's MNC but showed an impaired capacity of patient's MNC to release CSF (Table 2).

Pair	Cell Source	Test Cells in Feeder Layer		Colony Growth (only Donor BM)
A	Donor	10^6 MNC		100 % (98 Col)
A	0	0 (Autostimulation)		12 %
A	Donor	10^6 MNC	+ 2.10^5 Patient's MNC	104 %
A	Patient	10^6 MNC		37 %
B	Donor	10^6 MNC		100 % (198 Col)
B	0	0 (Autostimulation)		4 %
B	Donor	10^6 MNC	+ 2.10^5 Patient's MNC	105 %
B	Patient	10^6 MNC		24 %
B	Patient	10^6 MNC	(Monocytes enriched:15%)	15 %

Discussion: Abnormal control of myelopoiesis in SAA by lymphocytes and also monocytes has repeatedly been reported. Accumulating evidence points towards lymphocyte derived inhibition of stem cell growth. The nature of factors generated by such inhibitory lymphocytes is less well characterized than their cellular sources: Generation of inhibitory material is mediated by T-cells phenotypically defined as E $^+$gamma$^+$,OKT3$^+$ Ia OKM1 (3). Recently, however, a Ia$^+$ Tac$^+$ OKT8 phenotype has been described which mediates haemo-suppression by releasing gamma-Interferon (4). In the aforementioned study, inhibitory material other than gamma-Interferon was detected in T-cell supernatants (3). Thus, although certain T-cell subsets may generate soluble factors leading to haemopoietic suppression in vitro, the significance in patients with aplastic anemia remains to be defined.

Identical twins with SAA who ultimately require pretreatment with Cyclophosphamide to obtain engraftment with syngeneic bone marrow represent a classical example of "immune"-mediated aplasia. One would expect to detect inhibition in-vitro of normal donor derived stem cells by patient's bone marrow or blood derived cells. However, we were unable to detect such inhibition. This result is in some variance with data from Appelbaum (5) who described patient's MNC being inhibitory for either CFU-GM (not for BFU-E) in one case or inhibitory for BFU-E (not for CFU-GM) in another case. Inhibition against BFU-E was not testet in our study and it might well be that "Auto-Immunity" might be expressed only in the BFU-E assay.

Our failure to detect inhibition of normal, syngeneic donor bone marrow colony growth by unseparated patient bone marrow cells (in one case) and by blood derived MNC in both patients was paralleled by the finding of a decreased generation of CSF, the putative activator of myelopoieis. This defect could not be corrected by increasing the proportion of monocytes or by incubation of the patient's cells with Indomethacin (data not shown). A decreased generation of CSF by isolated MNC from patients with SAA, in our hands, is a regular finding (Figure 2).

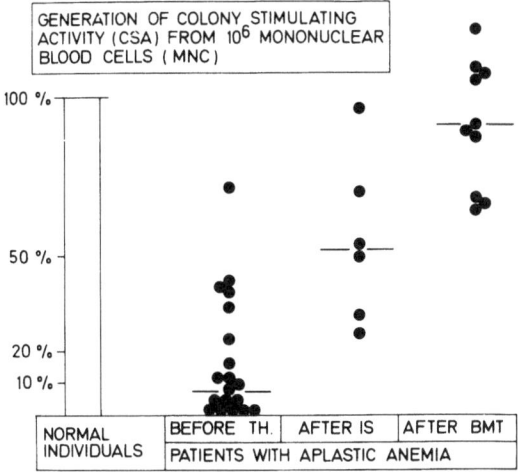

In untreated patients with SAA, the release of CSF by 10^6 MNC was uniformly diminished; in patients who recently had combined Immunosuppression with ATG and high-dose Methylprednisolone, the CSF release was higher albeit not normal. In patients who were successfully allografted, the release of CSF was in the normal range. Thus, a diminished release of CSF is apparently a regular finding in patients with SAA. In patients who had treatment with ATG/Methylprednisolone, the increased release of CSF might be due to a CSF inducing property of steroids (6). It might be argued, that the lower proportion of monocytes in the MNC fraction of patients with SAA could contribute to the decreased release of CSF. This possibility, however, is extremely unlikely, as we could not detect a correlation between the proportion of monocytes in the MNC fraction and the amount of CSF released. In recent experiments we found that the adherent but also the non-adherent fraction of MNC of patients with SAA is defective in their generation of CSF in vitro (7). A decreased generation of Interleukin I by monocytes and increased production of Interleukin 2 by T-cells has recently been reported in patients with SAA (4). Both molecules, however, are involved in the release of CSF by MNC (8).

We conclude from our in-vitro myeloid colony studies in 2 patients who ultimately required Cyclophosphamide to obtain engraftment of syngeneic donor bone marrow, that

1. The in vitro myeloid colony assay is not useful to detect this particular form of "immune"-mediated Bone marrow failure, and that

2. MNC from patients with SAA generate only a subnormal amount of CSF, the putative activator of myelopoiesis.

Thus, attacking of stem cells by some lymphocytes is apparently not the predominant mechanism of "immune"-mediated marrow failure. The adverse affection of haemopoiesis may rather be due to abnormal growth control expressed by impaired generation of positive regulatory signals.

References:
1. Singer J., et al., Blood 52:37-46 (1978)
2. Hinterberger W., et al., Scand J. Haematol. 33:244-251 (1984)
3. Bacigalupo A., et al., in: Aplastic Anemia. eds: Young, N., Levine, A., Humphries, R. Alan Liss Inc. New York (1984) 173-185
4. Zoumbos C., et al., N. Engl. j. Med. 312:257-264 (1985)
5. Appelbaum F., et al., Blood 55:1033-1039 (1980)
6. Nissen C., et al., Brit. J. Haematol. 53:301-310 (1983)
7. Hinterberger W., in press
8. Oppenheim J., et al., in: Basic and Clinical Immunology, eds: Fudenberg, Stites, Caldwell, Wells. Lange Med. Publications. 4.th Edition, page 86-103 (1984)

Exp. Hematol. (suppl. 17) 13:68 (1985)
© International Society for Experimental Hematology

CFU-GM Growth and LEU-7 Positive Cells in SAA Patients Treated by Combined ISS

W. Arcese, L. De Felice, M. Lopez, F. R. Mauro, F. Torti, M. Vignetti, A. Blanchi, C. Riguzzi, M. Luciani, T. Dentamaro, and G. Papa

Institute of Hematology, University "La Sapienza", Rome, Italy

INTRODUCTION

Several clinical and laboratory evidences support the hypothesis of an immune mechanism in the pathogenesis of SAA. At the onset of the disease a T-lymphocyte imbalance and activation have been found. Using in vitro culture technique, T-suppressor cells, acting directly or by soluble factors, have been more often identified as responsible for the hemopoietic suppression in SAA. However other mononuclear cells (MC) have been reported to inhibit hemopoiesis in normal and aplastic individuals. The clinical relevance of these studies is the potential for developing an in vitro test to identify immune-mediated SAA. Towards this end some correlations have been found. Considering that ISS is an effective therapy for a number of SAA pts, we performed a sequential study of the lymphocyte subset distribution and in vitro CFU-GM growth from bone marrow (BM) and peripheral blood (PB) of SAA pts treated by combined ISS.

MATERIALS AND METHODS

Patients: 5 SAA pts were randomized to receive combined ISS with 6-MPr plus horse ALS according to the EBMT protocol.

Lymphocyte Analysis: Lymphocyte subpopulations were recognized by the following monoclonal antibodies (MoAbs): OKT11, OKT8, OKT4, Leu-7. Reactivity with MoAbs was detected by indirect immunofluorescence. In vitro CFU-GM culture tests: Ficoll-Hypaque separated BM and PB MC were recovered and washed twice. 2×10^5 MC were plated immediately without any further treatment according to the Pike and Robinson technique. T-cell depletion: Mc were rosetted with SRBC treated with AET. 2×10^5 Ficoll-Hypaque separated rosetting cells were than plated as described above. ALS and Cyclosporin-A (CyA) incubations:10^6 MC were incubated with ALS (0.01 mg/ml) and CyA (1×10^{-3} mg/ml) for 1 hour at 37°C in 5% CO_2. The cells were washed three times and plated. Cytotoxic tests: Employing the following MoAbs: 35.1 (OKT11); 51.1 (OKT8); 66.1 (OKT4); 10.2 (Leu-1) (by J.A. Hansen - FHCRC-SE) and Leu-7, these assays were performed according to the method described elsewhere (1). For each culture experiment described above an autologous control was made. All culture tests were performed in triplicate and scored on day 10 for colonies (over 40 cells), macroclusters (20-40 cells) and small clusters (3-20 cells). Lymphocyte analysis and culture tests were carried out at diagnosis and on days 15, 30, 90 and 180 from ISS.

RESULTS

Lymphocyte Analysis: At the onset of the disease all pts showed an increasing BM T11 cells (mean 60±13%), that returned in the normal range only in 1 pt at day 30. 2 pts showed an inverted T4/T8 ratio in PB: 0.81; 0.38 (n.v. 1.8±0.5). In these 2 pts the absolute number of the T8 lymphocytes was not influenced by ISS, while T4 subset increased on day 15. At this day 4 pts showed a significant rise of the PB T4 cells with a mean peripheral absolute number passed from 746± 9.6 to 1608±664/mm^3 (n.v. 839± 179) (P .05). No important change of T4 cells percentage was observed in BM. Before ISS, BM Leu-7 cells were increased in all 5 pts (mean 30.8±4.2%). The absolute number of Leu-7 cells was significantly enhanced in the PB of 3 pts (mean 707±271 - n.v. 242±98) (P .01). On day 15, corresponding to the rise of the T4 cells, both BM and PB Leu-7 cells reduced in all pts. Leu-7 cells remained in the normal range at the other study days in 4 pts. No further changes of the other lymphocyte subsets were observed on the follow-up.

BM and PB in vitro culture: No enhancement of the in vitro CFU-GM growth was obtained after T-cell depletion when cell concentration was considered. After ALS and CyA incubations BM and PB growth pattern was not different from the controls. Before ISS an enhancement of the in vitro BM and PB growth (mean from 9.66±5.5 to 21±12.2) was obtained in 3 pts after Leu-7 MoAb incubation. However this enhancement was not statistically significant. This effect was absent after ISS. No changes of the in vitro growth was observed with the other MoAbs. On day 15, 3 pts showed a not statistically significant increasing growth of BM macroclusters and colonies (mean: from 1±1.7 to 4.6±2.5). A further enhancement was observed in the other controls during the follow-up. On day 15 the appearance of the CFU-GM growth was observed from PB of the same pts (mean: from 1.33±2.3 to 15.66±15). PB CFU-GM growth was reduced or absent in the following controls.

Clinical Course: 3 pts showed a complete or partial hematological reconstitution at 4, 3 and 2 mo from ISS and are surviving at 22, 16 and 15 mo respectively. Of the other 2 no responder pts the first died at 1.5 mo and the second is surviving at 5 mo from ISS.

COMMENTS

An expansion of the BM and PB Leu-7 subset has been observed in these 5 SAA pts. As effect of the ISS the normalization of Leu-7 cells observed in all pts on day 15 was associated with an increase of the PB T4 cells in 4 pts, 4 pts were evaluable for hematological response. No BM and PB CFU-GM growth and no rise of the T4 cells were detected in the no responder pt. Leu-7 cells contain almost all the NK cells that could exercise an inhibiting activity on human hemopoiesis as shown by other experiences. The reduction of the Leu-7 cell subset associated with an increase of T4 cells could positively influence the hemopoiesis as reflected by the enhancement of the BM and PB CFU-GM growth on day 15 from the start of the therapy.

REFERENCES

1 - Torok-Storb B. et al. (1984) Blood 63: 349-355.

Exp. Hematol. (suppl. 17) 13:69 (1985)
© International Society for Experimental Hematology

In vitro Inhibition of Hematopoiesis by T_3, HNK_1, T_8, DR Positive T Cells after Bone Marrow Transplantation

G. Vinci, J. P. Vernant, C. Cordonnier, A. Henri, H. Rochant, J. Breton-Gorius, and W. Vainchenker

INSERM U.91, Hôpital Henri Mondor, F-94010 Creteil, France

The possible inhibiting role of T lymphocytes on the in vitro hematopoiesis after allogeneic BMT have been investigated. In fact, T cells with a phenotype identical to inhibitory T cells in aplastic anemia or T CLL have been observed in allogeneic BMT. 20 patients were investigated in their capability of blood CFU-GM and BFU-E growth between 20 and 40 days after bone marrow transplantation, when PMN blood count is 1.000 -1.200/mm3. CFU-GM and BFU-E colonies were obtained by the plasma clot technique.

The number of colonies obtained was variable among the patients and always lower than in normal subjects; therefore we have hypothesized an inhibitory effect by blood mononucleated cells. Indeed, colony growth increased in 8 of 13 cases after removing the cells rosetting with sheep red cells (E^+C). In order to demonstrate that the increase of colony growth was not due to hemopoietic precursor concentration by E^+C depletion, rosette forming cells were added with increasing ratios to cells depleted of E^+C. Addition of E^+C at different ratio from 1:1 to 8:1 led to an inhibition of colony growth with a range from 30 to 100 %.

The phenotype of these suppressive cells was further analysed by complement-mediated lysis with MoABs and immunofluorescent labelling. The results demonstrated that the HNK_1 antigen was the most characteristic an-

tigen of these E^+C. Complement mediated lysis with HNK_1 MoAb significantly increased CFU-GM colony growth in the six patients studied. T_3 complement-mediated lysis had the same effect that HNK_1 MoAb. T_8 complement-mediated lysis had an intermediate effect.

Immunofluorescent labelling showed that almost all HNK_1^+ cells also exhibited an E receptor and were also labelled by the T_3 or T_8 MoAbs. In contrast, the percentage of DR positive, HNK_1^+ cells was extremely variable from patient to patient. These results afford some evidence that the subset of T cells inhibiting the "in vitro" hematopoiesis after allogeneic BMT has the following phenotype T_{11}^+, T_3^+, T_8^+, HNK_1^+ and DR^+.

No clear correlation between the inhibition of colony growth by T cells and the clinical status of patients was observed. Some evidences suggest that this inhibition of hemopoiesis by T cells in these patients is genetically restricted to the HLA locus since in cocultures with cells from unrelated normal subjects, no suppression was observed, whereas inhibition always occurred when donor cells or cells from an HLA identical member of the family were used as the target. This expansion of these suppressive T cells could be the consequence of an allogeneic reaction since no inhibition by T cells was observed in four autologous BMT and one syngeneic BMT.

Exp. Hematol. (suppl. 17) 13:70 (1985)
© International Society for Experimental Hematology

CFU-GM Growth after Bone Marrow Transplantation

J. A. Adams and A. J. Barrett

Charing Cross and Westminster Medical School, Department of Haematology, Westminster Hospital, Dean Ryle Street, London SW1, Great Britain

Bone marrow cultures were carried out after BMT on 80 samples from 9 patients transplanted for aplastic anaemia and 50 transplanted for acute leukaemia. Samples were assayed for CFU-GM content and in some cases for CFU-GM proliferation in short term suspension culture as previously described.[1]

CFU-GM numbers after BMT were in most cases lower than normal, however mean values increased with time after BMT and reached low normal values after 1-2 years. Patients grafted for aplastic anaemia tended to have lower CFU-GM numbers after BMT than those grafted for ALL.

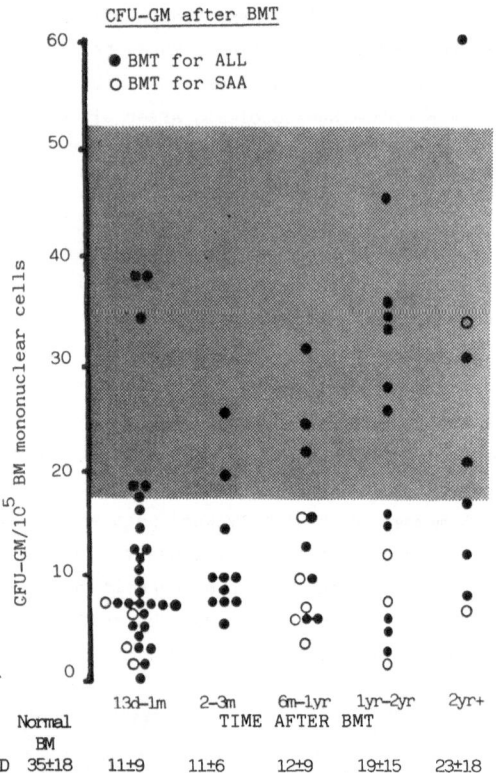

CFU-GM after BMT

● BMT for ALL
○ BMT for SAA

CFU-GM/10⁵ BM mononuclear cells

	Normal BM	13d-1m	2-3m	6m-1yr	1yr-2yr	2yr+
x̄±SD	35±18	11±9	11±6	12±9	19±15	23±18

TIME AFTER BMT

.Analysis using an unpaired t-test showed that the CFU-GM content of bone marrow more than two years after grafting was higher than BM 13d-1m after BMT (p < 0.02).

Samples tested in suspension culture consistently showed defective CFU-GM proliferation, with slight improvement with increasing time after BMT.

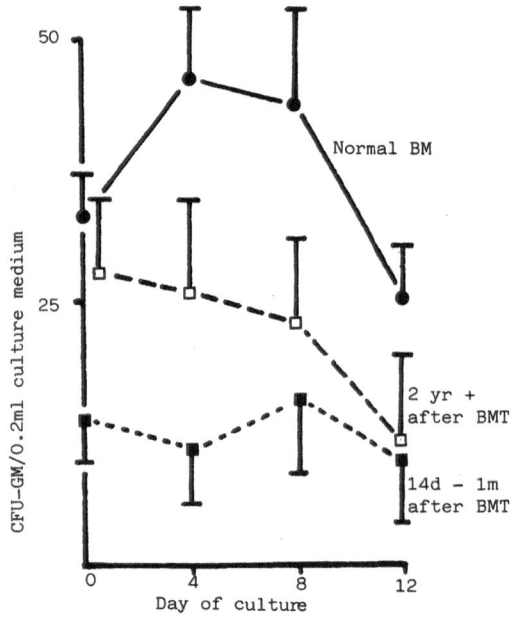

CFU-GM proliferation in suspension culture

CFU-GM/0.2ml culture medium

Normal BM

2 yr + after BMT

14d - 1m after BMT

Day of culture

The proliferative abnormality after BMT could be a result of recipient stromal cell damage caused by conditioning treatment, allogeneic difference or stem cell defects.

BM from ALL patients taken 14 days after grafting with twin donor BM did show this proliferative abnormality which was not corrected in vitro by co-culture with donor twin BM stromal cells. These results suggest the abnormality is not primarily due to stromal damage or allogeneic differences but also involves the stem cell and the persistence of the proliferation abnormality up to two years after transplant suggests the defect may be permanent

REFERENCES
1. Barrett A J, Adams J A (1981) A proliferative defect of human bone marrow after transplantation. Brit.J.Haem 49 159-165

Exp. Hematol. (suppl. 17) 13:71 (1985)
© International Society for Experimental Hematology

EB Virus Infection and Immunity in Bone Marrow Transplant Patients

D. H. Crawford [1], N. Mulholland [1], V. Iliescu [1], and R. Powles [2]

[1] ICRF Human Marrow Immunology Group and Department of Haematology University College, London
[2] Royal Marsden Hospital, Sutton, Surrey, Great Britain

INTRODUCTION

EB virus is a human herpes virus which infects most individuals subclinically during childhood, and thereafter remains in the body in a latent form. The virus can be found in the saliva and a few B lymphocytes in most seropositive individuals. This infection is thought to be controlled by memory T lymphocytes found in the peripheral blood which can be stimulated in vitro to become specifically cytotoxic for EB virus-infected target cells in a major histocompatibility complex (MHC) - restricted manner. Reactivation of this infection may occur in immunosuppressed individuals and is recognised by raised antibody levels to EB viral capsid antigen (VCA) and increased salivary EB virus secretion. An absence of circulating T cells which are specifically cytotoxic for EB virus infected cells has also been reported in immunosuppressed individuals, particularly renal transplant recipients receiving cyclosporin A (CSA). In some of these patients an uncontrolled, fatal B lymphoproliferation has been reported in which the B cells carry the EB viral genome. We have studied 10 patients over a six-month period, following a MHC matched, allogeneic bone marrow transplant (BMT), in order to monitor the reactivation of, and immunity to, EB virus infection in these patients.

METHODS

1. EB virus genome-carrying lymphoblastoid cell lines (LCL) were generated from peripheral blood mononuclear cells (PBM) obtained prior to BMT by infection with EB virus.
2. The presence of EB virus in saliva specimens obtained prior to and for up to 1 year post transplant was detected by culturing the filtered diluted specimens with umbilical cord blood mononuclear cells.
3. Serum antibody levels to VCA were determined by the routine methods.
4. EB virus-specific cytotoxic T lymphocytes in PBM were stimulated in vitro by coculture with X irradiated (XR) (4000R) autologous LCL (4 : 1) for 10 days.
5. E rosette positive cells from the stimulation cultures from 10 patients and control seropositive individuals were tested for cytotoxic activity in a 4 hour chromium (Cr) release assay using autologous and allogeneic LCL as targets, as well as K562 to detect natural killer (NK) cell activity. In some cases the E rosette positive cells were restimulated for a further 10 days with the XR autologous LCL (10 : 1) and then tested for cytotoxic activity.
6. 10 patients who received an MHC-matched allogeneic BMT were studied. The diagnosis in eight patients was acute myeloid leukaemia; one had acute undifferentiated leukaemia and one had a lymphocytic lymphoma. Age range 14 - 41; 6 male, 4 female. All received total body irradiation (9 - 10 Gy) prior to transplant and cyclosporin A (4 - 12.5 mg/kg. BD) for six months following BMT.

RESULTS & DISCUSSION

Serum anti VCA antibodies were present in all patients and bone marrow donors prior to BMT. The titres fell during the first 6 months post BMT and then rose to above pre-transplant levels in the majority of cases, although a level above the upper limit of normal was recorded in only one patient by 1 year post BMT.

Salivary virus was isolated in 10% of transplant patients studied prior to BMT in 10% of normal seropositive individuals, but in only 3% at 3 months post and 5% at 6 months post BMT.

EB virus-specific cytotoxic T cells could be stimulated from PBM from all normal serpositive control donors. In some cases the specific cytotoxicity was masked by NK cell activity after primary stimulation, but after secondary stimulation in vitro with autologous XR-LCL specific cytotoxicity could be clearly distinguished.

All 10 patients had recovered EB virus-specific cytotoxic T cell activity by 6 months post BMT and in 3 patients this activity could be detected by 3 months post BMT. In most cases the recovery of NK cell activity preceded the detection of EB virus-specific cytotoxicity.

The results show that in the 10 patients studied, who all received an allogeneic, matched BMT the recovery of cell mediated immunity to EB virus was complete by 3 - 6 months post BMT. No increased levels of salivary virus secretion or anti VCA antibody levels were detected during this period, indicating that the latent EB virus infection in these patients was adequately controlled.

Exp. Hematol. (suppl. 17) 13:72 (1985)
© International Society for Experimental Hematology

Frequency of Reactivation of Varicella-Zoster Virus (VZV) Infection with and without Symptoms After Bone Marrow Transplantation

B. Lönnqvist[1], P. Ljungman[1,4], P. Bolme[2], G. Gahrton[1], O. Ringdén[3], and B. Wahren[4]

[1] Division of Clinical Hematology and Oncology, Department of Medicine, Huddinge Hospital, Huddinge
[2] Department of Pediatrics, Huddinge Hospital, Huddinge
[3] Department of Transplantation Surgery, Huddinge Hospital, Huddinge
[4] National Bacteriological Laboratory, Stockholm, Sweden

Cytomegalovirus (CMV) is often reactivated in asymtomatic patients after bone marrow transplantation (BMT). It is less well known how frequently reactivation of varicella-zoster virus (VZV) without clinical disease occurs in these patients.

PATIENTS AND METHODS

Ninety-eight consecutively transplanted bone marrow recipients were investigated. Eighty-five patients had hematological malignancies (HM), 13 had severe aplastic anemia (SAA). Forty of the patients were part of a double-blind randomized study with prophylactic acyclorvir, and will be presented elsewhere. Nineteen patients received acyclovir and 21 placebo. Sera were sampled before BMT and consecutively in 80 of 83 patients surviving more than two months. Sera were analyzed for IgG and IgM antibodies by ELISA. The method used is specific for VZV and no cross reactions with antibodies to Herpes Simplex occur. Lymphocyte stimulation with VZV antigen was performed before BMT and repeatedly thereafter in 53 patients. Clinical reactivation was defined as the known classical picture of Herpes Zoster (HZ) or varicella (V). Subclinical reactivation was defined as a VZV IgM response or an IgG titer increase of more than fourfold or a return of lymphocyte reactivity after BMT, all without clinical signs of VZV disease.

RESULTS

Of 85 patients with HM, 6 were seronegative (VZV IgG <100) before BMT, and one of them developed uncomplicated V one year after BMT. Nineteen patients with HM developed HZ and 3 further patients clinical V in spite of seropositivity before BMT. Six of 13 patients with SAA developed HZ. One, who acquired the disease 55 months after BMT, had generalization of the disease at diagnosis. One patient with V got only a modifying dose of gammaglobulin after exposure, all others received antiviral therapy with vidarabine or acyclovir and all recovered. VZV disease was seen with the same frequency in all age groups. Seventeen of 21 adequately monitored patients with VZV disease had a significant antibody titer rise, in 16 patients to more than 10,000. Lymphocyte reactivity was seen in 12 of 13 studied patients after V and HZ. Five of 10 patients observed for more than 6 months later lost their VZV lymphocyte reactivity.

Subclinical Reactivation

Subclinical reactivation was seen in 21 patients. Three of them had also had episodes of clinical disease and the reactivation was registered as a second episode with positive serology. The type of titer changes is seen in Table I. Seven of 18 repeatedly tested patients without clinical disease regained VZV reactivity. Fever accompanied the titer rise in one patient and hepatitis in another. No other signs of disease were seen.

Table I:
VZV subclinical reactivation

	n	IgG >10000	Pos. IgM	Lymphocyte reactivity
IgG >fourfold titer increase	13	9	4	2
IgG ≤fourfold titer increase	8	1	3	5

The median ELISA titers before BMT did not influence the development of clinical disease or subclinical reactivation.

VZV and Chronic Graft-versus-Host Disease (ch. GVHD)

The relationship between VZV disease, subclinical reactivation and ch. GVHD was investigated. A higher frequency of VZV was found in patients developing ch. GVHD.

Table II:
VZV infection in patients with or without ch. GVHD

	No. of patients			
	Total	HZ	V	Subclinical reactivation
Patients with ch. GVHD	28	12 (43%)	2 (7%)	8 (28%)
Patients without ch. GVHD	70	13 (19%)	2 (3%)	13 (19%)
Total	98	25 (26%)	4 (4%)	21 (23%)

CONCLUSION

Of 83 patients surviving more than 2 months after BMT 77 had previous experience of VZV. Twenty-eight (36%) of these developed HZ or V. Twenty-one (28%) of 74 adequately followed patients showed signs of subclinical reactivation. Since 19 patients had been treated with prophylactic acyclovir during the first half year of maximal immunodeficiency, the percentages do not represent the maximum frequency of VZV reactivation of BMT.

Exp. Hematol. (suppl. 17) 13:73 (1985)
© International Society for Experimental Hematology

Early Diagnosis of Toxoplasmosis After Bone Marrow Transplantation

F. Derouin[2], A. Devergie[1], B. Beauvais[2], M. Lariviere[2], R. Melo[1], N. Lemercier[3], E. Vilmer[1], F. Isnard[1], J. M. Miclea[1], and E. Gluckman[1]

[1] Bone Marrow Transplant Unit, Department of Hematology, Hôpital Saint-Louis, Paris
[2] Parasitology Mycology Laboratory, Hôpital Saint-Louis, Paris
[3] Blood Bank, Hôpital Saint-Luis, Paris, France

Various opportunistic infections have been described in patients treated with allogeneic bone marrow transplantation (BMT). Acute disease with toxoplasma gondii is a significant cause of mortality and morbidity in transplant patients. The difficulty of diagnosis and the possibility of an effective treatment in case of early diagnosis prompted us to prospectively perform serial serological studies in BMT donors and recipients, in order to correlate the evolution of antibody titers and the clinical evidence of toxoplasmosis. We studied 80 consecutive patients. Antibody titers were measured before transplant in donors and recipient's sera. After transplant, they were measured every two weeks for 3 months and then every 3 months. All patients described here have been followed for at least 3 months. Both indirect immunofluorescence antibody test and direct agglutination test were performed on each sample.

RESULTS

1. Before transplant :

45 donors and 26 recipients had no detectable antitoplasms antibodies. Among 54 patients and 35 donors who had a positive serology before transplant, 5 recipients and 2 donors had antibody titers of more than 500 I.U./ml with IgM antibodies in 1 case. None of them had any evidence of clinical infection.
Among 26 seronegative recipients, 16 patients received a BMT from a seronegative donor and 10 from a seropositive donor. After BMT, 17 patients remained negative, 7 had a transient increase of antibodies just after transplant. This antibody detection appeared as a passive antibody transmission by donor or by blood transfusions as shown by the disappearance of these antibodies within 2 to 4 months ; only 2 patients had serological evidence of infection with a rise of IgG and IgM, without severe clinical symptoms. Both had received a transplant from a seronegative donor. An exogenous contamination is very likely, evenmore because it appeared several months after transplant when patients had resumed a normal life. Among 54 seropositive recipients, 29 patients received a BMT from a seronegative donor. In 21 patients, antibody titers began to decline after 3 months and was low or null at the 4th to 5th month. Three cases of cerebral toxoplasmosis were observed while antibody titers were low. In 5 patients, antibody titers decreased until complete negativation then a rise of IgG and IgM antibodies ($\geqslant 1/100$) was observed 3 to 6 months later. Clinically, 2 patients had fever and lymphadenopathies, 1 had asthenia and 2 were asymptomatic. 3 patients had unchanged titers early after transplant, followed by a delayed rise of specific IgG and IgM ; in one patient, this was followed by a fulminant disseminated toxoplasmosis which was diagnosed at autopsy. 25 patients received a BMT from a seropositive donor. In 4 cases, the antibody titers remained unchanged. In 13 cases antibody titers decreased until complete negativation within 1 to 8 months after BMT. In 8 cases, a delayed rise of IgG antibodies was observed. Clinically, one patient had fever and cervical lymphadenopathies compatible with the diagnosis of toxoplasmosis.

DISCUSSION

The analysis of the results shows the frequency of cerebral toxoplasmosis (4 out of 80 patients) and the frequency of serological modifications compatible with active infection since 18 patients (22,5%) had a secondary increase of antibody titers. The frequency of clinical and serological toxoplasmosis appears to be higher in patients seropositive before transplant. In addition to the possibility of reinfestation by toxoplasms, the mechanism of reactivation of latent cysts must be emphasized. According to our observations, prophylactic recommendations could be given. To prevent exogenous contamination, all patients should handle food properly, eat well cooked meat and avoid cat feces. In all patients and more specifically in seropositive recipients, antibody titers have to be followed regularly. Because diagnosis of toxoplasmosis in immunocompromised patients is difficult and often delayed, it seems that chemoprophylaxis could be recommended in patients susceptible to reactivation of latent cysts. For this purpose, administration of Spiramycine or Trimethoprim-Sulfamethoxasole coud be useful to limit the diffusion of the parasite from a reactivated focus. However, the association of Pyrimethamine and Sulfadiazine or Sulfadoxine seems the most effective treatment. In BMT patients, the high morbidity and mortality of cerebral toxoplasmosis should be considered on account of the potential toxicity of these drugs.

Exp. Hematol. (suppl. 17) 13:74 (1985)
© International Society for Experimental Hematology

Rapid Detection of Cytomegalovirus Antigens in Human Tissues

Gilbert C. Faure[1], Marie C. Bene[1], Pierre Bordigoni[2], and Francis Witz[3]

[1] Laboratoire d'Immunologie, Faculté A de Médecine de Nancy
[2] Service de Médecine Infantile 2. Hôpital d'Enfants, CHU de Nancy
[3] Clinique Médicale A, CHU de Nancy, France

Cytomegalovirus (CMV) is an ubiquitous pathogen implicated in a wide variety of disease syndromes. Its pathogenicity is especially dreaded in the first months after bone marrow transplantation (BMT), because of the immunodeficiency status of such patients. An early diagnosis of CMV infection therefore is necessary in this condition, while precise location of the infected organ is a must. Classical techniques such as virus cultures and specific antibody assays have limitations, the major one being the delays in the laboratory response. New techniques have been proposed to speed serologic diagnosis, by using more sensitive reagents and/or detection devices. Short-term cultures and in vitro detection of early virus-coded proteins in infected cells have been proposed (1). Progress in molecular biology also recently made possible the detection of viral nucleic acids in infected cells (2).

In this paper we report our experience in the tissular detection of CMV antigens (3,4), in samples from patients presenting with or suspected of generalized or localized CMV infection. Correlation was attempted with clinical, virological and pathological data.

PATIENTS AND METHODS

Twelve BMT recipients were included in a systematic study during a 6 months period of time after transplant. Two samples were obtained from different patients suffering from interstitial pneumonitis in a context of acute leukemia, and from intestinal disorders. Samples were obtained from clinically suspect organs through classical biopsy techniques. More systematic samples were collected from salivary glands and rectal mucosa, when such syndromes as graft versus host disease were evoked. Five bronchus and lung, 6 liver, 17 ileon or rectum, 10 salivary gland and 4 skin samples were analysed. All biopsies were collected in liquid nitrogen. After conservation in a deep-freezer, 3 um thick frozen-cut sections were obtained with a Slee (London, U.K.) cryostat. Two monoclonal antibodies directed to early and late nuclear proteins (Biotech Res. Lab. Rockville, MD, USA), were used in indirect immunofluorescence. Sections were stained unfixed, and FITC-sheep anti-mouse serum (Institut Pasteur Production, Paris, France) was used as second-step reagent. Adequate controls with irrelevant mouse serum or anti-mouse serum alone were satisfactory and assessed the specificity of positive labellings. Serological assays were performed in parallel to evaluate specific IgG and IgM antibodies.

RESULTS AND DISCUSSION

CMV antigens were visualized 9 times out of 42 tissular investigations. Good correlation was obtained three times between pulmonary detection and clinical features. In 2 cases, CMV appeared associated with other pathogens and may not have been responsible for clinical signs. CMV antigens were observed in the liver biopsy of one patient with clinical signs of CMV infection. They could not be found in a post mortem sample after indisputable diffuse CMV infection, but the tissue was profoundly altered. In two other instances when hepatic disturbances were attributed to GVH or ciclosporin cytotoxicity, no fluorescence was observed in biopsy samples. Digestive mucosa systematic sampling allowed positive findings in 3 samples from feverish and pancytopenic patients. Seroconversion followed several days later. Salivary glands, positive once in an infected patient, never allowed early diagnosis. Skin samples were always negative.

As a whole, a good correlation was established between these data and clinical as well as serological and/or pathological features. Some negative tests occurred in tissues where CMV infection is known to be focal; the samples available for immunohistological study might have been to small and obtained in a non infected area. In 2 lung samples, CMV was evidenced as associated with other pathogens considered responsible for clinical symptoms. This technique appears useful to establish an early and rapid diagnosis of CMV infection. It demonstrates the reality of viral material production, while viral DNA assessment can be made in the absence of viral replication. It is somehow limited by the size of the samples, and the necessity of getting tissular material. This fast and easy to perform methodology may however prove itself more effective than virus identification in situations where, because of timing and distance, sample inoculation is delayed.

REFERENCES

1. Griffiths P.D. et al., Lancet, 1984, ii, 1242-1245
2. Meyerson D. et al., J.Infect.Dis., 1984, 150, 272-277
3. Sacks S.L. et al., Gastroenterol., 1984, 86, 346-350
4. Volpi A. et al., J.Infect.Dis., 1983, 147, 1119-1120.

Exp. Hematol. (suppl. 17) 13:75 (1985)
© International Society for Experimental Hematology

Incidence and Significance of Cytomegalovirus Viremia in Bone Marrow Transplantation

E. Vilmer[1], M. C. Mazeron[2], C. Rabian[3], O. Azogui[1], A. Devergie[1], Y. Perol[2], and E. Gluckman[1]

[1] Bone Marrow Transplant Unit
[2] Laboratory of Microbiology
[3] Unité INSERM U.93, Hôpital Saint-Louis, Paris, France

INTRODUCTION

In immunosuppressed patients (pts), cytomegalovirus (CMV) viremia is an accurate marker for disseminated CMV infection as opposed to urine excretion or changes in antibody titers. A systematic study of CMV viremia was serially performed after allogenic transplantation (BMT) in 96 pts whose the clinical manifestations related to viremia were described. The occurrence of viremia was examined according to graft versus host disease (GVHD) and pts or donor pretransplant immunity against CMV.

PATIENTS AND METHODS

We studied 96 pts transplanted for a severe aplastic anemia (SAA) (67 pts) or a leukemia (29 pts), from 1979 to 1984. All the pts had an HLA identical donor except for 3 pts. Details of BMT procedure and conditioning have been published elsewehere (1). GVHD prophylaxis consisted of either Cyclosporine A (52 pts) or Methotrexate (33 pts) or both (10 pts). Granulocyte transfusions were not given prophylactically. CMV viremia assays, based on detection of cytopathic effect (1), were performed weekly until 10 weeks post transplant and thereafter according to clinical signs. The CMV induced lymphocyte proliferation had been assayed as already detailed (1).

RESULTS

Viremia was documented in 43 pts (51%) among 84 pts who survived at least 3 months post-transplant. This incidence was similar whatever the initial diagnosis. Twenty per cent of the overall isolations were positive, with a frequency peak during the 6th to 9th week post transplant. Various clinical signs may be related to viremia (fever, cytolytic hepatitis). Nevertheless, such manifestations were not associated with 40 % of positive isolations. Viremia was also detected in pts with CMV interstitial pneumonia or with other proven CMV infections in organs. Whereas the hematological engraftment was similar as regards to the presence or not, of CMV infection, secondary thrombocytopenia (platelet < 50 000 per mm³) which occurred at least 6 weeks post transplant were observed in 11 out of 37 pts with viremia and never found in 23 pts without any evidence of CMV infection.

Similar results were noticed for the secondary neutropenia (neutrophils < 1000 per mm³) (14/37 pts versus 3/23 ; p < 005). In few pts a central and/or peripheral mechanism of cytopenias were documented. The cytopenias possibly due to other causes, had not been taken into account. Finally viremia may be completely asymptomatic in a few cases (4 pts).

A significant difference was noted in the incidence of pts with viremia, in relation to the presence of CMV antibodies in recipients (R) or donor (D) before transplantation. Twenty six per cent of pts with viremia were found in the group D−/R− compared to 69% in the group D−/R+ or D+/R− (p < 005) and to 62% in the group D+/R+. The same significant difference was not observed when the lymphocyte proliferative response to CMV antigens was considered before transplant. Seventy two per cent of 25 pts who received granulocyte transfusion had viremia as compared to 42% of 60 pts who did not (p < 005). Viremia was never detected when the following criteria was associated : no granulocyte transfusion and no pretransplant sign of CMV infection diagnosed by serology and the proliferative response to CMV antigens. The incidence of severe (grade II or more) acute GVHD was higher in the 43 pts with viremia than in the group of 50 pts who had no viremia (48% versus 18% ; p < 005). A same difference was shown for the incidence of extensive chronic GVHD. Conversely, the incidence of viremia was higher in pts with severe GVHD compared to pts with minor or no GVHD (70% versus 34% ; p < 005). The CMV isolation occurred before, during or after the course of GVHD. Forty per cent of viremia were detected in pts who had already seroconverted. When the pt developped CMV lymphocyte response after graft, CMV was no longer recovered from blood.

DISCUSSION

This paper reports on the frequency of CMV viremia and on the correlation with particular clinical features such as GVHD or late cytopenias. Nevertheless, the difficult question is whether CMV is causally associated with a number of problems following BMT or just "a bystander effect". The systematic study of CMV viremia contributes to a better knowledge of the incidence and occurrence of CMV disseminated infection. Furthermore we are now able to rapidly diagnose CMV by means of an immunofluorescence system and monoclonal antibody to CMV early antigens. Such a virological marker may provide a basis for improving prophylactic treatment and for assessing the efficiency of antiviral drugs.

REFERENCE

VILMER E., MAZERON M.C., RABIAN C. et al. : Clinical significance of cytomegalovirus viremia in bone marrow transplantation . Transplantation 1985 (in press).

Exp. Hematol. (suppl. 17) 13:76 (1985)
© International Society for Experimental Hematology

Successful Treatment of Cytomegalovirus Pneumonitis After Allogeneic Bone Marrow Transplantation Using High Titre CMV Immunoglobulin (Cytotect)

H. A. Blacklock[1], P. D. Griffiths[2], P. R. Stirk[2], and H. G. Prentice[3]

[1] Department of Haematology, Hospital for Sick Children, Great Ormond Street
[2] Department of Virology
[3] Academic Department of Haematology, Royal Free Hospital, London, Great Britain

Cytomegalovirus (CMV) pneumonitis has had a mortality of >85% in allogeneic BMT recipients[1]. We have treated 9 episodes in 8 patients using Cytotect immunoglobulin (Biotest Pharma Company) which has a high titre against CMV (>1:50,000 Elisa). The treatment regimen used was 400 mg/kg IV days 0, 4, 8 and 200 mg/kg IV days 12 and 16.

The patients treated in five separate hospitals, ranged in age from one to 30 (median 25) years. Their diagnoses were AML (n=1), ALL (3), CGL (3) and Hurlers (1). Five were CMV sero-negative with negative donors, two were positive with positive donors and one was positive with a negative donor at the time of BMT. Two patients had Grade II acute GvHD and two Grade III. Each of the 8 were receiving immunosuppressive drugs at study entry (either Prednisolone, Cyclosporin A ± Prednisolone, or Prednisolone + Azathioprine) for the treatment or prevention of GvHD. Two patients developed their CMV infections despite receiving lower dose immunoglobulin prophylaxis, one Intraglobin (Biotest Pharma) and the other Cytotect. All patients except one were treated with antibiotics ± antifungals + acyclovir, with no clinical response, prior to study entry. Cytotect therapy was started 50 to 289 (median 125) days after BMT.

The diagnosis of CMV was made in all cases in the context of an interstitial pneumonitis on X-ray with hypoxia (three were on a respirator at the time of the first infusion and four were receiving oxygen by mask) and fever (n=7). The known duration of symptoms or radiological changes ranged from two to 60 (median 10) days. Four patients had open lung biopsies which revealed CMV histological changes ± immunofluorescence; two also had hepatitis. In this group, each of three tested at a suitable time after stopping the treatment, had seroconverted. The remaining four patients with five episodes of pneumonitis, had bronchial lavage with rapid detection of viral encoded early antigen fluorescent foci using specific anti-CMV monoclonals[2]. In each case the virus also grew from routine cultures of the washings two to four weeks later. These five episodes were associated with viral excretion from urine in three, viremia in two and positive saliva culture in one. One patient in this group had two separate episodes of pneumonitis, with CMV detected in the bronchial washings on both occasions, the first 70 days after BMT, the second 55 days later, after 30 asymptomatic days. There was no other evidence for CMV, and he did not seroconvert,

possibly because his donor marrow was T, and B, cell depleted using the panlymphoid monoclonal antibody CAMPATH, and he had received Cytotect immunoglobin prophylaxis until the onset of pneumonitis, followed by the high dose therapy (? preventing production of specific antibody as in the rhesus incompatibility situation). In none of the 8 patients (biopsy, culture or post mortem) was another cause identified for the pneumonitis.

Outcome: Six episodes in five of the eight patients were successfully treated, including one patient receiving respirator support, and two who had open lung biopsies. These patients are now alive and well 43-379 (median 171) days after beginning therapy. In these patients, although the progression of the pneumonitis was halted after the first Cytotect injection, resolution of the symptoms and signs (such as fever, and X-ray changes) did not occur until after four or five doses. Three patients died. The first on a respirator and hypotensive when beginning therapy, died after four days after study entry; the second also on a respirator died on day +7 from pre-existing renal failure - his lungs were stable after the Cytotect therapy was begun; the third patient who also had candidemia died on day +8. These preliminary results are encouraging with 62.5% survival of this patient group. Further clinical studies with Cytotect seems warranted. Rapid diagnosis and earlier institution of therapy particularly before respirator support is necessary, may improve these results further.

1. Hersman J, Meyers J D, Thomas E D, Buckner D, Clift R (1982) The effect of granulocyte transfusions upon the incidence of cytomegalovirus infection after allogeneic bone marrow transplant. Ann Int Med 196: 149-52

2. Griffiths P D, Panjwani D D, Stirk P R, Ball M G, Ganczakowski M, Blacklock H A, Prentice H G (1984) Rapid diagnosis of cytomegalovirus infection in immunocompromised patients by detection of early antigen fluorescent foci. The Lancet ii: 1242-5

Exp. Hematol. (suppl. 17) 13:77 (1985)
© International Society for Experimental Hematology

A Trial of Intravenous Immunoglobulin for Prevention of CMV Infection After Marrow Transplantation

T. R. Rogers, R. Joshi, S. White, P. Shaw, Y. Tryhorn, A. J. Barrett, P. G. Riches, K. Hugh-Jones, and J. R. Hobbs

Westminster Hospitals Bone Marrow Transplant Team, London SW1P 2AR, Great Britain

Introduction. A prospective controlled study was undertaken to establish whether intravenous immunoglobulin could prevent infectious complications arising in the first 100 days after bone marrow transplantation (BMT). Three previous open studies of passive immunisation have indicated a protective effect against cytomegalovirus (CMV) infection, which is the principal infective complication of BMT. An important part of the analysis in our study was to establish the effect of the immunoglobulin on the incidence of CMV infections.

Patients, materials and methods. Sixty consecutive candidates for BMT were admitted to the trial, including 37 with leukaemia, 20 inborn errors and 2 idiopathic aplasia patients. One patient died during induction prior to BMT. Patients were randomized to receive blind either an intravenous IgG preparation (Sandoglobulin) or placebo, which was administered at a dose of 500 mg/kg pre-BMT and on weeks 1, 4, 7 and 11 at 200 mg/kg. Adverse effects were recorded. Serum was collected pre-BMT from both donor and recipient to establish their CMV antibody status by complement fixation and ELISA methods, and urine culture was performed. These investigations were repeated at regular intervals after transplant, and in patients with symptoms of CMV infection additional cultures of pharyngeal aspirates, buffy coat and urine were taken.

Results. Trial therapy was well tolerated in all except two patients who received IgG; one developed severe hypertension during the first infusion and another acute respiratory symptoms and no further infusions were administered. The results of CMV studies are shown in the table. 44 out of 60 (73%) BMT recipients were seronegative pre-transplant. Active CMV infection was demonstrated in only 6 (10%) patients between days -7 and +100. In three patients, all children under 5 years old, CMV infection was found before BMT and these patients each developed fatal interstitial pneumonia post-transplant. Lung biopsies confirmed the presence of CMV pneumonia in two of these patients. Of the three patients who developed infection post-transplant, two were primary, and one a secondary infection. CMV pneumonia was confirmed on lung biopsy in two of these patients, while the other had an asymptomatic seroconversion. 5 patients had received immunoglobulin and one placebo, and CMV pneumonia was documented in 3 vs. one patient respectively.

Conclusion. Compared to the experience of centres in the United States,[1] the 10% incidence of CMV infection in our trial was low. Only one infected patient belonged to the leukaemia group. In the three

patients with active CMV infection before transplant immunoglobulin failed to prevent the subsequent development of interstitial pneumonia. As only one of the 44 seronegative patients developed CMV infection, no conclusion can be drawn about the role of immunoprophylaxis in this category. The Seattle team evaluated the role of I.M. immunoglobulin in 62 seronegative BMT recipients[2]. 10 globulin recipients versus 14 controls developed CMV infection, while in those who did not receive granulocyte transfusions 2 vs. 8 respectively developed CMV infection. Two other studies of I.V. immunoprophylaxis have shown a reduction in the incidence of CMV pneumonia[3,4]. The efficacy of the immunoglobulin therapy may well depend upon the titre of biologically active antibody to CMV, and the dose used and frequency of administration

CMV INFECTIONS

CMV status pre-transplant		Donor: Recipient: Number:	Neg. Neg. 28	Pos. Neg. 14	Pos. Pos. 7	Neg. Pos. 7
CMV infection	Pre-transplant:		0	0	1	2
	Post-transplant: (days 0 to +100)		0	1	2	0

References.
1. Watson, J.G. Problems of infection after bone marrow transplantation. J. Clin. Pathol., 36: 683-692 (1983).
2. Meyers, J.D., Leszczynski, J., Zaia, J.A. et al. Prevention of cytomegalovirus infection by cytomegalovirus immuneglobulin after marrow transplantation. Ann. Intern. Med., 98: 442-446 (1983).
3. Condie, R.M., O'Reilly, R.J. Prophylaxis of CMV infection in bone marrow transplant recipients by hyperimmune CMV gammaglobulin. Dev. Biol. Stand., 52: 501-513 (Karger, Basel 1982).
4. Winston, D.J., Pollard, R.B., Ho, W.G. et al. Cytomegalovirus immune plasma in bone marrow transplant recipients. Ann. Intern. Med., 97: 11-18 (1982).

Exp. Hematol. (suppl. 17) 13:78 (1985)
© International Society for Experimental Hematology

B-Cell Reconstitution After Allogeneic Bone Marrow Transplantation (ABMT)

M. Gobbi[1], F. Lauria[1], P. Tazzari[1], D. Raspadori[1], R. Conte[2], G. Bandini[1], A. Guarini[1], P. Paolucci[3], and S. Tura[1]

[1] Istituto di Ematologia "L. e A. Seragnoli"
[2] Centro Trasfusionale
[3] Clinica Pediatrica Policlinico S. Orsola, Bologna, Italy

It is well known that patients subjected to ABMT present a profound and long lasting immunological impairment. Although the pattern of the phenotypic expression and the function of T cells, as well as the immunoglobulin levels and the capacity to produce specific humoral responce after ABMT have been extensively studied (1), few informations have been produced on the B-cell lineage. In this study we analized the pattern of B-cell reconstitution in the bone marrow (BM) and peripheral blood (PB) in the firtst 3 months after ABMT.

PATIENTS AND METHODS

Sixteen patients, 10 males and 6 females, 13 to 46 years of age (median 29) received BM from HLA identical and MLR non responsive siblings. There were 10 CML, 7 in chronic phase and 3 in transformation, 3 AML in first CR, 2 ALL, 1 in first CR and 1 in 2nd CR, 1 multiple myeloma. Conditioning followed the "Seattle standard" plus additional drugs for CML and myeloma (details elsewere in this issue). All of them received immunosuppression with cyclosporine A from day – 1 to 120-180, prednisone was given when required as well as antibiotics and high dose i.v. immunoglobulins. Acute GVHD, confined to skin only occurred in 12 patients; one patient had severe GVHD and died at day 67. The clinical outcome of these patients is described elsewere in this issue. Immunological studies were performed 15,30,60 and 90 days after ABMT. The following parameteres were studied: T and B cell subpopulations in PB, serum immunoglobulin levels by radial immunodiffusion, cytoplasmic IgM^+ and membrane IgM^- (Pre-B) cells, as well as membrane IgM positive (B) cells and plasmacells in BM (for methods see reference (2)).

RESULTS

Table 1.

Days after ABMT	15	30	60	90
IgG mg/ml	980	1173	1022	945
IgA mg/ml	138	126	89	84
IgM mg/ml	56	114	51	199
Pre-B %	0,55	0,68	1,0	2,0
BM.B-Ly %	1,12	0,71	2,33	1,0
Plasma C %	2,62	0,33	0	0
PB B-Ly %	6,0	1,33	0,62	0,5

Table 1 summarizes the results; briefly: Pre-B cells fell to near 0 after 15 days and rose to 2% in 3 months. BM B cells remained very low (1%) throughout the period of observation, while the plasmacells, still detectable after 15 days (2,6%) fell to 0 within a month and were not appreciable during the 3 months of observation. Similarly, PB $SmIg^+$ lymphocytes reahed 6% (range 4-12) after 15 days and were detected sporadically throughout the 3 months. Serum IgG were in the normal range, while IgA resulted significantly diminished. IgM, after an initial decrease started to increase at the 3rd month. No significant differences were see between patient with GVHD and without.

DISCUSSION

The findings of this study allow to make some considerations. Firstly, the B-cell compartment is considerably late in its reconstitution since Pre-B and BM B lymphocytes are seen in appreciable numbers only 2 months after BMT. Secondly, it seems impossible to expect during this period an effective antibody production as both BM plasmacells and PB B-lymphocytes (B memory cells) are not detected. Thirdly, raises in specific antibody titers (i.e. to CMV, ABO antigens etc.) are probably due to the host residual B-cells and/or the transfused mature immunocompetent cells. Finally this data suggest that the deep immunodeficiency of the transplanted patients is more pronounced than one whould expect from serum immunoglobulin levels only.

REFERENCES

1) R.P. Witherspoon, L.G. Lum, R. Storb
   Immunologic reconstitution after human marrow grafting.
   Semin. Hematol. 21, 2-10, 1984.

2) M. Gobbi, F. Caligaris-Cappio, G. Janossy
   Normal equivalent cells of B cell malignancies: analysis with monoclonal antibodies.
   Br. J. Haematol 54, 393-403, 1983.

Study supported by C.N.R., Rome, Progetto Finalizzato Oncologia, contract n. 84.00834.44 and 84.00613.44.

Exp. Hematol. (suppl. 17) 13:79 (1985)
© International Society for Experimental Hematology

T Lymphocyte Reconstitution Following Bone Marrow Transplantation

P. Myrenfors, O. Ringdén, U. Persson, P. Larsson, B. Sundberg, and G. Johansson

Department of Transplantation Surgery and Clinical Immunology, Huddinge Hospital;
Department of Clinical Immunology, Karolinska Hospital, Karolinska Institute, Stockholm, Sweden

INTRODUCTION

Despite regeneration of normal T and B cell numbers, bone marrow transplantation (BMT) recipients remain immunosuppressed for long periods after transplantation. By using monoclonal mouse antibodies, it is possible to enumerate T cell subsets: helper/inducer (OKT4) cells and cytotoxic/suppressor (OKT8) cells. After BMT a reversed 4/8 ratio has been reported. The role of graft-versus-host disease (GVHD) seems controversial.

PATIENTS AND METHODS

Fifty-four BMT recipients, 44 with hematologic malignancies, 9 with severe aplastic anemia and one with Gaucher's disease were included in the study. Median age of the patients was 15 years, with a range from 1 to 57. Conditioning was performed according to the Seattle protocol, with minor modifications (Ringdén et al. 1982). Prophylaxis against GVHD was by methotrexate or cyclosporin. Using fluorescein-labelled monoclonal mouse antibodies, T cell subsets OKT3 (Pan T cells), 4, 8 and 11 cells were determined by Ortho spectrum laser flow cytometry. Proportions, absolute counts and 4/8 ratios were calculated.

RESULTS

OKT 4/8 ratio before BMT was 2.1±0.3. This was decreased to 1.2±0.2 (p<0.02) in patients with grade 0-I acute GVHD, and from 2.0±0.2 to 0.4±0.1 in patients with grade II-IV GVHD (p<0.001). At 3 weeks, the ratio in patients with grade II-IV GVHD was lower than in those with grade 0-I (p<0.01). This is due to a decreased % OKT4 cells and an increased % OKT8 cells in patients with grade II-IV GVHD, Table 1.

At 3 weeks GVHD	0-I	II-IV	p
% OKT4	39±3	24±3	<0.01
% OKT8	36±4	51±4	<0.01

During CMV infection the OKT4/8 ratio decreased, compared to one month before CMV infection or to patients without CMV infection, Table 2.

	1 mo before CMV	at CMV	Pts with no CMV
4/8 ratio	1.0±0.2**	0.3±0.1	0.9±0.2**
% OKT4	38±4***	13±1	28±4**
%OKT8	44±4*	62±6	36±3***
total 8 cells x 10^9/l	242±69*	599±131	215±35**

t-test * <0.05; ** <0.01; *** <0.001 compared to patients at diagnosis of CMV

In long-term survivors it was found that patients who had experienced CMV infection had increased proportions, and absolute counts, of OKT8 cells compared to patients without CMV infection (p<0.01). Patients with chronic GVHD had a lower OKT4/8 ratio, lower OKT3 and OKT4 counts and an increased proportion of OKT8 cells compared to patients without chronic GVHD. During the first 6 months patients treated with methotrexate and cyclosporin had the same OKT4/8 ratio. Between 6-12 mos. patients receiving cyclosporin had a decreased ratio of 0.5±0.1, compared to 1.1±0.1 in patients previously treated with methotrexate (p<0-01).

DISCUSSION

The OKT4/8 ratio is lowered when the marrow is reconstituted, compared to before BMT. In patients with acute GVHD the ratio is reduced. This is due to a decreased % OKT4 and increased % OKT8 cells, which seems logical since the effector cells in acute GVHD are thought to be cytotoxic T cells. In contradiction to our findings, Atkinson et al. (1982) reported that the OKT4/8 ratio was not affected by GVHD. In healthy individuals there is a reversed ratio during CMV infection (Carney et al. 1981). In our BMT patients, this imbalance is profound and persists for a long time after transplantation.

CONCLUSION

OKT4/8 ratios were decreased during acute GVHD, CMV infection and chronic GVHD. This was due to a decreased proportion of OKT4 cells and an increased proportion of OKT8 cells.

REFERENCES

Atkinson K, Hansen JA, Storb R, Goehle S, Goldstein G, Thomas DE (1982) T-cell subpopulations identified by monoclonal antibodies after human marrow transplantation. I. Helper-inducer and cytotoxic-suppressor subsets. Blood 59:1292-1298

Carney WP, Rubin RH, Hoffman RA, Hansn WP, Healey K, Hirsch MS (1981) Analysis of lymphocyte subsets in cytomegalovirus mononucleosis. J Immunol 126:2114-2116

Ringdén O, Lönnqvist B, Lundgren G, Gahrton G, Groth CG, Möller E, Båryd I, Johansson B, Pihlsted P, Gullbring B (1982) Experience with a cooperative bone marrow transplantation program in Stockholm. Transplantation 33:500-504

Address: O Ringden, Department of Transplantation Surgery, Huddinge Hospital, S-141 86 Huddinge, Sweden

Exp. Hematol. (suppl. 17) 13:80 (1985)
© International Society for Experimental Hematology

Ontogeny of Human T Lymphocytes: Phenotypic and Functional Characteristic

Catherine Royo, Odette de Bouteiller, and Jean-Louis Touraine

INSERM Unit 80, Hopital Edouard Herriot, Pavillon P, F-69374 Lyon Cedex 8, France

For both fetal liver and bone marrow transplantation, knowledge on T-cell ontogeny is crucial. Human liver, bone marrow, thymus, and spleen mononuclear cells from 7 to 24 week-old fetuses were studied for T-cell antigens and for T-cell functions.

An immunofluorescence analysis, with a panel of monoclonal antibodies(MoAbs) (OKT3, OKT4, OKT6, OKT8, OKT9, OKT10, OKT11, OKIa1, anti β2-microglobulin and HNK-1), was carried out for the identification of human T-cell subsets during fetal development. Antigen expression was measured by cytofluorometry (Ortho 50H) Less than 5% of lymphoid cells from the liver and the bone marrow expressed T3,T4, T6, T8 or T11 antigens. Most thymocytes of more than 12 weeks expressed these antigens, and many of them have a simultaneous expression of T4, T6 and T8 antigens. The percentage of cells expressing HLA Class I was low in the liver(17%) while it was found to be 90% as a mean in the thymus and in the spleen. In all organs, a large percentage of cells expressed the T10 antigen, which didn't appear to be specific for a lymphocyte subpopulation. From these results, it appears that T-cell specific antigens are rapidly expressed by lymphoid cells after they had colonized the thymus. Following their intrathymic differentiation, cells migrate to peripheral lymphoid organs, but only few of them return to the liver or the bone marrow.

The cell surface density of T10 and HLA Class I antigens was significantly increased by an 18h preincubation with 30U/ml of α_2 interferon (DNAX, Palo Alto, Ca.).

Proliferative responses to Concanavalin A(ConA), Phytohemagglutinin(PHA) and Pokeweed Mitogen(PWM), in relation with fetal age, were investigated. Fetal liver cells demonstrated a high degree of spontaneous proliferation and responded only slightly to ConA in 10 week-old fetuses. Fetal thymocytes had a significant mitogen responsivness, from 13 weeks onwards. Indices of stimulation were: ConA: 42.9; PHA: 19.7; PWM: 13.1. A very high response was consistently found at 14 weeks, then it decreased to plateau at levels comparable to those of children's thymocytes. The response of spleen cells to mitogens appeared a few weeks after that of thymocytes. Our results suggest different behaviors of T lymphocytes at distinct stages of development. Thymus colonization with lymphoid stem cells or prothymocytes from the fetal liver occurs between the 7th and the 11th week of gestation. From 13 weeks onwards, there is a transient homing of T-cells in the thymus. After 16 weeks of gestation, T lymphocytes leave the thymus and complete maturation is then achieved at the periphery.

Interleukin-2 (IL-2) production and IL-2 receptor expression by fetal cells were induced by mitogen activation. Fetal mononuclear cells from 20,21 and 24 week-old fetuses were cultured (2×10^6 cells/ml) with either ConA (10µg/ml) or PHA (1:400). Control cultures were left without mitogen. At set time intervals(24h, 48h and 72h), culture supernatants were harvested and assayed at various dilutions, for the presence of IL-2, on the clone IL-2 dependent T-cell line, CTLL2. IL-2 receptor expression was measured by cytofluorometry, using an anti-Tac MoAb and an FITC goat anti-mouse immunoglobulin antiserum. Activation was required to induce IL-2 production and IL-2 receptor expression. Activated fetal liver and bone marrow cells failed to produce IL-2 and to express IL-2 receptors. By contrast, thymus and spleen cells, at the same ontogenetic stages, were able to produce IL-2, upon mitogen stimulation. The quantity of IL-2 produced was comparable to that released by adult peripheral blood lymphocytes(PBL), although it was occasionnally lower. The optimal IL-2 production was obtained either at day 1 or at day 2 of culture, depending on the fetal donors. ConA and PHA also induced IL-2 receptor expression on fetal thymocytes and splenocytes, as determined by the Tac MoAb. This effect was comparable at day 1,2 and 3 of the culture with mitogen. It was lower than in the control adult PBL.

Other experiments were designed to determine (a) the capacity of fetal B-cells to differentiate into plasma cells and (b) the capacity of fetal T-cells to help B-cell differentiation. In brief, it was found that splenocytes from 20-24 week-old fetuses could synthetize intracytoplasmic immunoglobulins in the presence of either adult or fetal T-cells, upon PWM stimulation. T lymphocytes from the thymus or the spleen of the same fetuses were able to exert an helper activity, the magnitude of which was only slightly below that of adult peripheral blood T cells.

In conclusion, ontogenetic studies show the importance for the T-cell development of the 11-20 week period. After the 20th week of gestation, T-cells and B-cells are present in relatively large numbers and their differentiation characteristics suggest that they are close to the stage when they can respond to antigenic challenges. Allogeneic responses are acquired even earlier, before the 15th week of gestation.

Exp. Hematol. (suppl. 17) 13:81 (1985)
© International Society for Experimental Hematology

A Sequential Study of Histological and Immunological Changes in the Skin After Bone-Marrow Transplantation

D. Guyotat [1], G. Mauduit [2], C. Dauriac [1], B. Chouvet [2], J. Kanitakis [2], H. Vu Van [1], J. Thivolet [2], and D. Fiere [1]

[1] Unite fonctionnelle de greffes de moelle and
[2] Clinique dermatologique et immunologique, Hôpital Edouard-Herriot, F-69378 Lyon, France

Graft-versus-host disease remains a major complication in allogenic bone-marrow transplantation (B.M.T.), and skin is frequently involved (1). Skin biopsy is the most satisfactory technique for diagnosis, but does not provide early diagnosis, and lesions are not always specific. Immunopathological studies of the skin after B.M.T. have been performed mainly in patients presenting G.V.H.D. (2, 3), and it is difficult to assess wether the abnormalities that have been described are related to G.V.H.D. or to the transplant procedure itself. In an attempt to describe early modifications and to eventually precise their relations to G.V.H.D., we have studied serial skin biopsies in recipients of allogenic and autologous B.M.T.

PATIENTS AND METHODS

13 adult patients transplanted for leukemia or aplastic anemia were studied. The conditionning regimen was cyclophosphamide and total body irradiation. Cyclosporin A was given in all but one patients as G.V.H.D. prophylaxis; immunodepletion with anti cytotoxic-T-cell antibody and complement was additionally performed in 3 patients. G.V.H.D. was scored according to Glucksberg (1). 2 patients undergoing autologous transplantation for lymphoma with the same conditionning regimen were also studied.

Skin biopsies were taken on days -10, 4, 11, 18, 25, and 32 in all patients with allogenic transplantation, regardless to occurence of G.V.H.D., and on days -10 and 4 or 18 in recipients of autologous transplantation. Skin specimens were cut into 2 pieces which were either fixed into buffered formalin and processed for histological analysis or snap frozen into liquid nitrogen and stored. Immunological analysis was performed with indirect immunofluorescence method using OKT 3, Leu 3a, Leu2a, BL 6 (specificity to common thymocytes and Langerhans cells, gift of J. Brochier, INSERM U 80, Lyon, France), BL 2 (to HLA-Dr antigens, J. Brochier).

RESULTS

Clinical and histological results

10 out of 13 patients had cutaneous acute G.V.H.D. In 8 cases, histological changes preceeded clinical onset. G.V.H.D. was scored as grade 1 in 7 patients, grade 2 in 1 patient, grade 4 in 2 patients with liver and intestinal involvment and fatal outcome on days 39 and 45.

Immunopathological studies

Weak dermal infiltration with OKT3+ cells was seen in 4 patients. Marked Leu3a+ cells infiltration in dermis and epidermis was seen in both patients with severe G.V.H.D. but did not preceed clinical lesions. These findings confirm those of Janossy (3) and are consistent with the hypothesis that these cells with cytotoxic phenotype are implicated in G.V.H.D. 4 other patients had occasional dermal or epidermal infiltration with Leu 3a+ cells but they only had minor G.V.H.D.

The second finding in our study is the absence of Langerhans cells in all patients (except one who had only a decrease in their number) during the early post-transplant period (up to days 25 or 32). This was shown with both BL 6 and BL 2 antibodies and confirmed in two patients by electron microscopy. As it was observed after autologous B.M.T. as well, we believe it is due to the conditionning regimen and not to G.V.H.D. Langerhans cells reconstitution was not delayed by G.V.H.D. as observed by Perreault (4).

Dermal infiltration with Dr + cells was seen in all cases. Intercellular epidermal staining with anti-Dr antibody was noted in three patients (one of them with severe G.V.H.D.), but each time on one biopy only. This has been described in patients with G.V.H.D. (3) but also in patients with lichen planus and does not seem to responsible for G.V.H.D.

In conclusion, the only change correlated with G.V.H.D. was a dermo-epidermal infiltration with Leu 2a+ cells. Other findings such as Langerhans cells absence and keratinocytes Dr staining were seen regardless to occurence of G.V.H.D.

REFERENCES

1. GLUCKSBERG H, STORB R, FEFER A, ET AL. Clinical manifestations of graft-versus-host disease in human recipients of marrow from HLA-matched sibling donors. Transplantation 18:295-304, 1974.
2. TSOI MS, STORB R, JONES E, ET AL. Deposition of IgM and complement at the dermo-epidermal junction in acute and chronic cutaneous graft-versus-host disease in man. J Immunol 120:1485-1491, 1978.
3. LAMPERT IA, JANOSSY G, SUITTERS AJ, ET AL. Immunological analysis of the skin in graft-versus-host disease. Clin Exp Immunol 50:123-131, 1982.
4. PERREAULT C, PELLETIER M, LANDRY D, ET AL. Study of Langerhans cells after allogenic bone-marrow transplantation. Blood 63:807-811, 1984.

Exp. Hematol. (suppl. 17) 13:82 (1985)
© International Society for Experimental Hematology

Analysis of Skin Reactivity with Monoclonal Antibodies After Allogeneic Bone Marrow Transplantation

Noel Milpied [1], , Brigitte Dreno [2], Brigitte Bureau [2], and Jean-Luc Harousseau [1]

[1] Service d'Hematologie Clinique (Prof. J. L. Harousseau)
[2] Service de Dermatologie (Prof. H. Barriere) C.H.U., F-44035 Nantes Cedex, France

Pathologic changes and pattern of cell reactivity with a panel of monoclonal antibodies using immunofluorescence staining was assessed on frozen skin biopsies systematically performed Day 14 to 21,100,365 and when clinical skin changes occured after 11 allogeneic bone marrow transplantations. The purpose of this study was to identify any immunopathological feature specific for Acute Graft vs Host Disease (AGVH) and predictive of Chronic form of the disease (CGVH).

PATIENTS AND METHODS :

Eleven patients, age 12 to 42 (median : 24), entered this study. Primary diagnosis was CML in 2 patients, ANLL in 7 and ALL in 2. Nine patients received cyclophosphamide (60 mg/kg/d,2 days) and Total Body Irradiation (10 Gy at 0.035 Gv/mn with lung shielding at 8 Gy). Two received an association of cyclophosphamide, etoposide (200 mg/m2 2 doses), carmustine (200 mg/m2 1 dose) and TBI. Marrow was harvested from identical sibling. Nine patients received cyclosporin-A (3 mg/kg IV from day-1) and two methotrexate as AGVH prophylaxis. Six mm size punch biopsies were systematically performed on D 14-21, 100, 365 and when clinical skin change occured at the site of eruption. Each biopsy was divided in two parts. One was embedded in paraffin, sections were stained with hematoxylin-eosin for standard pathology. The other was snap frozen in liquid nitrogen for indirect immunofluorescence labelling using a panel of monoclonal anti bodies : IOT1[+] (pan T), IOT4[+] LEU3* (helper T cells), IOT8[+]-LEU2* (suppressor T cells), IOT6[+] (thymocytes-Langerhans'cells-LC) IOB1[+] (B cells), IOT2a[+] (HLA-DR) and KL1[+] (keratin polypeptides 55-57 kd).

RESULTS :

EARLY BIOPSIES : D14-21. Pathology showed ballonisation, vacuolisation of some keratinocytes and dermo-epidermal junction changes. No T6+ epidermal (LC) or T cells were detected in the epidermis. In the dermis some cells were Ia+ of which only 10% were LEU3+ with double labelling, other Ia+ cells being histiocytic or dentritic cells. The same immuno-pathological features were found on biopsies performed within the same period after 3 similarly conditionned autologous marrow grafts.Of the 11 allogeneic grafted patients, 6 furthermore developped AGVH grade II to IV.

INTERMEDIATE BIOPSIES : D21 to D100. Nine patients exhibited skin changes. In 6, pathology was consistant with AGVH: Infiltrate of mononuclear cells in the upper dermis ballonisation, vacuolisation and in some instances satellite cell necrosis of the keratinocytes. According to the LERNER's classification (1) grading of the lesion was II in 2 cases, III in 3 and IV in 1. The cells in the infiltrate were IOT1+ and IOT2a+. In the dermis, double staining showed 40% Ia+-LEU3+ cells and 20%

Ia+-LEU2+. In the epidermis, no T6+ nor LEU3+ cells could be detected. In all cases keratinocytes were strongly I a+, expressivity of keratinocyte polypeptides was severely altered with absence of KL1 staining sometime at all level of epidermis. In 3 patients, pathology did not showed AGVH features. Immunopathology showed discrete Ia+-LEU3+ infiltrate, no Ia+ keratinocytes and only minimal changes in the expressivity fo keratin polypeptides.

LATE BIOPSIES : D100. Nine patients were evaluated, 8 had normal clinical and pathological skin aspect, 1 had ongoing AGVH lesions. Il 3 (1 with no previous AGVH and 2 with), epidermal LC (T6+ Ia+) were present. One developped CGVH later. Il the other 6 (2 without, 3 with resolved and 1 with on-going AGVH), no LC could be found. Five subsequently developped localised or extensive CGVH. In all cases, LEU3+ cells were spared in the dermis only.

Only 3 patients have been evaluated on D365. They all exhibited normal pathologic skin aspect. Number of T6+-Ia+ epidermal LC were normal.

These sequential skin biopsies performed after allogeneic bone marrow transplantation allowed us to show, as others (2,3) that :
- Early disappearance of LC is therapy related since the same feature occurs after autologous transplantation..
- Ia positivity of keratinocytes is, in this setting, specific of AGVH but not predictive since it was not present in 6 patients one to two weeks before onset of AGVH.
We also showed that :
- Keratin polypeptide expressivity is severely altered during AGVH. Are these alterations secondary to immune disturbances occuring during AGVH or themselves the cause of antigenic modifications triggering these disturbances is not know at the moment.
- A relationship between tempo of recovery of LC epidermal cells and CGVH may exist, the absence of LC af D100 becoming an additional predictive feature for the onset of CGVH. These studies are continued in an attempt to confirm these preliminary results.

+ : Immunotech
* : Beckton-DICKINSON

REFERENCES

1).LERNER KG et al:Transplant Proc 1974,6,367-371.
2).SLOANE JP et al:J.Clin.Pathol 1984,37,919-930.
3).LAMPERT IA et al:Nature 1984,293,149.

Exp. Hematol. (suppl. 17) 13:84 (1985)
© International Society for Experimental Hematology

Self/Non Self Education and HLA-Restricted Cell Cooperation After Haploidentical Bone Marrow Transplantation

J. P. De Villartay, A. Fischer, and C. Griscelli

Groupe de Recherches d'Immunologie et de Rhumatologie Pédiatriques, INSERM, U. 132, Hôpital Necker-Enfants Malades, Paris, France

Animal models of major histocompatibility complex (MHC) incompatible bone marrow transplantation (BMT) have gained considerable insight into the understanding of self education mechanism. It has been shown that the Ia molecules expressed on intrathymic cells dictate the self recognition pattern of engrafted MHC-incompatible T cells and thus tolerance to host cells (1, 2). The precise mechanism (s) of self education remains however, unknown. The correction of the severe combined immune deficiency (SCID), by T cell depleted BMT provides an unique model for the study of tolerance education to host and donor HLA antigens as well as of self acquisition.

Five patients have been successfully transplanted 400 to 650 days ago and have been included in this study (3). They have received haploidentical BM cells depleted of T cells by E-rosetting and have been treated by cyclosporin A for 60 days post transplant. Four patients have experienced the development of full T and B cell immune functions while the fifth has developped partial T cell and no B cell functions. In this patient, T cells only are of donor origin whereas in the four others T cells are of donor origin, B cells and monocytes are of both donor and host origin. As seen in other patients (4) engrafted T cells were unreactive to recipient blood mononuclear cells (PBM) in a mixed leukocyte reaction (MLR) assay in contrast to donor cells in all patients. No suppression could be found accounting for this tolerance to the host HLA antigens.

Surprisingly, we have observed in all cases that PBM isolated post transplant from the recipient and shown by HLA typing to be of donor origin, were significantly reactive to irradiated donor PBM. This "auto" reactivity was proven to be mediated by T lymphocytes and to be a transient phenomenon observed within the first 4 months post transplant. In the unique patient who experienced donor T cell engraftment only, this auto reactivity is persisting 16 months post transplant. Furhtermore, by weekly stimulation with irradiated donor PBM, it was possible to grow an IL_2-dependent T cell line from this patient. A low number of these T cells were shown to be able to block specifically the allogeneic reactivity of donor cells to unrelated cells. These autoreactive T cells were found to recognize HLA-DR and DQ determinants, and not to exert any cytotoxic activity. These observations have led to a model of self tolerance education that could be used as a working hypothesis for further studies. The assumption is made that immature T cells have a full potential repertoire for HLA class II antigens. Early post transplant, only host Ia^+ cells are present inducing by an unknown mechanism tolerance to host Ia antigens, then following the differentiation of donor Ia^+ cells (monocytes ?) then tolerance to both host and donor Ia antigens is achieved. If the differenciation of Ia^+ cells of donor origin does not occur, then Ia^+ activated T cells of donor origin will be seen as non self and their function blocked by "auto reactive" T lymphocytes. This would lead to a persisting immunodeficiency as seen in one patient.

Whether such tolerance is acquired in the thymus cannot be deduced from these data, although in animal models, tolerance education to host Ia antigens has been located in the thymus (1).

In patients with full immune development, it has been possible to demonstrate that engrafted T cells are able to help B cells for in vitro antibody production to influenza virus, expressing either donor or host HLA class I antigens but not other HLA class II antigens (5). Similarly engrafted T cells can kill influenza-infected cells expressing either donor or host HLA class II antigens but not other HLA class I antigens (5). These data are suggestive for a central role of HLA class II (and I) expressing cells in self education, the presence of both host-derived and donor-derived HLA class II+ cells leading to restriction of T cell responses by both sources of HLA antigens (2, 4, 5). Further studies of similar patients and other types of mixed chimerism following haploidentical BMT should help in a better understanding of the fine mechanisms of self education.

1. ZINKERNAGEL, R.M., Immunol. Rev., 42, 225-270, 1978.

2. LONGO, D.L., and DAVIES, M., J. Immunol., 130, 2525-2527, 1983.

3. FISCHER, A., DURANDY, A., DE VILLARTAY, J.P. & al., Transplant Proc. (in press).

4. CHU, E., UMETSU, D., ROSEN, F., & al., J. Clin. Invest., 72, 1124-1129, 1983.

5. DE VILLARTAY, J.P., FISCHER, A., and GRISCELLI, C., In Human T cell cell clones. M. Feldmann ed. Humana Press. (in press).

Exp. Hematol. (suppl. 17) 13:83 (1985)
© International Society for Experimental Hematology

HLA-DR Expression by Keratinocytes in Acute Cutaneous Graft-Versus-Host Disease

A Diagnostic Aid

Beatrix Volc-Platzer[1], Th. Radaskiewicz[2], Isabella Mosberger[2], W. Hinterberger[3], Waltraud Schmidmeier[4], and G. Stingl[1]

[1] Department of Dermatology I
[2] Institut of Pathology
[3] Department of Internal Medicine I, University of Vienna
[4] St. Anna Children's Hospital, Vienna, Austria

The emergence of acute graft-versus-host disease (GvHD) is a potentially life-threatening complication in patients receiving allogeneic bone marrow transplantation (BMT) and therefore requires accurate diagnosis and rapid treatment. For this purpose clinical and histopathological evaluation of skin rashes occurring after BMT are of great value but, occasionally, yield only equivocal results.

In search of additional diagnostic tools we performed a highly sensitive 3-step immunoperoxidase technique (1st incubation was performed with the respective monoclonal antibodies, as 2nd step reagent we used a Peroxidase-conjugated rabbit anti-mouse immunoglobulin and for the 3rd incubation a Peroxidase-conjugated swine anti-rabbit immunoglobulin (Dakopatts)) on frozen sections of skin biopsies from 12 patients undergoing allogeneic BMT for leukemia or aplastic anemia (AA). Conditioning regimens consisted of cyclophosphamide (Cy) and total body irradiation (TBI) for leukemia patients and of Cy for AA patients (according to the established regimens), who - in order to prevent graft-rejection - also received donor buffy coat cells. GvHD prophylaxis was attempted by the use of methotrexate. Skin biopsies were performed prior to and sequentially after BMT on days +1, +10, +21, +60 and +100.

Our studies yielded three major findings: 1) a numerical decrease of OKT6 positive epidermal Langerhans cells (LC), 2) the appearance of cells bearing natural killer (NK) cell markers (Leu 7) in the epidermis and 3), class II alloantigen expression by keratinocytes (KC) in cutaneous GvHD.

Neither decrease in the number of OKT6 positive LCs nor appearance of anti-Leu 7 reactive cells are helpful in securing the diagnosis of cutaneous GvHD. LCs are decreased already prior to BMT in leukemia patients, and are further decreased between days +10 and +21 independantly from cutaneous GvHD. The emergence of anti-Leu 7 positive cells in the epidermis may well be an important diagnostic parameter but, due to the paucity of BMT patients studied, we cannot exclude the possibility that these cells might also infiltrate the epidermis in viral or drug induced skin rashes.

We believe, however, that the expression of class II alloantigens on KC, which under normal circumstances bear only class I alloantigens (wheras in normal epidermis class II alloantigens are found on LCs only (Fig. 1)), is of preeminent importance in the diagnosis of acute cutaneous GvHD. This is evidenced by the fact that within all skin biopsies from the patients with acute cutaneous GvHD (from 12 BM grafted patients 8 developed acute cutaneous GvHD) HLA-DR antigens on KC could be observed (Fig. 2), and, equally important, that none of the patients receiving allogeneic BM but never developing any signs of acute cutaneous GvHD, never displayed HLA-DR expressing KC.

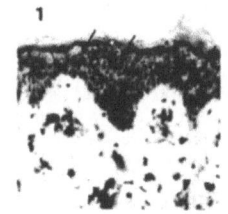 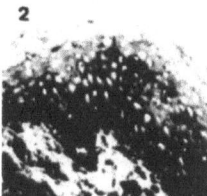

Fig. 1 Normal human epidermis pre BMT: only LCs bear class II alloantigens

Fig.2 Acute cutaneous GvHD KC display surface-bound HLA-DR α / β chains (visualized by the mAB anti HLA-DR, 1:100 Becton Dickinson, CA)

The contention that in acute cutaneous GvHD the lymphokine mediated phenomenon of HLA-DR antigen biosynthesis by KC visualized by immunohistology is occasionally superior to conventional H&E light microscopical procedures is derived from observations made in a child, who received allogeneic BM as treatment for AA and on day +14 developed a maculopapular rash highly suggestive of acute cutaneous GvHD. Whereas routine histopathology did not allow diagnosis of cutaneous GvHD, the immunohistological procedures revealed the presence of HLA-DR α + β chains in and on KC and HLA-DR γ chains within the cytoplasm of the very same KC, a fact evidencing biosynthesis of class II alloantigens by KC (Volc-Platzer et al., 1984, J.Exp.Med. 159: 1784). Routine histopathology typical of acute cutaneous GvHD could be observed five days later.

Thus we conclude that HLA-DR expression by KC provides an additional helpful tool in the diagnosis of acute cutaneous GvHD.

Exp. Hematol. (suppl. 17) 13:85 (1985)
© International Society for Experimental Hematology

HLA Mismatched Bone Marrow Transplantation for Severe Combined Immunodeficiency and Other Non Malignant Disorders

A. Fischer, A. Durandy, J. P. De Villartay, S. Blanche, E. Vilmer, and C. Griscelli

Groupe de Recherches d'Immunologie et de Rhumatologie Pédiatriques, INSERM, U. 132, Hôpital Necker-Enfants Malades, Paris, France

The use of haploidentical, T cell-depleted bone marrow has recently be shown to be an efficient procedure to cure severe combined immuno deficient (SCID) patients (1-4). Several methods have been proposed for the removal of mature T lymphocytes from the bone marrow. The most frequently used consists in soy bean agglutination of T lymphocytes followed by E-rosetting (1, 2). This has be proven to prevent GVHd, to allow T cell reconstitution and in one half of the cases B cell reconstitution. This method is however associated with several failures of engraftment requiring multiple grafts (1, 5). Specific anti-T cell monoclonal antibodies plus complement have also been used with success (3) although the further occurence of GVHd has not been totally eliminated. We have chosen to use the E-rosetting method for T cell depletion because of its simplicity and low cost (4).

Thirteen patients aged 3 to 42 months with SCID (ADA deficiency : 3, alymphocytosis : 2, absence of T cells : 3, abnormal T + B cells : 5) have received T cell depleted bone marrow from partially mismatched related donors (HLA B locus different : 2, HLA DR different : 1, HLA B, DR different : 1, HLA A, B, DR different : 9). Patients with residual T cells or ADA deficiency have received an immunosuppressive regimen consisting of Busulfan (8 to 16 mg/kg) and cyclophosphamide (200 mg/kg).

T cell depletion by rosetting with neuraminidase-treated sheep red cells was efficient since it resulted in 2 log reduction of T cell numbers. One X10^8 BM cells/kg were approximately infused. Since a few number of T cells excaped the depletion procedure, cyclosporine A was given from day -1 to +60 by continuous intravenous infusion in order to maintain a through plasmatic level around 100 mg/ml.

In all patients but 2, engraftment was observed following the first BMT attempt. The last 2 patients did receive a second transplant following an immunosuppressive regimen. Engraftment was achieved in one, and one patient has been grafted too recently to be evaluated.

An acute GVHd occured in four patients (2 grade I and 2 grade II) and was always transient. No chronic GVHd has been observed.

Nine of 13 patients are alive 25 to 700 days post transplant. Three patients died within the first 3 months from interstitial pneumonitis that were already present prior to BMT and one at day 95 from a polyclonal B cell proliferative syndrome of donor origin. It is striking to note that death occured in the three patients with ADA deficiency. Five patients are home and doing well more than one year post BMT. Four of them have stable full T cell immune functions and full or partial B cell immune functions (antibody responses post vaccination) while the fifth has T cell functions only.

Among the four others (day +25 to +100 post BMT) two patients have partial T cell reconstitution. These results are comparable to those achieved with the other methods used (1-3, 5) and suggest that the E-rosetting procedure may allow an easier engraftment.

Using the same approach, we have tried to perform haploidentical BMT for patients with other congenital disorders (Wiskott Aldrich syndrome : 1, phagocytic cell disorder with adhesive protein deficiency : 1, osteopetrosis : 1, Chediak Higashi : 1). The patient with the Chediak Higashi syndrome died early post transplant from viral infection without evidence of engraftment. Partial engraftment has been achieved in the patients with the Wiskott Aldrich syndrome (D 220+) and with the osteopetrosis (D 240+). However, the former developped a T cell lymphoma currently treated by chemotherapy. Finally, the patient with the complex phagocytic cell disorder experienced full engraftment and phagocyte cell functions correction after having received an conditioning regimen consisting of cyclophosphamide and total body irradiation (D 250+). None of these patients suffered from GVHd.

These results indicate that haploidentical BMT using E-rosetting T cell depletion and a short course of cyclosporin A can be successfull in treating SCID providing that no severe infection occured prior to BMT and/or that SCID is not due to ADA deficiency. Moreover this procedure gives encouraging results for other inherited diseases although engraftment is not always achieved and can be delayed. Efforts are still required in order to improve the engraftment such as the use of stronger conditioning regimens and in order to reduce the risk of secondary lymphomas.

1. REISNER, Y., KAPOOR, N., KIRKPATRICK, D. & al., Blood 61, 341-348, 1983.

2. FRIEDRICH, W., GOLDMANN, S.F., VETTER, V., & al., Lancet, i, 761-764, 1984.

3. REINHERZ, E.L., GEHA, R., RAPPEPORT, J.M., & al., Proc. Natl. Acad. Sci. 79, 6047-6051, 1982.

4. FISCHER, A., DURANDY, A., DE VILLARTAY, J.P. & al., Transplant Proc. (in press).

5. O REILLY, R.J., BROCHSTEIN, J., DINSMORE, R., & al., Semin in Haematol. 21, 188-221, 1984.

Exp. Hematol. (suppl. 17) 13:86–87 (1985)
© International Society for Experimental Hematology

Thirty International Cases of Bare Lymphocyte Syndrome: Biological Significance of HLA Antigens

Jean-Louis Touraine, Gian-Luigi Marseglia, and Herve Betuel

INSERM Unit 80, Hôpital Edouard Herriot, Pavillon P, F-69374 Lyon Cedex 8, France

INTRODUCTION

Lack of expression of class I HLA antigens and combined immunodeficiency were observed in the initial patient in whom the Bare Lymphocyte Syndrome(BLS) was described (1). Since then, a total number of 30 patients have been reported, worldwide, with "bare lymphocytes", i.e. cells devoid of either class I or class II HLA antigens at their surface. Twenty-eight of these patients have a combined immunodeficiency disease and several of them have been previously described (2,3). Complete informations have been gathered on clinical manifestations from twenty patients and they are described herein. Immunological data from most of these patients are also given. They show a complete lack of any cellular or humoral response to soluble antigens whether the defect predominates on class I or on class II HLA antigens. In addition to these twenty patients, two individuals have been found to have "bare lymphocytes" without significant immunodeficiency (4). However, in these two siblings, the defect in HLA expression was only partial and it may have been insufficient to interfere with the immune development.

HISTORY OF THE BLS

-1974 : Discovery of the syndrome (lack of cellular expression of class I HLA antigens + combined immunodeficiency) in an Algerian infant. *J.L. Touraine & H. Bétuel.*

-1976 : Identification of 2 other cases in a Turkish family (findings comparable with those in the Algerian patients, although β-2-microglobulin was normally detected on B-cells). *R.K.B. Schuurman & J.J. Van Rood.*

-1979 : Additional case of Bare Lymphocyte Syndrome in the initial, Algerian family. *J.L Touraine*

-1972-82 : 11 new cases reported (defective expression of either class I or class II HLA antigens + combined immunodeficiency). *C. Griscelli, W. Kuis.*

-1983 : Identification of two siblings with " Bare Lymphocytes" without immunodeficiency. *R. Payne & L.M. Young.*

-1984 : 13 additional patients with lack of expression of HLA antigens and combined immunodeficiency included into the international Registry held in Lyon, France.

CLINICAL MANIFESTATIONS IN PATIENTS WITH BLS

Data from the twenty fully reported cases are summarized below :
Ages at onset : 1 to 8 months

Consanguineous union : 10/20
North Africain origin : 15/20
Sex : 16 males, 4 females
First manifestations :
  - diarrhea.......................14
  - respiratory tract infection..... 8
  - oral candidiasis............... 9
Main clinical symptoms observed during the course of the disease :
  - protacted diarrhea..........................18
  - failure to thrive..........................19
  - respiratory manifestations...................19
  - interstitial pneumonia (Pneumocystis, CMV).... 6
  - iterative infections.......................17
  - severe infections...........................16
  - severe viral infections (CMV, Herpes, Adenovirus, Coxsackie...)...............10
  - cholangitis.................................. 2
  - generalized BCG infection.......0/7 vaccinated
  - GvHD after blood transfusion....0/2 transfused
  - neurologic disturbances..................... 4
  - paralysis after live polio vaccine administration............................... 1
  - auto-immune hemolytic anemia................. 1
Ages at death : 7 to 66 months
Ages of alive patients : 8 months to 12 years

MAIN IMMUNOLOGICAL DATA IN PATIENTS WITH BLS

Cellular immunity :
  - number of total lymphocytes consistently below 1500/mm^3 of blood.....................1/20
  - number of total T lymphocytes:decreased.... 7/20 (but, more frequently, selective decrease of OKT4+ lymphocytes)
  - mitogen-induced proliferation: significantly decreased.................... 1/20
  - antigen-induced proliferation: absent......20/20
  - delayed-type skin hypersensitivity: absent or extremely reduced...............20/20
  - proliferation of patients'cells in mixed leukocyte reaction: significantly decreased.4/14
  - cell-mediated lymphocytotoxicity: significantly decreased.....................3/11
Humoral immunity :
  - number of total B lymphocytes: decreased... 0/16
  - hypogammaglobulinemia..................... 20/20
  - antibody production post-vaccination: virtually absent......................... 20/20
  - allo-hemagglutinins: decreased........... 7/7

Altogether, the most consistent and impressive feature in patients with BLS appeared to be the complete lack of any cellular or humoral response to soluble antigens.

IMMUNOGENETIC DEFECT IN PATIENTS WITH BLS

Three sub-types of BLS have been observed :
- BLS-type I: predominant defect
  of class I expression.............. 5 patients
- BLS-type II: predominant defect
  of class II expression............ 4 patients
- BLS-type III: combined defects of both
  class I and class II expression....11 patients

No major clinical or immunological difference has been seen between these sub-types. The most severe forms were found in BLS-type I and type III. Cytotoxic reactions were not more significantly reduced in BLS-type I. Helper activities were as much inhibited in BLS-type I as in type II.

When patients with type III were repeatedly investigated, their lymphocytes were occasionnally found to express trace amounts of HLA antigens of one class, suggesting borderline forms with either type I or type II.

EBV-transformed B-lymphoblastoid cells from patients with BLS-type I also lacked HLA&β2m expression when initially studied(fig.1). After several weeks in culture, however, a proportion of cells expressed β2m and HLA, then all cells became positive(3).

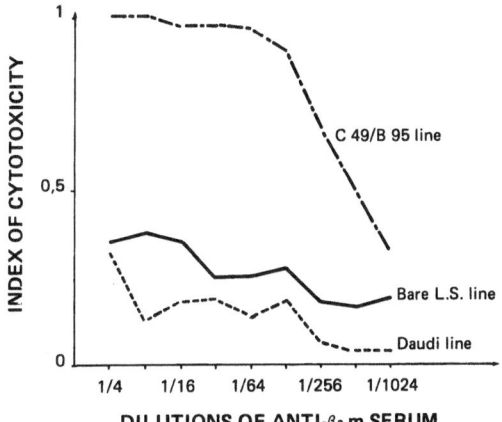

Fig.1. Lack of expression of β2m on Daudi and BLS cell lines in comparison with a "normal"cell line.

This phenomenon of acquired HLA expression by the BLS line suggests the presence of HLA structure genes in the patients'cells.

Genetic analyses in two families(2,5) confirmed that BLS is associated with genes different from those of the major histocompatibility complex (MHC) region. One such family is depicted in Table I.

Table I. HLA genotypes in one family with BLS-type I

Father A :	A24	BW35	DR5
B :	AW30	B5	DR3
Mother C :	A2	BW35	DR6
D :	A11	BW21	DR4

2 children with BLS : AC, BD
6 other healthy children : AC, BD, AD, BC

The existence and the intra-familial mode of transmission of BLS, therefore, reveals the presence of gene(s) not borne by the N°6 chromosome but controlling the expression of HLA antigens. A family of distinct genes controlling the expression of various parts of the MHC region can be postulated, hence the various types of the syndrome.

The effect of α-interferon, initially investigated by A. Durandy et al. (6), has been more recently analyzed on a variety of BLS cells. The results are schematically expressed in Table II. Interferon, given in vitro or in vivo, increased the expression of class I HLA antigens when these antigens were present, even in significantly reduced amount, at the cell surface before interferon treatment. No modification,however, was found on cells completely devoid of HLA antigens.

Table II. Effect of α-interferon on HLA expression in BLS-type I.

Lymphocytes from	Expression of β2m and HLA antigens at the cell surface	
	Cells without IFN	Cells with IFN for 3 days
Normal	+	++
Incomplete BLS	±	+
Complete BLS	0	0

CONCLUSIONS

The BLS demonstrates the major part played by HLA antigens in interactions of lymphocytes with other cells. Responses to antigen are severely impaired by the lack of HLA molecules. "Education" of T-cells in the thymus may also require HLA antigens. A normal expression of HLA antigens is therefore needed not only for T-cell effector functions but also for a full T-cell differentiation which includes the acquisition of the repertoire for antigen recognition. Genetic analyses have established that the BLS is transmitted independently of the N°6 chromosome, thus encovering other genes involved in the regulation of expression of either class I or class II HLA antigens.

REFERENCES

1. Touraine J.L., Bétuel H., Souillet G., Jeune M.:Combined immunodeficiency disease associated with absence of cell-surface HLA-A and B antigens. J. Pediatr. 1978, 93, 47-51.
2. Touraine J.L.: The bare lymphocyte syndrome: Report on the Registry. Lancet, 1981, 1, 319-321.
3. Touraine J.L., Bétuel H., Touraine F.: The Bare Lymphocyte Syndrome. In: Progress in Immunodeficiency Research and Therapy I, C. Griscelli and J. Vossen eds, Elsevier, Amsterdam, 1984, 27-34.
4. Payne R., Brodsky F.M., Peterlin B.M., Young L.M.: "Bare lymphocytes" without immunodeficiency. Human Immunol. 1983, 6, 219-227.
5. Schuurman R.K.B., Van Rood J.J., Vossen J.M., Schellekens PtH., Felkamp-Vroom Th.M., Doyer E., Gmelig-Meylinf F., Visser H.K.A.: Failure of lymphocyte-membrane HLA-A and B expression in two siblings with combined immunodeficiency. Clin. Immunol. Immunopathol. 1979,14, 418-434.
6. Durandy A., Virelizier J.L., Griscelli C.: Enhancement by interferon of membrane HLA antigens in patients with combined immunodeficiency with defective HLA expression. Clin. Exp. Immunol. 1983, 52, 173-178.

Exp. Hematol. (suppl. 17) 13:88 (1985)
© International Society for Experimental Hematology

Acquired Deficiency of Fibrinogen (Fbg) and Factor VII (F VII) During and Following Immunosuppression for Severe Aplastic Anemia (SAA) with Antithymocyte Globulin (ATG) and High-Dose Methylprednisolone (MP)

M. Fischer, R. Dudczak, W. Hinterberger, C. Korninger, K. Lechner, E. Neumann, H. Niessner, and I. Pabinger

1st Department of Internal Medicine, University of Vienna, Austria

Introduction: While determing clotting and fibrinolysis proteins by conventional laboratory test kits before, during and after ATG/MP treatment we found a yet undescribed reversible deficiency of Fbg and F VII.
Patients and Methods: 2 males and 3 females (a:22-49; median 42) with SAA (1 idiopathic,4 druginduced) were treated with ATG (ATGAM,Fa.Upjohn,15 mg/kg, day 1-8),6-Methylprednisolone (20 mg/kg,day 1-4, thereafter reduction to the half every 4 days) and Oxymetholon (1.5 mg/kg).Pat 3 died from pseudomonas septicemia on day 23.Pat 1,2,4 and 5 were followed up for 490,444,281 and 80 days,res.,and stayed free of bacterial infections.Pat 1 and 4 recovered completely,Pat 2 was a treatment failure and Pat 5 is too short to be evaluated.
Results: A decrease of Fbg (Fig 1) and F VII (Fig 2) was seen in all 5 patients during and following ATG/ MP.In Pat 3 Fbg increased during septicemia between days 10 and 23 (shown as dotted lines to the tops of the ranges).The nadirs of Fbg and F VII reached 41.5% and 48.7%,res.,of the pretreatment values (Tab).Normal levels of Fbg (200mg%) were reached between days 28 and 80,of F VII (75%) between days 9 and 95.Ethanol gelation test was always negative,biological half life of Fbg measured in Pat 2,4 and 5 was normal,Fibrin(-ogen)-Degradation Products (FDP) and Fibrinopeptid-A (FPA) were normal.All the other clotting and fibrinolysis proteins did either not change or increased (Tab).
Discussion: We do not have any explanation for this contrasting observation.Excluded were:1)Hepatic impairment (serial liver function tests were normal,other liver derived clotting factors increased).2)Hyperfibrinolysis (Antiplasmin and Plasminogen increased,FDP were not elevated).3)Disseminated intravascular coagulation (DIC) (Ethanol test was always negative,FPA was not elevated).4)Abnormal Fbg (good agreement of functional and immunological values of Fbg).The best explanation for this finding is a selective impairment of the synthesis of Fbg and F VII (Decrease of F VII and Fbg according to their half lives,normal half life of labeled Fbg).The pathogeneic mechanism is unknown yet.To avoid an increase of bleeding tendency in thrombocytopenic patients serial measurements of Fbg and F VII during ATG/MP are recommended.

Supported by Grant 4100 of the "Fonds zur Förderung der Wissenschaftlichen Forschung in Österreich" and by the "Kommission für Leukämieforschung und Knochenmarktransplantation" of the Austrian Academy of Sciences

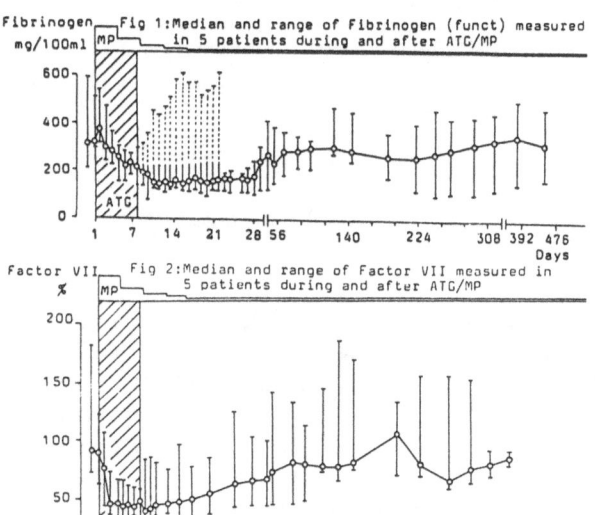

Fig 1: Median and range of Fibrinogen (funct) measured in 5 patients during and after ATG/MP

Fig 2: Median and range of Factor VII measured in 5 patients during and after ATG/MP

Table 1. Median values of clotting factors (calculated from the highest or lowest values measured before, during or after treatment in the individual patients)

		pretreatment median(range)	during or after treatment median(range)	normal range
Fibrinogen Clauss	mg/dl	315 (220-580)	131 (90-221)	200-400
Ag	mg/dl	372 (250-480)	150 (121-225)	200-400
Factor II:C	%	87 (85- 98)	125 (98-150)	75-110
V:C	%	145 (105-170)	410 (325-550)	75-110
VII:C	%	82 (68-155)	40 (31- 55)	75-110
VIII:C	%	207 (202-320)	580 (347-830)	60-180
IX:C	%	95 (80-159)	201 (174-241)	60-140
X:C	%	102 (90-140)	150 (120-215)	75-110
XI:C	%	102 (94-104)	165 (112-189)	60-140
XII:C	%	111 (78-150)	241 (113-322)	60-140
XIII (S)	%	110 (80-130)	113 (90-130)	75-125
(A)	%	107 (68-108)	96 (88-133)	75-125
Prekallikrein:Ag	%	81 (78- 97)	100 (66-124)	75-125
AT III (funct)	%	76 (69-105)	152 (95-162)	84-116
Ag	%	82 (70- 92)	163 (96-164)	82-120
Protein C: Ag	%	75 (60- 89)	195 (167-352)	70-140
Plasminogen: Ag	%	92 (84-109)	136 (103-167)	75-125
Antiplasmin (funct) %		98 (97-107)	158 (140-190)	75-125

Exp. Hematol. (suppl. 17) 13:89 (1985)
© International Society for Experimental Hematology

Improvement of Severe Aplastic Anemia (SAA) Following Treatment with Cyclosporin-A (CY-A) After Failure of Antithymocyte Globulin (ATG) and High-Dose Methylprednisolone (MP)

M. Fischer, W. Hinterberger, K. Lechner, K. Geißler, and E. Neumann

1st Department of Internal Medicine, University of Vienna, Austria

Case History: A 42 a female with a 2 years history of AA deteriorated to transfusion dependency and was admitted for combined immunosuppression (IS). Blood counts before IS were: Red cells 2.9×10^{12}/l (posttransfusion value), Reticulocytes 40×10^9/l, Platelets 11×10^9/l, PMN 0.5×10^9/l. IS consisted of ATG (ATGAM, Fa. Upjohn, 15 mg/kg day 1-8), 6-Methylprednisolone 20 mg/kg day 1-4, reduction to the half every 4 days to a maintenance dose of 0.5 mg/kg until day 164. Oxymetholon (1.5 mg/kg) was stopped on day 42 because of increased liver encymes. Cell support was given to maintain hemoglobin levels 8g/dl and platelets 20×10^9.

During and after IS the bleeding tendency increased. The requirement for red cell and platelet transfusions remained unchanged until day 150 and only a gradual improvement was seen afterwards (Figure). Severe mental disturbance (Paranoia) between days 128 and 178, possibly attributed to high-dose MP, precluded a second course of ATG/MP.

Cyclosporin-A (Cy-A) Treatment: On day 197 after IS, Cy-A 7.5 mg/kg/day was administered orally with dose adapted to the (RIA-) trough levels between 200 and 400 ng/ml.

Approximately 100 days after the institution of Cy-A, the transfusion requirement for platelets and red cells decreased and the patient is self sustaining from day 297 after ATG/MP up to now (day 521 after ATG/MP). Withdrawal of Cy-A on day 500 did not cause deterioration of blood counts. All bone marrow derived cell lines at present continue to increase without any further treatment. The last blood count was (day 521): Platelets 45×10^9/l, Haemoglobin 11.1g/dl, Reticulocytes 97×10^9/l, Leucocytes 3.7×10^9/l.

Discussion: In this case, treatment with ATG/MP followed by CY-A led to a small but clinically relevant improvement of haemopoesis. While there was probably a minimal improvement between days 150 and 197 before CY-A treatment, the patient became definitely transfusion independent approximately 100 days after CY-A was started. In contrast to a previously reported case (1), the improvement in our case occurred rather later and more slowly. Due to the minimal improvement before Cy-A a late effect of ATG/MP cannot be excluded but seems, on the other hand, unlikely, since haematologic self sustaining was reached not earlier than 9.9 month after ATG/MP. We consider it more likely that CY-A contributed to this late improvement.

Reference: 1) New. Engl. J. Med. 310, 10, 665

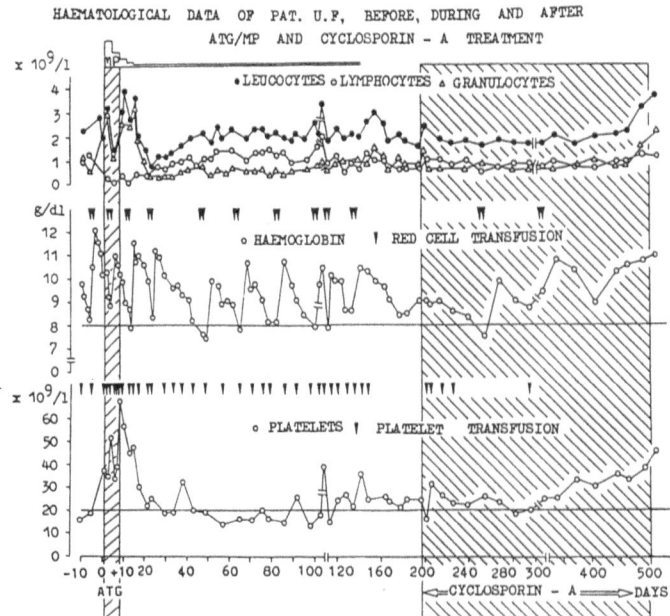

HAEMATOLOGICAL DATA OF PAT. U.F. BEFORE, DURING AND AFTER ATG/MP AND CYCLOSPORIN - A TREATMENT

Supported by Grant 4100 of the "Fonds zur Förderung der Wissenschaftlichen Forschung in Österreich" and by the "Kommission für Leukämieforschung und Knochenmarktransplantation" of the Austrian Academy of Sciences

Exp. Hematol. (suppl. 17) 13:90 (1985)
© International Society for Experimental Hematology

Bone Marrow Transplantation (BMT) for Severe Aplastic Anemia (SAA): Results Obtained in 19 Patients

Waltraud Schmidmeier [2], W. Hinterberger [1], A. Hajek-Rosenmayr [3], P. Höcker [4], B. Volc-Platzer [5], G. Grabner [6], R. Hawliczek [7], A. Laszkowicz [8], W. Mauritz [9], W. Graninger [10], H. Gadner [2], K. Lechner [1], M. Fischer [1], G. Stingl [5], K. Lenz [1], and E. Deutsch [1]

[1] First Department of Medicine, University of Vienna
[2] St. Anna's Children Hospital, Vienna
[3] Institute for Blood Group Serology, Vienna (National Blood Group Reference Laboratory, WHO and National Tissue Typing Reference Laboratory, Council of Europe)
[4] Blood Transfusion Service, University of Vienna
[5] First Department of Dermatology, University of Vienna
[6] Second Department of Ophthalmology, University of Vienna
[7] Department of Radiotherapy and Radiobiology, University of Vienna
[8] Second Department of Surgery, University of Vienna
[9] Department of Anesthesiology, University of Vienna
[10] Department of Chemotherapy, University of Vienna, Austria

Patients: 10 adult patients and 9 children with SAA underwent allogeneic (17) or syngeneic (2) BMT. The median age was 17 years (range 4-37), all patients were pretransfused with a median of 7 units of red blood cells (range: 2-50), 15 of 19 patients had received platelet support with a median of 8 single donor platelet transfusions (range 1-29). The median duration of disease was 12 weeks (3-150). 9 cases were classified as idiopathic, 5 had a history of hepatitis, 2 were previously exposed to Chloramphenicol and 2 cases were due to Novaminsulfone and Phenylbutazone, respectively. 1 patient had Fanconi-anemia. 17 of 19 patients were pretreated with low-dose steroids, 5 patients were also pretreated with androgens, without any success. Prior to BMT, 16 patients had suffered from febrile episodes, all patients had experienced minor or major bleeding complications.

17 donors were healthy, HLA-matched, MLC non-reactive siblings, 2 donors were syngeneic twins. In 3 donor-recipient pairs a low, reproducible stimulation was seen in MLC (SI: 2.25, 2.72 and 4.77, respectively).

Bone Marrow Transplantation Procedure: All allogeneic recipients were preconditioned with 4x50 mg/kg Cyclophosphamide. For prophylaxis against graft rejection, all adult patients and 5 children received donor buffy coat cells on 4 consecutive days after BMT. Since buffy coat donation in 4 children donors appeared inacceptable, the respective recipients were preirradiated with 300 rad TBI (3 cases) or 400 rad TLI (1 case). A total number of $2.0-5.8 \times 10^8$ nucleated bone marrow cells was given. Methotrexate was given as prophylaxis for allogeneic recipients, according to the Seattle protocol. Acute GVH-reactions were treated with 2 mg/kg Prednisolone/days. If no improvement was seen after 3 days, a combination of ATG (ATGAM, 15 mg/kg) and Cyclosporine A (i.v., beginning with 10 mg/day) was given for at least 20 days (ATGAM) or 6 months (Cyclosporin-A).

Clinical Results: 15 of 19 patients are currently alive 131-1135 days after BMT (median: 654 days). UPN 1 (grafted 1978) died from candida septicemia (day 4), UPN 2 (grafted 1980, Fanconi-anemia) died from left ventricular failure (day 14), UPN 3, grafted 1981, died from GVH-D of the gut and Pseudomonas septicemia (day 85). UPN 12, grafted 1984, rejected his donor marrow twice. This patient had accidentally received maternal platelets prior to BMT. In spite of TLI (400 rad) and a low Stimulation Index (1.20), the patient died in aplasia after the second graft (from the same donor) was likewise rejected (day 140). Both syngeneic recipients failed to engraft after the first bone marrow infusion. Permanent engraftment was achieved after

Cyclophosphamide (4 x 50 mg/kg) conditioning was given prior to the second bone marrow infusion from the same donor (Hinterberger et al, this issue). In the 3 recipient-donor pairs having an elevated stimulation index, prompt engraftment occurred. 4 patients developed acute GVH-D grade IV. It was the cause of death only in UPN 3, in whom high dose steroid monotherapy (1000 mg Prednisolone/day) was unable to control the disease. 3 of 4 patients, however, recovered completely upon combined Prednisolone, ATG and Cyclosporine treatment. 6 patients developed chronic GVH-D (3 de-novo, 3 progressive disease). 5 of 6 patients responded to immunosuppressive therapy consisting of Prednisolone/Azathioprine or Prednisolone/Cyclosporine. The oldest patient in this series (37 years) had "limited" disease GVH-D, involving skin and mucous membranes, but progressed to blindness after bilateral corneal perforation in spite of vigorous immunosuppressive therapy Grabner et al, this issue)

Discussion: Our data confirm that BMT is a very effective treatment for SAA with stable haemopoietic chimarism obtainable in about 75% of patients. Transplant related problems, as seen in larger series, were also reflected in our group of patients: Rejection, which occurred in one patient who was pretransfused with maternal platelets, was not predicted by an elevated stimulation index. The pretransplant clinical condition determined the outcome in UPN 1 and UPN 2: Both patients were in such a poor clinical condition, that, nowadays, BMT would have been performed either much earlier in the course of the disease or would rather be withheld. Chronic GVH-D is, at present, a major problem. New treatment approaches, capable of modulating auto-immunity of donor lymphocytes, are urgently needed. Also, reduction of the risk of rejection by techniques other than donor buffy coat infusions are likewise needed. A progress, in our hands, was the introduction of Cyclosporin-A for the treatment of established acute GVH-D (in combination with ATG) and for the long term control of chronic GVH-D.

Supported by Grant 4100 of the "Fonds zur Förderung der Wissenschaftlichen Forschung in Österreich" and by the "Kommission für Leukämieforschung und Knochenmarktransplantation" of the Austrian Academy of Sciences

Exp. Hematol. (suppl. 17) 13:91 (1985)
© International Society for Experimental Hematology

Agranulocytosis After BMT

R. Arnold, T. Schmeiser, W. Heit, E. Kurrle, H. Heimpel, and B. Kubanek

Department of Internal Medicine III, Department of Transfusion Medicine, D-7900 Ulm, Federal Republic of Germany

Introduction

Agranulocytosis is a rare event with a total incidence of 5 cases per 1 million inhabitants per year. We observed agranulocytosis in 3 out of 33 patients after allogeneic bone marrow transplantation. We analyzed several factors to find an explanation for this observation.

Material and Methods

From May 1980 to August 1983 33 adult patients underwent allogeneic bone marrow transplantation for treatment of severe aplastic anaemia (n = 8), acute leukaemia (n = 21) or chronic granulocytic leukaemia (n = 4). A mean of 2.56 x 10 nucleated cells/kg bone marrow were transplanted. In all cases the marrow was unpurged. All patients had a permanent take as demonstrated by different markers. For GvHD prophylaxis methotrexate was given. Standard antibiotic therapy consisted of a combination of betalactam antibiotics and aminoglycosides.

Results

Drug exposure and incidence of agranulocytosis: During the phase of severe granulocytopenia 26/33 patients developed infections. The mean dose of broad spectrum penicillin per treated patient was 272 (45-717) g. In addition, cephalosporins with a mean dose of 121 (18-400) g were given to 19/26 treated patients. No case of agranulocytosis was observed.

After haemopoietic reconstitution 21/32 patients received antibiotics for treatment of infection mostly in association with acute or chronic GvHD (n = 18). 19/21 patients received broadspectrum penicillins with a mean dose of 279 (75-941) g. Cephalosporins were given to 16/21 patients with a mean dose of 123 (30-560) g. Three out of 32 patients developed an agranulocytosis on day +74, day +95 and day +215 after BMT. Bone marrow aspirations on day +75, day +99 and day +218 after BMT revealed the typical picture of agranulocytosis with a lack of granulocytes, megakaryocytes and myelocytes and a marked shift to the left with promyelocyte predominance. Agranulocytosis was associated with the exposure of broadspectrum penicillins in two patients and with cimetidine in one patient. Furthermore all 3 patients had acute or chronic GvHD and were treated with prednisolone. Patients with agranulocytosis received in total a higher dose of broadspectrum penicillin in comparison to patients without agranulocytosis (822 vs. 375 g). Cimetidine was given to 9 patients. The mean dose was not different between patients without agranulocytosis and the patients with agranulocytosis (18.4 g vs. 20.4 g). All patients recovered from agranulocytosis after the exposure to the incriminated drug was discontinued.

Discussion

Betalactam antibiotics and cimetidine are incriminated to be causatively involved in agranulocytosis. The observation of a high incidence of agranulocytosis in transplanted patients might be explained by the increased exposure rate to antibiotics and drugs which can cause agranulocytosis in comparison to other hospitalized patients. One can speculate that GvHD present in all our patients with agranulocytosis could be an additional risk factor for agranulocytosis.

Inborn Errors of Metabolism

Exp. Hematol. (suppl. 17) 13:92 (1985)
© International Society for Experimental Hematology

Experience with Busulphan and Cyclophosphamide as Pre-Graft Conditioning Regime in Inborn Errors of Metabolism

P. J. Shaw, K. Hugh-Jones, A. J. Barrett, S. J. S. Desai, and J. R. Hobbs

Westminster Bone Marrow Transplant Team, London, Great Britain

INTRODUCTION

We have used Busulphan and Cyclophosphamide for conditioning 39 patients prior to bone marrow transplantation. We report the early toxicity of the regime.

PATIENT POPULATION

Thirty-nine patients were admitted for bone marrow transplantation, with a mean age of 3 years. Eighteen patients had HLA- and MLC- matched donors; 21 were mismatched donors. Twenty-seven of the patients had one of the mucopolysaccharidoses; 7 had thalassaemia; 5 had other lysosomal storage disorders.

CONDITIONING REGIME

This usually consisted of Busulphan in a dose of 80 mg/m^2/day for 4 days, followed by Cyclophosphamide 2 g/m^2/day for 4 days. This resulted in a large variation in dose when expressed as mg/kg.

RESULTS

Because 7 patients needed a second transplant, the 39 patients received 46 courses of conditioning. The total Busulphan dose ranged from 8 to 21 mg/kg. There was no toxicity attributable to the Busulphan. The only side effect was occasional vomiting, following which the vomited dose was repeated. Lung fibrosis has been associated with long term low dosage Busulphan. Although several of our patients had pulmonary complications, such as infection, none had lung problems which could be related to the Busulphan dose.

The usual total Cyclophosphamide dose was 8 g/m^2, with a range of 160 to 440 mg/kg. Most patients tolerated the regime well, but problems were encountered with some patients who were less than 0.5 m^2 in surface area. Four patients had clinically significant effects related to Cyclophosphamide administration. One patient suffered a fatal cardiac arrest. Three others had to have their planned dose reduced because of a reduction in ECG voltage. These 4 were planned to receive a mean total dose of 386 mg/kg of Cyclophosphamide. All 4 had an average pulse rate on day 3 of Cyclophosphamide administration, 25 to 30 beats/minute greater than the day prior to starting the drug. Of 23 patients who received significantly less Cyclophosphamide, when calculated in mg/kg (an average of 321 mg/kg, p <0.01), only 2 had an increase in pulse on day 3 of more than 20 beats/minute.

CONCLUSION

From our experience with this regime, our present policy is to use a total Busulphan dosage of 16 mg/kg. We limit the Cyclophosphamide dose to 300 mg/kg and pay particular attention to the ECG and pulse in patients who are less than 0.5 m^2.

Exp. Hematol. (suppl. 17) 13:93 (1985)
© International Society for Experimental Hematology

Allogeneic Bone Marrow Transplantation for Chronic Myelogenous Leukemia
Pescara Team Experience

G. Di Girolamo, P. Di Bartolomeo, D. Natale, A. Iacone, G. Muzil, G. Prosperini, and G. Torlontano

Cattedra di Ematologia e Divisioni di Ematologia e Radioterapia, Chieti-Pescara, Italy

Median survival of patients with chronic myelogenous leukemia (CML) is estimated about 36 months and have not changed substantially in the last two decades. Allogeneic bone marrow transplantation (BMT) has been demonstrated to be the only therapeutical approach capable of eradicating the Ph'-positive clone and offering a sustained possibility of cure. We report here our experience about BMT in CML.

Beetween March 1982 and October 1984, 10 patients with CML underwent BMT. At the time of transplantation 7 patients were in first chronic phase (CP) and 3 patients were in accelerated phase (AP), defined according to criteria published by the International Bone Marrow Transplant Registry (1). They ranged in age from 4 to 53 yr, median 27 yr. Median interval between diagnosis and BMT was 35 mo (range 3-93 mo). Marrow cytogenetics in 9 cases showed 46 chromosomes with a single Ph'-chromosome. One patient (unique patient number, UPN, 8) had undergone splenectomy prior to transplantation. Conditioning regimen consisted of daunorubicin (60 mg/m^2) on day –8, cyclophosphamide (120 mg/Kg) on day –7 and day –6 and total body irradiation (1000 cGy at a dose rate less than 3 cGy/min in a single dose in 3 cases or in 5 fractions over 3 days in 7 cases, without lung shielding). Four patients also received two fractions of 500 cGy to the splenic area during irradiation. All marrow donors were HLA-identical and MLC-nonreactive siblings. The marrow dose ranged from 1.9 x10^8 to 6.8 x10^8 nucleated cells /Kg recipient weight. All patients received cyclosporin A as prophylaxis against graft-versus-host disease (GvHD) and oral acyclovir as prophylaxis against herpetic infections and were nursed in laminar-air-flow rooms from day –10 to the discharge (approximately day +30).

Prompt engraftment and complete hematological remission were seen in all cases. Ph'-chromosome disappeared from all 9 patients who had it before BMT. Six of the 10 patients developed acute GvHD, that was grade I in 3 patients, grade II in 1 patient and grade III in 2 patients. The median onset was 21 days after transplantation (range 13-31 days). One of these patients (UPN 11) subsequently developed limited chronic GvHD. Three patients died, two of them had grade III acute GvHD and died of viral infection, the third patient had grade I acute GvHD and died of severe venocclusive disease of the liver. The remaining 7 patients are alive and well in clinical, hematological and cytogenetic remission 228-789 days after BMT. An unusual clinical and cytogenetic outcome occurred in a patient (UPN 18). This patient showed evidence of full engraftment, as assessed by ABO blood type conversion and disappearance of Ph'-chromosome, until 12 mo post grafting. As from this time a progressive decrease in hemoglobin level and leucocyte and platelet counts was evident. At the same time bone marrow cytogenetic examinations revealed reappearance of the Ph'-chromosome and others abnormalities (trisomy of chromosomes 8 and 19, isochromosome of 17, double Ph'-chromosome). These findings were taken as evidence of relapse. The patient was treated with blood transfusions and prednisone therapy. Three months later, 2 consecutive cytogenetic examinations showed a normal karyotype, that was associated with good hematological conditions.

In conclusion, several investigators have demonstrated that allogeneic BMT is capable of inducing sustained complete hematological and cytogenetic remissions with the potential for cure in a substantial percentage of patients. The best results have been obtained in young patients transplanted in CP and with a short interval between diagnosis and transplantation (2-5). In our experience, successfull BMT performed in 3 patients older than 40 yr shows that BMT is a reasonable therapeutic modality also for adult patients and/or with a long interval between diagnosis and transplantation (5).

References :
1) IBMTR report. Lancet 1984, i, 665.
2) Champlin R, Mitsuyaru R, Elashoff R, et al. Recent advances in bone marrow transplantation. Alan R. Liss, New York 1983, pag 141.
3) Goldman JM, Baughan ASJ, McCarthy DM, et al. Lancet ii, 623.
4) Clift RA, Buckner CD, Thomas ED, et al. Lancet 1982, ii, 621.
5) Di Bartolomeo P, Di Girolamo G, Natale D, et al. XX Congress ISH, Buenos Aires, September 1-7, 1984.

Supported by CNR "Oncology", Grant n° 84.0830.44

Exp. Hematol. (suppl. 17) 13:94 (1985)
© International Society for Experimental Hematology

Functions of Monocytes After Allogeneic Bone-Marrow Transplantation (BMT)

P. Bordigoni[1], M. Marchand[2], F. Witz[2], and D. Olive[1]

[1] Hôpital d'Enfants, Nancy
[2] Centre Regional de Transfusion Sanguine, Nancy, France

INTRODUCTION

In an attempt to determine whether monocyte dysfunction to the increased susceptibility to infections after BMT, monocyte **adherence, random migration, chemotaxis, reduction of NBT and chemiluminescence** were evaluated after 23 allogeneic, HLA identical marrow grafts. The relationship to a number of clinical parameters was also examined.

MATERIAL AND METHODS

- STUDY OF POPULATION : we investigated at various intervals (day 20 to 360 after BMT) 14 leukemias (ALL : 9 - ANLL : 3 - CML (CP) : 2), 4 Non Hodgkin's lymphomas, 2 aplastic anemias, 1 neuroblastoma and 1 inherited disease.

- PATIENTS' MANAGEMENT : 12 received Cyclophosphamide (CPM) + fractionated total body irradiation (FTBI) (12 - 13,2 Gy), 2 CPM + TBI (6 Gy), 5 high dose cytosine arabinoside + FTBI (13,2 Gy), 2 Melphalan + FTBI (13,2 Gy), 2 Busulfan + CPM. 17 of them were treated with Cyclosporin (Cy A) as GVHD prophylaxis, and 6 with Cy A + Methotrexate. Methylprednisolone (MP), 60 mg/m²/d or 1 g/m²/d $\pm$ ATG was given for acute GVHD treatment (15/23 patients). Prednisone (1 mg/kg/d) $\pm$ Azathioprine was given for chronic GVHD treatment (10 patients).

- MONOCYTE STUDY : the following functions were studied : adherence to glass, NBT reduction, chemiluminescence for : Zymosan (Zy), extracts from soluble products of candida albicans (CA) and staphylococcus aureus (SA) by cytochrome C reduction, random migration and chemotaxis to Zy activated serum, FMLP, CA and SA, by migration under agarose. Abnormal values are defined as less than 75 % of corresponding normal control subjects (< 35 % of normal : severely depressed - 35 - 75 % : moderately depressed). Statistical comparison was made using a paired Student's t test.

RESULTS :

- normal values for NBT and adherence
- moderately depressed values for : **random migration** (mean : 50 + 12,9 %) in 7/23 (26 %) patients and 7/48 experiments (exp.). **Chemotaxis** (mean : 49,8 + 13,7 %) in 7/23 (30,4 %) patients (Zy : 19,5 % - CA : 15 % - SA : 16,2 % - FMLP : 12,8 %) and

25/47 (17 %) exp. 4 defects was secondary events appearing between day 88 and day 300, 3 was primary events (maturational delay ?) (d 29 to d 97) with subsequent return to normal. **Chemiluminescence** (mean : 53 % $\pm$ 13,2) in 5/23 (21,7 %) patients (Zy 14,8 % - CA : 18,7 % - SA :17,6 %) and 10/60 (16,6 %) exp. 4 defects was secondary events appearing between day 76 and day 320, 1 is primary event (day 58) with subsequent return to normal (day 97).

DISCUSSION : (1 - 2 - 3)

In this group, 20 - 30 % of all tested monocytes showed moderate functional defects essentially of chemotactic response, random migration and chemiluminescence, whatever the stimuli (soluble or particulate). It is noteworthy that the defects were rarely seen within the first 80 days after BMT. The recovery of monocyte functions was generally very prompt, mature by day 30. Most of the defects occured between day 80 and day 360 in patients who had previously demonstrated normal recovery of monocyte functions. The patients with chronic GVH seem to have a tendency for a higher incidence of altered chemotaxis and chemiluminescence.

These defects were not correlated with any of the other clinical parameters explored, namely acute GVHD, incidence of infections, ATG and/or corticosteroids therapies, GVHD prophylaxis. This data suggest that monocyte dysfunction cannot be incriminated as a predominant factor responsable for the high incidence of bacterial and fungal infections particularly within the 80 first days after BMT.

REFERENCES :

1 - CLARK RA, JOHNSON FL, KLEBANOFF SJ, THOMAS ED (1976). Defective neutrophil chemotaxis in bone marrow transplant patients. J Clin Invest, 58 : 22 - 31.
2 - VAN DEN BROEK PJ, VAN DER MEER JWM, LEIJH PCJ, ZWAAN F, VAN DEN BARSELAAR M, VAN FURTH R (1981). Functions of granulocytes after allogeneic bone marrow transplantation. Blut, 42 : 252 - 253.
3 - WINSTON DJ, TERRITO MC, HO WG, MILLER MJ, GALE RP, GOLDE DW (1982). Alveolar macrophage dysfunction in human bone marrow transplant recipients. Am J Med, 73 : 859 - 866.

Exp. Hematol. (suppl. 17) 13:95 (1985)
© International Society for Experimental Hematology

Polymorphonuclear Chemotaxis After Allogeneic Bone Marrow Transplantation

F. Bernaudin [1], C. Cordonnier [2], E. Escudier [3], J. P. Vernant [2], and J. F. Bernaudin [3]

[1] Service de Pédiatrie CHIC, Creteil
[2] Departement d'Hématologie, Hôpital Henri Mondor, Creteil
[3] Departement d'Histologie, Faculté de Médecine, Creteil, France

Infection is a frequent cause of death in patients receiving bone marrow transplantation (BMT). Defects of neutrophil functions have been suspected to contribute significantly to the impairment of host defenses. However conflicting results arose from different works dealing with the study of neutrophils chemotaxis (1-3,5). For that reason we undertook the present study in 50 patients using an under agarose method.

Patients
The study was performed in 50 patients who received allo (n=47), syngeneic (n=1), autologous (n=2) BMT for hematologic malignancies : AML (n=18 ; first CR 14, subsequent or partial R=4) ; ALL (n=17, first CR 11, subsequent or partial R=6 ; CML (n=14 ; chronic phase 6 ; accelerated or blastic phase 8), NHL (n=1 second CR). The mean age was 28 -9 years, and the ratio male/female = 30/20. The pregraft preparation consisted of cyclophosphamide and TBI. The patient at risk received MTX to prevent GVHD. Acute GVHD was treated with steroid therapy and chronic GVHD with steroid and/or azathioprine. Antithymocyte globulin was not used. Patients in relapse were excluded. The control group consisted of 18 healthy adults.

Methods
Seventy five studies were performed, 19 patients were serially studied.
- Erythrocytes in heparinized blood were sedimented in 4,5 % dextran T500 and the leukocyte supernatant was centrifuged at 500 g for 8 mn. The cellular pellet was washed twice in PBS and resuspended in PBS at a concentration of $10^5 \mu l^{-1}$;
- The random migration and stimulated locomotion induced by FMLP (10^{-7} M), autologous (auto S) and pooled human AB serum (AB S) were tested using an under agarose method. The distance migrated by the leading front neutrophils and the score of migrating cells were counted using an ocular grid. The data were compared using the student t-test.

Results
The random migration was significantly decreased until d.90 (p<0,001 until d.30, p < 0,01 d.30 to d.90) and became normal after. Stimulated locomotion was significantly decreased until d.30 whatever the attractant used

(p < 0,001 with auto S). The response to FMLP, auto-S, AB-S, were respectively 65 %, 42 %, and 51 % of controls. After d.30 stimulated locomotion was not impaired (fig.)

Discussion
Impaired chemotaxis before d.30 has been already reported (1,3,5). In the present study however, the stimulated migration was more defective with auto S than with AB-S ; a search for a defect in chemotactic factors in serum of recently engrafted patients is in progress. Chemotaxis in patients with GVHD was normal, no study however was performed before the treatment of GVHD. In patients receiving steroids for GVHD, chemotaxis seems to be improved when compared with patients without steroids. Although, this difference was not significant, it could raise a possible suppression by steroid therapy of a previously reported (1) inhibitory factor associated with GVHD.
In spite of individual variations, the absence of significant difference in chemotaxis after the 3d month in engrafted patients when compared to controls, suggests that other factors are involved in the development of infections.

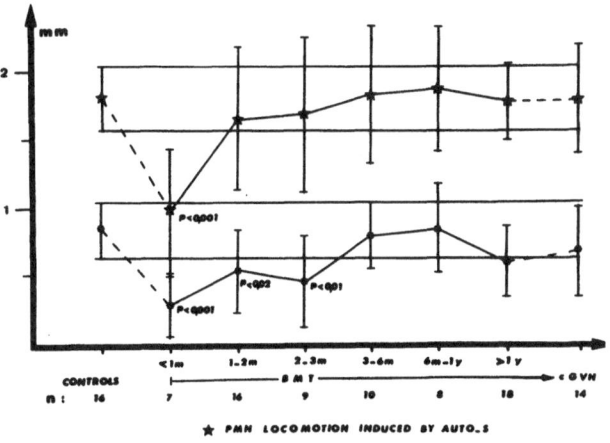

★ PMN LOCOMOTION INDUCED BY AUTO_S
● SPONTANEOUS PMN LOCOMOTION

1. R.A.CLARK and al J.Clin.Invest. 1976.58.22
2. M.C.TERRITO and al Br.J.Haemat. 1977.35.245
3. R.SOSA and al Exp.Hematol. 1980.8.10.1183
4. P.J.VAN DEN BROEK and al Blut.1981.42.253
5. R.DOPFER and al Exp.Hematol.1983,11,S13,110

Exp. Hematol. (suppl. 17) 13:96 (1985)

Folic Acid Deficiency After Bone Marrow Transplantation

H. Link [1], P. Ostendorf[1], P. Wernet [1], K. Wilms [1], and D. Niethammer [2]

[1] Medizinische Klinik,
[2] Kinderklinik, Eberhard Karls Universität, D-7400 Tübingen, Federal Republic of Germany

INTRODUCTION

Megaloblastic and dyserythropoetic bone marrow pathologies which cannot be explained by drug effects are found frequently after bone marrow transplantation (BMT). The high proliferation rate of transplanted hematopoetic cells, total-body irradiation, mucositis, diarrhea, total parenteral nutrition and anorexia may all contribute to low folic acid levels, which could help account for such pathologies.

PATIENTS AND METHODS

This study incorporates the data of 32 patients with leukemia, 8 with severe aplastic anemia and 1 with neuroblastoma. All of them were isolated in laminar air-flow units and underwent total enteral decontamination. Each patient was given Cotrimoxazol (30 mg/kg per day), except for those receiving Cyclosporin A, in which case it was omitted between Day 0 and 14. Conditioning for BMT was performed as previously published (Wilms 1982). 27 patients were given Methotrexate (MTX) and 10 patients Cyclosporin A (CsA) as GvHD-prophylaxis. 36 patients received 200-600 µg of folic acid (FA) intravenously and 25 patients were also given 5 mg FA orally per day after BMT in addition. The total serum concentrations of bound and unbound FA were determined using a radioimmunological test.

RESULTS

The FA-values of all the patients fell significantly ($p < 0.002$) from 10.35 ± 8.0 ng/ml before BMT to 4.34 ± 2.8 ng/ml after BMT. If no oral FA was administered, the values were lower (2.58 ± 3.06 ng/ml, $p < 0.01$). The FA values of patients with megaloblastic marrow after BMT were lower (2.74 ± 1.79 ng/ml) than those of patients without such changes (5.38 ± 2.78 ng/ml, $p < 0.05$). The 18 patients with FA deficiency (<3.0 ng/ml) had more megaloblasts, binucleate erythropoetic cells, Howell-Jolly bodies, giant myelocytes and metamyelocytes ($p < 0.05$). FA deficiency did not slow down the recovery of granulocytes, thrombocytes and reticulocytes.

DISCUSSION

Dyserythropoetic marrow changes after BMT can be explained in part by a maximum increase in hematopoesis (Marmont 1979), by sideroblastic hematopoesis (Nichols 1984) or by a reappearance of fetal hematopoesis (Rozman 1982). In such cases, though, megaloblastic changes are usually missing (Marmont 1977). The finding that megaloblastic and dyserythropoetic bone marrow, which occur more frequently with FA deficiency, can be reduced by FA dietary supplementation suggests a direct contributory effect of FA deficiency to such pathologies. MTX might have caused some of the megaloblastic changes, but they also occured in 8 of the 14 patients not treated with MTX. The regeneration of bone marrow cells and of the gut mucosa requires large amounts of FA (Halsted 1979). Fewer megaloblastic changes appear with the oral substitution of at least 5 mg. The optimal dose, however, is still unknown. FA acid deficiency is caused by the use of sterilized food and the destruction of the intestinal flora by enteral decontamination (Herbert 1962). Furthermore, total-body irradiation causes mucositis and enteritis, which prevent the absorption of FA (Selhub 1983) and also block intestinal folate uptake (Shaw 1979). Intestinal resorption disorders occur during GvHD (Atkinson 1984). Thus, 14 of the 18 patients with FA deficiency had also developed acute GvHD as opposed to only 14 of the 23 patients with normal values. Although the quantitative regeneration of hematopoesis hardly seems to be impaired by FA deficiency, avoiding FA deficiency is vital in order to prevent the impairment of the cellular functions of lymphocytes (Gross 1975) and granulocytes (Youinou 1982) and of erythropoesis.

REFERENCES

Wilms K. et al (1982) Klin Wochenschr 60:1279-1287
Marmont AM. et al (1979) Nouv Rev Fr Hématol 21:133-148
Nicholls MD. et al (1984) Brit J Haematol 56:153-156
Rozman C. et al (1982) Brit J Haematol 50:63-73
Marmont, AM. et al (1977) Brit. J. Haematol. 36:511-518
Halsted CH. (1978) in Botez MI, Reynolds EH (eds): Folic Acid in Neurology, Psychiatry and Internal Medicine. New York, Raven p 133
Herbert V. et al (1962) Trans Assoc Am Phys 75:307-320
Selhub J. et al (1983) Pharmacol Ther 20:397-418
Shaw MT. et al (1979) Cancer Treat Rev 6: 141-151
Atkinson K. et al (1984) Brit J Haematol 56:223-232
Gross RL. et al (1975) Am J Clin Nutr 28:225-232
Youinou PY. et al (1982) Am J Med 73:652-657

Exp. Hematol. (suppl. 17) 13:97 (1985)
© International Society for Experimental Hematology

Megakaryocytopoiesis Stimulating Factors are Highly Increased in Sera from Patients After Bone Marrow Transplantation

K. Geißler, W. Hinterberger, M. Fischer, and K. Lechner

1st Department of Medicine, Division of Haematology and Blood Coagulation, University of Vienna, Vienna, Austria

Introduction: The relative roles of various humoral factors on megakaryocytopoiesis in man remain still unclear. However, in vivo and in vitro studies support a bi-level regulation of megakaryocyte formation. Hoffman et al. have observed, that sera from patients with hypomegakaryocytic thrombocytopenia significantly enhanced the formation of megakaryocytic progenitor cell (CFU-Meg) derived colonies in an in vitro clonal assay suggesting a humoral feedback regulation acting in vivo. In order to investigate this feedback regulation after bone marrow transplantation (BMT), we tested sera from 2 patients with SAA, from 3 patients with CML and from one patient with AML in complete remission (CR), who underwent allogeneic BMT, for their capacity to stimulate megakaryocytic colonies from normal bone marrow a) before BMT, b) during severe aplasia following BMT, c) at the time of beginning engraftment, d) after haematological reconstitution.

Patients: SAA patients received cyclophosphamide (50 mg/kg) on each of four consecutive days. CML and AML patients received cyclophosphamide (60 mg/kg) on two days combined with TBI (1000 rad midline tissue with lung shielding to 800 rad).

Methods: CFU-Meg were cultured in a clonal assay for committed progenitor cells (CFU-GM, BFU-E) and pluripotent progenitor cells (CFU-MIX) as well, using a modification of the technique described by Fauser & Messner.

Results: Fig.1 shows the capacity of sera from 6 BMT patients to stimulate megakaryocytic colonies from the same normal bone marrow before and at variable times after BMT. Values are means ± SD of duplicate cultures. Sera from 3 normal controls induced only 0-1 CFU-Meg per 10^5 normal BM-cells. Likewise, sera from 3 CML patients and 1 AML patient in CR before BMT stimulated 0-1 CFU-Meg per 10^5 normal BM-cells. In contrast, sera from 2 SAA patients before BMT promoted the growth of 19 and 22 CFU-Meg per 10^5 normal BM-cells. Sera from 6 patients posttransplant obtained during severe aplasia and at the time of beginning engraftment activated between 3 and 30 (md=20) megakaryocytic colonies per 10^5 normal BM-cells. The stimulatory capacity declined in all patients after haematological reconstitution.

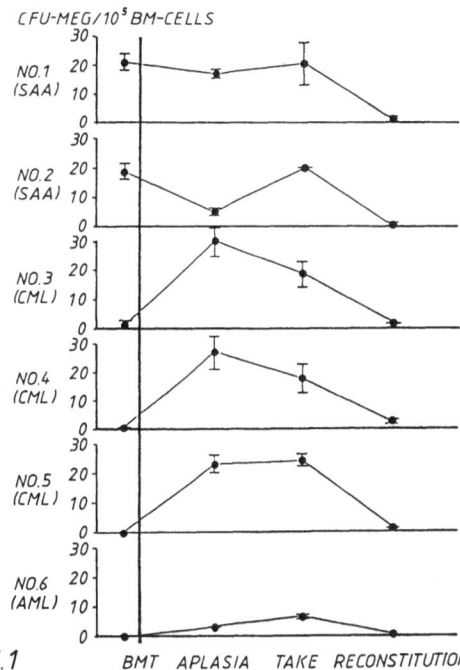

FIG.1

Y-axis label: CFU-MEG/10^5 BM-CELLS

Rows: NO.1 (SAA), NO.2 (SAA), NO.3 (CML), NO.4 (CML), NO.5 (CML), NO.6 (AML)

X-axis: BMT APLASIA TAKE RECONSTITUTION

Conclusions: Megakaryocytopoiesis stimulating factors are highly increased in sera from BMT patients in the period of severe thrombocytopenia. This finding suggests undisturbed stimulatory conditions during severe aplasia following BMT. Cells producing these factors are likely to be resistant to irradiation and cyclophosphamide.

References:

Fauser AA & Messner HA (1978) Granuloerythropoietic colonies in human bone marrow, peripheral blood and cord blood. Blood, 52:1243-1248

Hoffman R, Mazur E et al (1981) Assay of an activity in the serum of patients with disorders of thrombopoiesis that stimulates formation of megakaryocytic colonies. N Engl J Med 305:533-538

Williams N & Levine RF (1982) The origin, development and regulation of megakaryocytes. Br J Haemat 52:173-180

Supported by Grant 4100 of the "Fonds zu Förderung der Wissenschaftlichen Forschung in Österreich" and by the "Kommission für Leukämieforschung und Knochenmarktransplantation" of the Austrian Academy of Sciences

Exp. Hematol. (suppl. 17) 13:98 (1985)
© International Society for Experimental Hematology

Assessment of T-Cell Depletion from Bone Marrow Grafts

L. J. Knott[1], D. C. Linch[1], H. M. Jones[1], A. Goldstone[1], A. C. Newland[2], and R. J. Levinsky[3]

[1] University College and Middlesex Hospital, London
[2] The London Hospital, London
[3] Institute for Child Health, London, Great Britain

Whereas T cell colony forming cells (T-CFC) derived from the peripheral blood are E+, many bone marrow derived T-CFC appear to be E-. It has been suggested therefore, that these marrow E- T-CFC are pre-thymic T cell progenitor cells capable of proliferation and maturation without a thymic micro-environment.

We have cultured T cells from bone marrow and peripheral blood E- and E+ fractions using a modification of the method of Lowenberg and De Zeeuw (1979)[1]. Cells were cultured at 2×10^5/ml in Iscove's Modified Dulbecco's Medium + 20% autologous serum containing optimal concentrations of reagent grade PHA. T cell numbers before and after 5 days of culture were assessed by E-rosetting and staining with monoclonal antibodies. The T cell growth is expressed as an expansion index (EI):

$$EI = \frac{No.\ T\ cells\ post\text{-}culture}{No.\ T\ cells\ pre\text{-}culture}$$

The EI is greatest in bone marrow E- fractions, compatible with the view that the T cells grown derive from an E- bone marrow progenitor cell. However, the assay was non-linear, there was no evidence of immature T cell markers and the T cells had a similar phenotype to those grown from peripheral blood. Studies of re-addition of different T cell populations to E- bone marrow cells indicate that T cells proliferate optimally in the presence of marrow accessory cells and the absence of inhibitory T cells.

We conclude therefore that the T cells grown from T-depleted bone marrow derive from the small number of contaminating mature T cells, freed of T cell suppression. This assay can thus be used as a sensitive measure of T cell contamination and we have studied marrows depleted of T cells by CAMPATH 1 lysis and E-rosetting, or by soybean lectin and E-rosetting prior to transplantation (Table 1).

[1] Lowenberg, B. and De Zeeuw, H.M.C., Am. J. Haematol, 6, 35. 1979.

Table 1   T cell growth following culture of T cell depleted bone marrow cells

T-depletion procedure	Pre-culture		Post-culture
	%E+	Stimulation Index[a]	EI
CAMPATH 1 + C'			
1	2	ND	110
2	2	1.7	9
3	4	1.6	4
4	0.5[b]	2.1	20
5	0.5[b]	ND	146
6	0.5[b]	ND	6
CAMPATH 1 + C' +E-ROSETTING			
1	1	1.4	13
2	1	1.2	18
3	1	2.0	0
4	0.5[b]	1.1	14
5	0.5[b]	ND	2
SOYBEAN LECTIN + E-ROSETTING			
1	1	<1	220
2	2	<1	125
3	1	<1	100
4	3	1.6	180
5	1	<1	72

a Stimulation indices determined by PHA mitogenic responses and mixed lymphocyte cultures.

b E-rosette counts of <1% are given an arbitrary value of 0.5% this being designated the limit of sensitivity.

Prolific T cell growth was obtained from marrows treated with soybean lectin and E-rosetting whereas very few T cells were grown from the CAMPATH 1 and E-rosette treated marrows. Conventional techniques for assessing T cell depletion are relatively insensitive and we have seen fatal GVHD with 0.2% T cell contamination and a negative proliferative response to PHA. The culture of T cells from these marrows may therefore prove to be a valuable means of monitoring the T cell depletion procedures.

Exp. Hematol. (suppl. 17) 13:99 (1985)
© International Society for Experimental Hematology

Analysis of Early T4/T8 Ratio Following Allogeneic Bone Marrow Transplantation: Correlation with Acute Cytomegalovirus Infection and Acute Graft-Versus-Host-Disease

C. Dauriac, D. Guyotat, H. Vu Van, J. P. Magaud, and D. Fière

Unité Fonctionnelle de Greffe de Moëlle Osseuse, Hôpital E. Herriot, F-69374 Lyon Cédex, France

One frequent complication of allogeneic bone marrow transplantation (BMT) is graft-versus-host-disease (GVHD). GVHD occurs in 25 % to 75 % of patients with HLA identical, MLC-unreactive donors and T lymphocytes in the marrow graft are likely to mediate this reaction.

In addition, another frequent complication of BMT is active cytomegalovirus, (CMV) infection which may itself be immunosuppressive, because a reversal in the normal ratio of helper (T4[+]) to suppressor (T8[+]) T lymphocytes is often described.

Some evidence is now available that indicates an imbalance in T cell subsets in patients after BMT.

In this report, marrow graft recipients were monitored before BMT and every 15 days during the first three months after BMT and T cell subsets bearing the T4 and T8 markers were enumerated using monoclonal antibodies. Patterns of ratio T4[+]/T8[+] were correlated with acute GVHD and active CMV infection.

MATERIALS AND METHODS
Patients :
9 patients (6 males and 3 females) ranging in age from 16 to 40 years old were transplanted with bone marrow from related siblings, identical for human leukocyte antigens (HLA), and negative in the MLR. The 3 patients with acute myelogenous leukemia in first remission, the 3 patients with acute lymphoblastic leukemia in first remission, the 2 patients with chronic myelogenous leukemia in first chronic phase were prepared with cyclophosphamide (60 mg/kg/day x 2) and 1 000 rad total body irradiation. 1 patient with severe aplastic anemia was prepared with cyclophosphamide (50 mg/kg/day x 3) and 600 rad total lymphoïd irradiation.
All patients received a median dose of 2 X 10[8]/kg nucleated bone marrow cells and cyclosporin-A (CyA) for GVHD prophylaxis. In addition, for 3 older recipients, bone marrow was depleted of lymphocytes by monoclonal antibodies (CD8) and cytolytic complement.
Before BMT, all patients were investigated with the enzyme-linked immunosorbent assay (ELISA) for IgG antibodies to CMV, and all were seropositive.
Acute GVHD was systematically treated with methylprednisolone (1 g/day for 3 days).

Analysis of T Cell subpopulations :
Heparinized venous blood samples of all recipients were obtained before BMT and every 15 days after BMT.

T cell subpopulations (T4[+] and T8[+]) were isolated from blood using monoclonal antibodies and immunoenzymological technique (indirect immunoperoxydase).

Virus isolation :
Urine and peripheral blood leukocyte fractions of recipients were cultived before BMT and every week after BMT on human embryonic lung (HEL) fibroblasts, permissive for CMV replication. CMV isolates were identified by characteristic cytopathic effects. Cell cultures were maintained for 1 month.

RESULTS
Acute GVHD occured in all patients and was identical as to time of onset and grade (I or II). It appeared later in 2 of 3 recipients who had been treated with monoclonal antibodies and cytolytic complement, but the grade was the same as for the other patients.

The T4[+]/T8[+] ratio distinguished 2 BMT groups during the first 3 months post-BMT :
- 7 of the 9 patients (two of whom had ex-vivo bone marrow treatment) had T4[+]/T8[+] < 1. Of the 7, all developed acute CMV infection within 3 months of BMT which was isolated in blood or urine samples.
- The 2 remaining patients (of whom 1 had ex-vivo bone marrow treatment) had T4[+]/T8[+] ratios > 1. Blood and urine were monitored also every week and none of the 2 experienced acute CMV infection during the first 3 months after BMT

Shifts in the T4[+]/T8[+] ratio seem to be linked more to acute CMV than to acute GVHD.

REFERENCES
Carney W.P., Rubin R.H., Hoffman R.A., Hansen W.P., Healey K. and Hirsch M.S. Analysis of T Lymphocyte subsets in cytomegalovirus mononucleosis. J. Immunol. 126 : 2114-2116, 1981.

Gratama J.W., Naipal A., Oljans P., Zwaan F.E., Verdonck L.F., de Witte Th., Vossen J.M.J.J., Bolhuis R.L.H., de Gast G.C. and Jansen J. T Lymphocyte repopulation and differentiation after bone marrow transplantation. Early shifts in the ratio between T4[+] and T8[+] T lymphocytes correlate with the occurrence of acute graft-versus-host-disease. Blood 63 : 1416-1423, 1984.

Exp. Hematol. (suppl. 17) 13:100 (1985)
© International Society for Experimental Hematology

Functional Capacity of Lymphocyte Subsets after BMT

N. Ødum[1], B. Hofmann[1], B. K. Jakobsen[1], N. Jacobsen[2], P. Platz[1], L. P. Ryder[1], and A. Svejgaard[1]

[1] Tissue Typing Laboratory of the Department of Clinical Immunology,
[2] University Clinic for Infectious Diseases, State University Hospital (Rigshospitalet), DK-2200 Copenhagen, Denmark

INTRODUCTION

Lymphocytes from patients early after bone-marrow transplantation (BMT) are in most cases predominantly of the Leu2[+] (cytotox/suppressor) phenotypes and are almost non-responsive to mitogens. In contrast, normal Leu3[+] (helper) depleted, Leu2[+] enriched lymphocyte suspensions retain about 50% of the mitogenic response compared to that of unseparated cells [1]. We selected 15 donor BMT patient combinations with different Leu3[+]/Leu2[+] ratios post BMT (range: 0.03 to 2.56). These post BMT lymphocytes were tested for functional suppressor activities against donor- and recipient pre-BMT lymphocytes.

SUBJECTS AND METHODS

Patients and marrow donors

Fifteen patients receiving allogeneic marrow (8 with acute lymphoblastic leukemia, five with myelogeneous leukemia, one with T-lymphoblastic lymphoma (non-Hodgkin type), and 1 with aplastic anemia. The age of the patients ranged from 7 to 35 years (median: 23 years). Ten were males and 5 females. The transplantation regimen followed the Seattle protocol with the modifications [2] that the patients were treated with germ-free regimen using laminar air flow and skin and gastrointestinal decontamination, and given cyclosporine as prophylaxis against acute GvHD. Thirteen of the marrow donors were HLA genotypically identical with the recipients, whereas 2 patients received marrow from HLA haploidentical, MLR compatible family donors.

Lymphocyte isolation and tissue culture procedures

Heparinized blood was obtained from family marrow donors (D) and the recipient (R) before BMT and from the recipients twice after BMT: C1 in average 79 days and C2 178 days after BMT. Procedures for isolation and culture of lymphocytes were those previously described [1,3]. The response of D and R lymphocytes to mitogenic (PHA, Con A, and PWM) - and allogeneic (MLR) stimulation was measured (i) in test co-cultures with post BMT (C1 or C2) cells (irradiated 7600 rad or non-irradiated) and (ii) in control cultures with autologous (D or R) cells (irradiated 7600 rad or non-irradiated). The response to mitogens of post BMT lymphocytes were measured in co-cultures with irradiated donor cells and in culture with and without exogeneous IL2 (TCGF; Lymphocult T-Biotest) 10% vol/vol added. The results are given as median cpm of triplicates. The inhibition was calculated by the formula:

$$\text{Suppression} = \left(\frac{\text{control cpm} - \text{test cpm}}{\text{control cpm}}\right) \times 100\%$$

Cells from at least 3 HLA-DR different healthy staff members were included as allogeneic stimulators (x-

irradiated 2400 rad).

RESULTS

None of the post BMT cells were capable of suppressing the donor response to PHA, Con A, and PWM. Likewise, no suppression of pre BMT (R) lymphocyte response to mitogens was found (data not shown). In contrast, as shown in Fig. 1, post BMT lymphocytes with low Leu3/Leu2 ratios seemed to suppress the MLR response of donor cells to HLA-DR different third party cells.

Correlation of T-helper/T-suppressor ratio and suppression of MLR after BMT

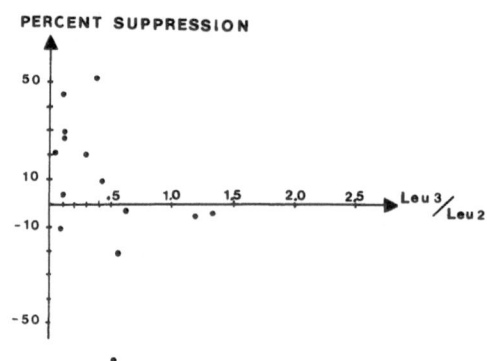

In fact, this correlation is significant for the 15 donor-recipient combinations tested (p<0.01, Kendall). Addition to IL2 or irradiated donor cells to post BMT lymphocytes partly restored the mitogen response. These findings indicate, that the early post BMT cells lack production of IL2 but are capable of responding to IL2. The suppression of the allogeneic but not the mitogenic response might be explained by differences in the mode of activation: e.g. the allogeneic response must involve the T-cell receptor while the mitogenic response may not. The common observation of an almost extinct transformation response of the early post BMT cells could be due to both immaturity (mitogens) and active suppression (MLR); the latter, however, only detectable in more sensitive assays.

REFERENCES

1. Hofmann et al. (1985) Scand. J. Immunol., in press.
2. Møller et al. (1984) Scand. J. Infect. Dis.,**16**,43.
3. Thomsen et al. (1982) Tissue Antigens **19**,25.

Exp. Hematol. (suppl. 17) 13:101 (1985)
© International Society for Experimental Hematology

Regeneration of Pre-B and B Cells in Bone Marrow of Children Transplanted for Acute Leucemia

G. E. M. Asma, R. Langlois van den Bergh, and J. M. Vossen

Department of Pediatrics, University Hospital Leiden, The Netherlands

INTRODUCTION

Pre-B cells are characterized by a scanty amount of intracytoplasmic μ chains. They lack intracytoplasmic light chains and surface immunoglobulins ($c\mu^+/sIg^-$). They precede B cells in the B cell line. B cells are defined as lymphoid cells expressing sIg. After birth pre-B cells are only found in the bone marrow (BM). A combined immunofluorescence staining was used for the simultaneous detection of pre-B and B cells in BM aspirates from BM graft recipients.

PATIENTS AND METHODS

Twelve patients (9 female and 3 male) were studied who had been successfully transplanted with BM from HLA-identical, MLC-negative siblings. Eight patients suffered from ALL (G.T., M.Bij., M.d.K., H.v.V., C.P., E.v.S., T.v.d.S., S.L.) and 4 from ANLL (S.C., M.K., M.B., B.T.). All patients were transplanted in complete hematological remission: the ALL patients in 2nd or 3rd remission, the ANLL patients in 1st remission. The age of the patients at the time of BMT ranged from 5 to 17 years. Pretreatment before BMT consisted of cyclophosphamide (120 mg/kg i.v.) or the VVRapid Regimen (M.Bij., C.P., S.L.) plus TBI. After BMT all patients received MTX to prevent GvHD.

Normal values for BM pre-B and B cells were determined in BM aspirates of 17 healthy BM donors, ranging in age from 3 to 24 years.

Immunofluorescence staining and microscopic analysis were performed as previously described (Asma et al., 1984).

RESULTS

Eight patients were investigated before BMT. In 5 the numbers of pre-B plus B cells expressed as % of nucleated BM cells (NBMC) were below the normal range (10-31/100 NBMC) and in 3 these numbers were normal; in all an abnormal ratio of pre-B to B cells was found (fig. 1). After BMT 8 out of 12 patients showed a temporary "overshooting" of BM pre-B cells, with pre-B to B cell ratios > 1. The other 4 patients (S.C., G.T., M.Bij., M.d.K.) showed a more gradual regeneration of BM pre-B cells with virtually no "overshooting" and pre-B to B cell ratios < 1 (fig. 1).

DISCUSSION

Before BMT, values for BM pre-B and B cells were mostly outside the normal range, i.e. especially the ratio of pre-B to B cells was always abnormal. The anti-leukemic treatment of these children before BMT causes a BM depression. The kinetics of BM regeneration after this depression may be influenced by the kind and duration of the anti-leukemic therapy and the time that has elapsed between the cessation of this therapy

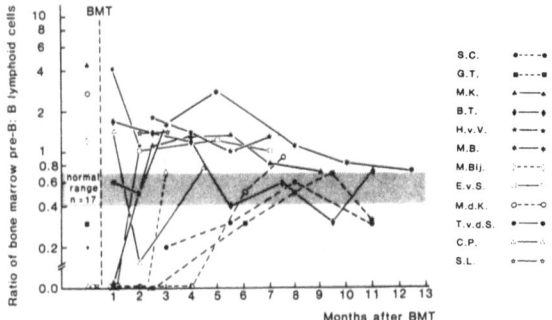

Fig. 1: Pre-B and B cells in BM from BM graft recipients

and the assessment of pre-B and B cell values.
After BMT, patients can be divided into two groups. In patients of group I (8) the pre-B cells outnumbered temporarily the B cells. This reflects the situation during B cell ontogeny. We found that in human fetal liver (up to 16 weeks of gestation) and in human fetal BM pre-B cells always outnumbered B cells (Asma et al., 1984). Group II consists of 4 patients. In this group numbers of pre-B cells were always lower than those of B cells. Group I probably reflects the normal pattern of regeneration of BM pre-B and B cells after BM suppression. The only obvious clinical differences between patients of group I and II, which could play a role in the delayed regeneration of pre-B cells observed in patients of group II, were: additional disease (S.C.: thalassemia major) and the duration of corticosteroid medication after BMT: > 74 days in patients of group II compared with < 54 days in patients of group I.

Although the number of patients studied is small there seems to be a certain correlation between the pattern of regeneration of the B cell system and the ability to mount an in vivo antibody response to recall antigens (diphtheria or tetanus toxoid and poliomyelitis virus). A significant increase in antibody titers after booster vaccination was found in 6 patients of group I, but only in 1 patient of group II (data not shown).

REFERENCES

Asma, G.E.M., Langlois van den Bergh, R. and Vossen, J.M. Development of pre-B and B lymphocytes in the human fetus. Clin. exp. Immunol 56: 407 (1984).

Exp. Hematol. (suppl. 17) 13:102 (1985)
© International Society for Experimental Hematology

T-Cell Functional Evaluation Following Bone Marrow Transplantation

Dominique Charmot, Daniel Olive, Dominique Maraninchi, and Claude Mawas

Centre d'Immunologie INSERM-CNRS de Marseille-Luminy, Case 906, F-13288 Marseille Cédex 9, and
Unité de Transplantation Médullaire, Institut Paoli-Calmettes, 239, boulevard de Sainte Marguerite, F-13273 Marseille Cédex 9, France

INTRODUCTION

After bone marrow transplantation (BMT), patients have a combined humoral and cellular immune deficiency, related to delayed repopulation by CD4 positive cells (2), deficit in IL-2 production (3), and suppressor cells (4), but not to defects of the monocytes (5). We have performed longitudinal studies of the alloreactive responses of allogenic and autologous BMT patients. The generation of allospecific cytolytic T cells is found normal or even higher than reactivity of donor cells, in spite of reduced MLR and production of IL-2. However, this generation is IL-2 dependent, as evidenced by the inhibition of their generation by anti-IL-2 receptor monoclonal antibodies (mAbs). Beside a quantitative CD4 cell subset defect, a qualitative CD8 cell subset difference is suggested.

MATERIALS AND METHODS

Patients. Blood samples from 24 allografts and 12 autografts were collected and frozen at regular intervals.

Cellular assays. Allogenic proliferation (MLR) and generation of effector cells (CML) were done according to published techniques (6).

mAbs used. Anti-IL-2 receptor mAbs, anti-LFA-1, anti-CD8, and anti-CD1 were locally derived (7). An anti-CD4 mAb was kindly provided by J. Brochier (Lyon, France).

RESULTS AND DISCUSSION

Allogenic BM reconstituted patients, with or without acute or chronic GvH and autologous BMT patients, used as responder cells in an MLR assay, show responses weaker than in the controls: cells from the HLA-identical donor, pre-BMT cells or unrelated donor cells. Table 1 is an example of such an MLR. Results are expressed as cpm x 10^{-3} of thymidine incorporation.

	Allogenic BMT		Autologous BMT
	Donor cells	Patient cells (day 52 after BMT)	Patient cells (day 60 after BMT)
Medium	2.0	.7	.4
stim.cells: 1	20.0	4.0	1.8
2	19.7	6.6	3.9
3	16.7	8.5	2.3
4	18.7	7.0	.4

IL-2 production has been studied (12 allogenic and 4 autologous). With one exception, all the measures were found lower than in the controls (data not shown). Allogenic cell-mediated lympholysis following BMT shows an CML activity after in vitro allosensitization much stronger than in the different controls. This CML was specific. Table 2 shows an example ; results are expressed as % of specific chromium-51 release at a given effector to target ratio (E/T).

	E/T	Specific target	Unrelated target
CTLs from			
Patient 1	1/1	33%	0%
Donor 1	93/1	21%	0%
Patient 2	1/1	38%	3%
Donor 2	74/1	28%	0%

This pattern of responses was found independent of the nature of the graft, the clinical status and the pre- and post-transplant regimen. Using different mAbs to phenotype these effector cells, we conclude that they are CD8 positive T cells (data not shown). The high level of the CML could simply be attributed to a relative enrichment in CD8 patient cells. Donor cells were pretreated with anti-CD4 mAb plus C', before setting up the culture. The CML activity was always reduced. Thus the mere depletion in CD4 cells is not sufficient to mimick the CML activity observed with patient cells. This suggests that there must exist some qualitative differences between post BMT cells and the genetically identical donor cells. To test the IL-2 dependency of these effector cells, we performed the sensitization in presence of a 1:60 dilution of an anti-IL-2 receptor mAb. The results show that the CML is totally abolished in patient and donor cultures indicating the IL-2 dependency of the CTL generation (data not shown).

The extensive comparison we performed on BMT patients indicated qualitative differences in the patient CD8 subset, beside the CD4 subset deficit. Taken together, these observations could explain in part the coexistence in the BMT patients of a severe immunodeficiency and the ability to mount a GvH.

REFERENCES
1. Storb, R and E.D. Thomas. 1983. Immunol.Rev. 71:78.
2. De Bruin, H.G. et al. 1981. J. Immunol. 127:244.
3. Azogui, O., E. Gluckman and D. Fradelizi. 1983. J. Immunol. 131:1205.
4. Tsoi, M.S. et al. 1981. Nature 292:355.
5. Tsoi, M.S. et al. 1984. Transplantation, in press.
6. Charmot, D. et al. 1980. Tissue Antigens 15:297.
7. Olive, D. et al. 1984. In : Proceedings of the 16th Leucocyte Culture Conference. A. Mitchison and M. Feldman, Eds., Humana Press, in press.

Exp. Hematol. (suppl. 17) 13:103 (1985)
© International Society for Experimental Hematology

Hematopoetic and Immunological Reconstitution Following Allogeneic Bone Marrow Transplantation Using Methotrexate or Cyclosporine A as Graft Versus Host Prophylaxis

M. Haen, E. M. Schneider, P. Ostendorf, and P. Wernet

Medizinische Universitätsklinik, D-7400 Tübingen, Federal Republic of Germany

The early phase after allogeneic bone marrow transplantation (BMT) is complicated by life-threatening infections and by graft versus host disease (GVHD).Up to now little is known about the behaviour of the regenerating immunocompetent cells involved in these complications. The study presented here, tries to correlate distinct lymphocyte subpopulations to events clinically observed after BMT.

PATIENTS AND TREATMENT CHARACTERISTICS

48 patients were treated with allogeneic BMT for various hematological disorders (severe aplastic anemia, SAA; acute leucemia, AL; chronic granulocytic leucemia,CGL). 24 patients received methotrexate (MTX) as GVHD-prophylaxis, 22 patients received cyclosporin A (CSA), and 3 patients received no GVHD-prophylaxis because of a syngeneic donor. All patients were prepared for bone marrow transplantation according to the Seattle protocol (1). CSA was continuously administered from day -1 up to about 400 days. Prophylaxis with MTX was performed from day +1 to 95. All patients received 2.0 - 4.0 x 10!8 bone marrow cells. Peripheral blood mononuclear cells (PBMC) of 19 patients were tested with monoclonal antibodies for surface markers. Immune response to different immune stimulative agents was tested repeatedly during follow up.

RESULTS:

The earliest onset of peripheral blood leukocyte (PBL)-recovery was seen around day 10 in syngeneic BMT patients and in allogeneic BMT patients treated with CSA(mean day 10.73 +/- 2.37). In contrast PBL recovery of MTX-treated patients was significantly delayed (day 16.75 +/- 2.91; p 0.001). At the beginning of GVHD CSA-treated patients presented with a so-called positive T4:T8 ratio more than 1.0. A few days later this ratio converted to values below 1.0. Disappear-ance of the acute GVHD was followed by reconstitution of the ratio to initial values, respectively. Similiar findings could be monitored following viral infections. Limited chronic GVHD and/or bacterial infections did not markedly affect T4:T8 ratios.On the other hand in MTX-treated patients a positive T4:T8 ratio was never seen at the onset of the acute GVHD and in the absence of viral infections (table 1). The further follow up to show a possible reconstitution of the T4:T8 ratio was hampered by the fact, that all these patients later suffered from persistent viral infections. Results obtained with experiments designed to evaluate T- and B-cell immune response capacity after BMT showed al-most normal responses to PHA, Con A, and alloantigens, whereas PWM was non-stimulatory in most cases. These results were consistent for the beginning of acute GVHD and in correlation to positive T4:T8 ratios.In case of reoccurance of GVHD and/or during viral infection rising T8 versus T4 levels impair in vitro responsiveness, in certain cases even to background proliferative responses.

DISCUSSION

The hypothesis drawn from our results is that in acute GVHD T4 positive helper T cells seem to induce proliferation of T8 positive effector T cells.The clinic of acute GVHD therefore would be caused by T8 positive effector T cells.We draw this conclusion from the behaviour of the T4:T8 ratio in our CSA-treated patients early at the onset of GVHD where we could see a shift from a positive to a negative T4:T8 ratio. The same mechanism explains the rapid restoration of a high but immunologically not committed T4 pool after effective treatment of the acute GVHD.Furthermore this applies to the overcome of viral infections which is also characterized by T8 positive effector populations. Concerning the situation in MTX-treated patients where the initial positive T4:T8 ratio at the onset of acute GVHD cannot be seen, CSA blocks distinct T-T interactions with apparent specific protection of T4 cells (2). The known requirement of T4 cells for hematopoietic differentiation (3) can furthermore explain the earlier regeneration of PBL in CSA-trereated patients as a direct CSA effect.

REFERENCES

(1) Wilms,K. et al (1982) Klin Wschr 60, 1279
(2) Cohen,D.J. et al (1984) Ann Int Med 101, 667
(3) Mangan,K.F. et al (1982) Blood 59,990

	PATIENT	DAY 10 - 30	30 - 50	50 - 100	> 100
MTX	E.R.	0.6 +	0.28●★	0.15●★★	
	G.S.	0.74 +	0.05 ↔●		
	G.W.	0.6 +	0.27○△		0.5△
	H.S.	0.33 +		0.39 +	
	G.B.	1.8 −	0.44 +	0.78★	1.0★
	H.S.	0.7			0.25
	W.K.	0.36 +	0.1●		
CSA	B.K.	1.2 +			0.27●
	G.K.	2.6 +	0.54−	3.0	0.85●
	B.O.	(17) 2.2 + (23) 0.7 +	0.3●★		0.23●
	T.S.	(10) 1.0 + (24) 0.13 +			
	S.W.	(17) 2.3 +		·− 0.16★	0.55★
	W.B.	(18) 6.7 + (27) 0.72 +	0.5 −	3.25 −	0.45★

Table 1: OKT4:OKT8 ratios in PBMC at different times after BMT of patients treated with MTX or CSA for GVHD prophylaxis Patients treated with CSA developped GVHD earlier than MTX patients. The former are also marked by primarily higher T4 counts compared to T8, although the ratio declined below 1.0 soon after onset of GVHD. Numbers in brackets indicate the exact date of testing. MTX patients had an T4:T8 ratio less than 1.0 immediate at onset of GVHD. Viral complications and relapse phase furthermore decreased T4 cells and increased T8 cells. (+ acute GVHD, ● Virus infection, ★ chronic GVHD, △ relapse, — none of the above)

Exp. Hematol. (suppl. 17) 13:104 (1985)
© International Society for Experimental Hematology

Immunisation Against Hepatitis B in BMT- and Leukemia-Patients

C. Rosendahl[1], Ch. Bender-Götze[1], F. Deinhardt[2], H.-J. Kolb[1], and R. Haas[1]

[1] Münchener Arbeitsgemeinschaft Knochenmark-Transplantation,
[2] Max-von-Pettenkofer-Institut, Universität München, D-8000 München, Federal Republic of Germany

INTRODUCTION

Hepatitis B infections in immunocompromised leukemic children or in BM recipients mostly take an inapparent course. However, a considerable proportion of these patients become chronic carriers and one third is considered infectious (HBsAg and HBeAg positive). To prevent this carrier status most centers immunise their patients by administration of hepatitis B immunoglobulin (HBIG) which confers only incomplete protection.
Since 1982 when the hepatitis B vaccine became available, we have tried to achieve a continuous protection of our patients by passive-active immunisation.

PATIENTS AND METHODS

We have administered passive-active immunisation to all children with acute leukemia (n=26) and all BMT patients (n=11) of the Munich university hospitals. Since we expected an impaired antibody response in these patients, the vaccination regimen was modified:
The usual dose of 20 µg HBsAg was doubled and given 4 instead of 3 times. The simultaneous injection of HBIG together with the first active vaccination was intended to protect the patients until their own antibody production had begun.

RESULTS

Figure 1 shows the anti-HBs development in children with leukemia and in BM recipients after passive-active immunisation against hepatitis B. The almost non-existing antibody response is demonstrated in comparison to a curve showing the anti-HBs response of healthy adults.

DISCUSSION

Our results clearly demonstrate that the active component of the immunisation has not improved the intended protection and therefore cannot be recommended for leukemic patients or BM recipients. Despite its deficiencies passive immunisation seems to represent the only prophylactic treatment of some value.
THus we developed a new vaccination strategy following the idea that immunity against hepatitis B could possibly be achieved by transplanting primed memory cells from the donor to the recipient.
With this intention we vaccinate the BM donors twice before transplantation expecting that the recipient will respond to a further vaccination with a booster of antibody production. This new immunisation strategy for BMT patients is shown in figure 2:

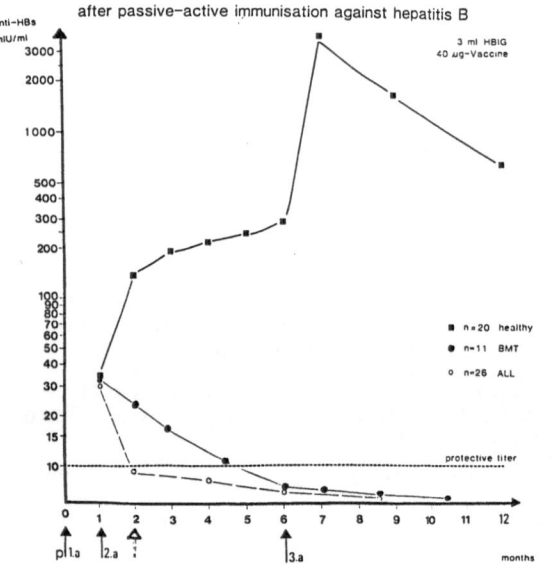

Comparison of anti-HBs development in healthy subjects and in ALL/BMT patients after passive-active immunisation against hepatitis B

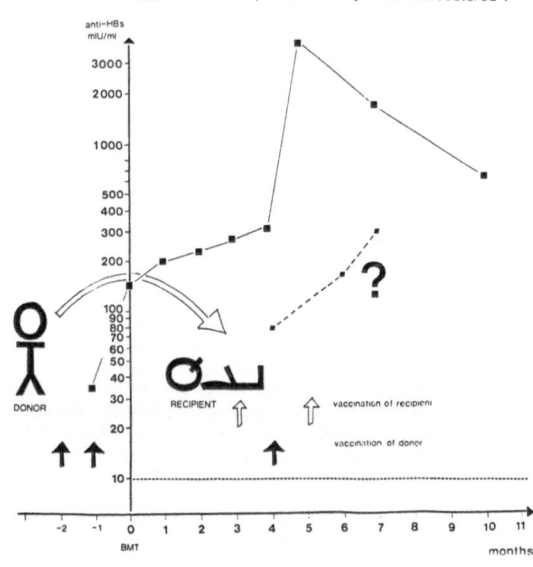

Can transferred primed memory cells be boostered ?

Exp. Hematol. (suppl. 17) 13: 105 (1985)
© International Society for Experimental Hematology

Prophylaxis Against Cytomegalovirus Infection After BMT with Gammaglobulins

H. Vu Van [1], D. Fiere [1], J. Chomel [2], D. Thouvenot [2], D. Guyotat [1], L. Dutou [3], C. Ginestet [3], M. Lacroze [3], and M. Aymard [2]

[1] Service Hématologie, Hôpital Edouard Herriot, F-69374 Lyon Cédex 8
[2] Laboratoire Universitaire de Virologie, Lyon
[3] Service de Radiotherapie, Centre Léon Bérard, Lyon, France

Prophylaxis with high-titered anti CMV globulins was studied in 2 pilot trials using 2 different schedules. Results were compared with a historical group without prophylaxis.

PATIENTS AND METHODS

All patients received BMT from HLA matched siblings. 40 leukemic patients were treated with CPM and single dose TBI (lungs shielding, dose rate< 5cGy/mn). 3 patients with SAA were treated by CPM and TLI or TAI. The gammaglobulins (Veinoglobuline*, Institut Mérieux, Lyon) were prepared from pooled human placentas. The contents of undenatured IgG were 40% (of the IgG1-2 and 4 subclasses). Different batches were checked for anti CMV antibody titers: They were found between 1:3200-1:12800 in Elisa, 1:256-1:1024 in Immunofluorescence, and 1:320-1:1060 in Neutralizing tests. Group0 (13 pts) was a historical group without prophylaxis. Group1 (15 pts) received at days 25,50 and 75 three IV infusions of Veinoglobuline* (200mg/kg/day). Group2 (15 pts) received Veinoglobuline* (200mg/kg/d) once per week from day0 until day100. In groups1-2 the virological surveillance associated virus cultures (in urine and buffy coat) and serolgy by CF and Elisa IgG-IgM assays, and was done weekly until day 120 and then bi-weekly then monthly. When a interstitial pneumonia occured, samples from bronchoalveolar lavage (or autopsy) were analyzed for virus, fungi, pneumocystis and other organisms.
The pre-transplant serology was found negative in only 3 patients out of 30 in groups1-2 (CF titers <1:8 and Elisa titers <1:100). In group0, 7 patients out of 13 had CF titers <1:8. No patient had CMV isolation before BMT.

RESULTS (see Table1)

High risk patients (in relapse or 2nd or subsequent remissions) were significantly more frequent in group 0 : 9 out of 13 vs 5 out of 30 in groups1+2 (0.01<p< 0.05).
Severe grade 3-4 GVHD were less frequent in group 2 receiving CiA than in groups 0 and 1 receiving exclusively or predominantly MTX (0.01<p<0.05).
In group0 6 IP were observed and all cases were fatal (2 cases with CMV in lungs).
In group 1, 6 IP occured (2 pts with CMV in lungs, 1 pt with CMV only in blood/urine), and 3 cases were fatal : 1 case with CMV and aspergillus, 2 idiopathic IP. In group 2, no IP was observed , the difference is

significant compared to groups0 and 1. Deaths by IP decreased significantly in group2, and in both groups 1+2 compared to group0.
3 cases of encephalitis were observed in groups1-2, 1 case was fatal. They were probably CMV related as CMV was isolated in urine/blood (absent in lumbar puncture). The other causes of early deaths were : 5 GVHD, 1 toxic cardiopathy (group2), 1 VOD and 1 hepatitis (group0). 8 other patients further relapsed with leukemia .18 other patients are alive and well (range 6 months - 4 years).

DISCUSSION

Our study was not a randomized trial, and the influence of the modulation of GVHD by CiA could not be exclu ded . In spite of these remarks our results suggested that prophylaxis with high titered anti CMV gammaglobu lins, administered in the intensive schedule as in the group 2 could be efficient. Although the total rate of CMV infection was not influenced, the mortality by IP could be decreased by passive immunization.

GROUPS	0	1	2
n pts	13	15	15
GVHD grade3-4	7	9	1*
CMV in urine/blood	ne	8	10
Seroconversion IgM Elisa	ne	4	6
Interstitial Pneumonias			
- total cases	6	6	0*
- cases with CMV	2	3	-
- fatal cases :	6	3**	0**
. CMV	2	1	
. aspergillus	1	(+ aspergillus)	
. pneumocystis	1		
. idiopathic	2	2	
Encephalitis (CMV?)		1	2
(fatal case)		(1)	(0)
Other causes of early deaths			
. GVHD	2	2	1
. other causes	2		1

Table1. Virological and clinical outcome
* 0.01<p<0.05 group2 vs groups 0 and 1
** 0.01<p<0.05 group 2 vs group 0
          groups 1+2 vs group 0
(Fisher's tests)

Exp. Hematol. (suppl. 17) 13:106 (1985)
© International Society for Experimental Hematology

Oral Prophylaxis of Herpes Infections with Acyclovir (ACV) After BMT

Clinical Study with Plasma Level Determination by Use of a New High-Performance Liquid Chromatography Method

K. Schüch, G. Ehninger, A. Vallbracht, I. Kumbier, and P. Ostendorf

Medizinische Klinik und Hygiene-Institut der Universität, D-7400 Tübingen, Federal Republic of Germany

INTRODUCTION

Virus infections are one of the major complications after BMT. Herpes simplex (HSV) and varicella zoster (VZV) infections occur in up to 80% of pts. (Harkness 1980). ACV a new specific antiviral agent has shown high activity in the treatment of VZV- and HSV-infections (Mitchell 1981).

We report the results of our study with oral ACV prophylaxis and control of bioavailability by a new HPLC-method.

METHODS

Twenty pts. had undergone BMT: 19 received allogeneic BMT (8 with acute leukemia, 7 with CML, 4 with SAA), 1 pt. with neuroblastoma received autologous BMT. Six pts. had virus infections in the pre-BMT period (2 CMV-sepsis, 1 VZV-pneumonitis, 1 HSV-keratitis, 2 HSV-mucositis). Eighteen pts. had elevated antibody titers. The age range was 4-24 years (median 16). All were isolated in LAF-units for at least 28 days with total enteral decontamination. The conditioning regimen with cyclophosphamide and total body irradiation followed the Seattle protocol, except the patient with neuroblastoma. GvHD prophylaxis was done in 6 pts. with methotrexate, and in 14 with cyclosporin A (age over 10 years). Oral ACV dose was 400 mg four times daily from day -12 to day +84 (below 6 years 200 mg per dose). All pts are concomitantly treated with anti - CMV - hyperimmunoglobulin and cotrimoxazol.

1 ml blood was drawn 3 hours after oral drug administration. To 0.5 ml plasma 0.5 ml of saturated ammoniumsulphate were added and centrifuged after 12 hours. 50 μl were injected into the HPLC system. Separation was obtained with a μBondapak C 18 column. The optimum isocratic system for the resolution of ACV was found to consist of methanol: water : 0.05 m ammoniumdihydrogenphosphat buffer (9:88.5:2.5, v/v/v) containing 5 mM 1-heptanesulfonic acid, detection at 254 nm.

RESULTS

During ACV prophylaxis 6 out of 20 pts. had evidence of virus infections. In 2 of 3 pts. with clinical diagnosis of HSV-mucositis virus was isolated in urine or throat. Two pts. had rise in HSV-titer (CFT) and 1 in CMV-titer (CFT). No ACV was present (detection limit 20 ng/ml) in plasma of 3 pts. Two of them had non compliance, a lack of ACV resorption developed in 1 pt. under conditioning regimen. ACV concentrations below 200 ng/ml were measured in the other 3 pts. After cessation of ACV prophylaxis HSV virus was isolated in urine or throat in 5 out of 7 pts. with mucositis .

Except in 1 pt. bioavailability of oral ACV was unchanged during treatment period. No drug related side effects were observed. Laboratory tests did not show liver or renal toxicity. Take and hematologic reconstitution were unchanged.

DISCUSSION

This study showed that the oral administration of ACV was safe as also reported by Anderson 1984. Bioavailability was not affected by concomitant administration of other drugs and diarrhoe in 2 pts., however a loss of ACV resorption during BMT procedure was documented in 1 pt. Non compliance was observed in 3 pts.

The effective prophylaxis or treatment of i.v. ACV in BMT is demonstrated by Saral (1981), Wade (1982) and Osterwalder (1984). In our study with oral ACV no severe virus infection occured during prophylaxis in pts. with a high risk.

REFERENCES

Harkness J. et al (1984) Transpl Proc 16:1016
Mitchell C. et al (1981) Lancet I:1389
Anderson H. et al (1984) Br J Cancer 50:45
Saral R. at al (1981) N Engl J Med 305:63
Wade J. et al (1982) Ann Int Med 98:265
Osterwalder B. et al (1984) Schweiz Med
    Wschr 114: 14

Exp. Hematol. (suppl. 17) 13:107 (1985)
© International Society for Experimental Hematology

Value of Serum C-Reactive Protein Measurement in the Management of Bone Marrow Recipients

S. A. Walker, T. R. Rogers, P. G. Riches, S. White, and J. R. Hobbs

Departments of Chemical Immunology and Medical Microbiology, Westminster Hospital, London SW1P 2AR, Great Britain

Serial serum levels of the acute-phase protein C-reactive protein (CRP) were measured by rate nephelometry on a Beckman ICS analyser (Beckman Instruments Inc, California, USA) and analysed in relation to episodes of documented infection and graft-versus-host disease (GVHD) in the early transplant period (less than 3 months post BMT)[1] and in the late post transplant period (later than 3 months post BMT)[2]. CRP levels were higher in patients with major bacterial infections, with or without GVHD, than in those with viral or fungal infections or GVHD without bacterial infection. Most of the fungal infections seen were localised, however, and so CRP levels were measured during the course of severe systemic fungal infections in two further BMT patients.

The first patient developed severe acute GVHD and fatal systemic aspergillosis post BMT but CRP levels never rose above 55 mg/l (the upper limit of normal being 10 mg/l).

The second patient (see figure below) had continuously elevated CRP levels and *Candida albicans* was grown from repeated blood cultures. Her condition deteriorated, failure of engraftment made a second BMT necessary and she died of systemic candidiasis, proven at post-mortem.

It would seem, therefore, that systemic yeast infections can cause high serum CRP levels comparable to those seen in major bacterial infections. This is supported by the results of a Finnish study in which extremely high CRP levels were seen in immuno-compromised patients with fungal septicaemias and deep-seated fungal infections, the majority of which were caused by *Candida spp*[3]. This is not unexpected since *Candida albicans* polysaccharide extract is known to stimulate production of the monokine Interleukin 1 (IL1) from macrophages[4], initiating the hepatic synthesis of CRP. It is possible that other fungi (as illustrated above in the patient with severe systemic aspergillosis) are less effective initiators of IL1 production, perhaps because of differences in cell wall composition, and hence do not cause marked rises in serum CRP levels.

We conclude, therefore, that the measurement of serum CRP levels during BMT is valuable in the diagnosis and monitoring of most major bacterial infections, even in the presence of GVHD, but, in addition, raised levels may indicate systemic or deep-seated yeast infections. Raised serum CRP levels in any patient responding well to appropriate antimicrobial therapy should fall rapidly towards normal.

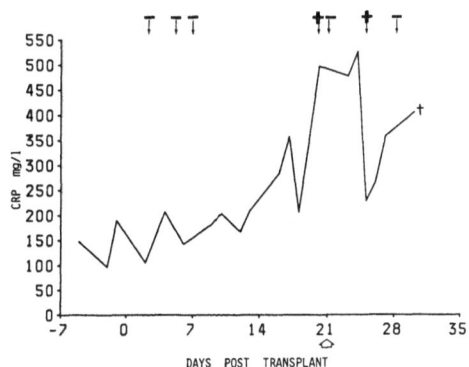

SERUM CRP LEVELS IN A BMT PATIENT WITH CANDIDIASIS

day 0 indicates day of first marrow infusion
⌂ indicates day of second marrow infusion
+ positive ⎫ blood culture
- negative ⎭

REFERENCES

1) Walker SA,Rogers TR,Riches PG,White S,Hobbs JR. Value of serum CRP measurement in the management of BMT recipients. Part 1:early transplant period. J Clin Pathol (1984):*37*;1018-1021

2) Walker SA,Riches PG,Rogers TR,White S,Hobbs JR. Value of serum CRP measurement in the management of BMT recipients. Part 2:late post transplant period. J Clin Pathol (1984):*37*;1022-1026

3) Kostiala I. CRP response induced by fungal infections. J Infection (1984):*8*;212-220

4) Lombardi G,Piccolella E,Vismara D *et al.* *Candida albicans* polysaccharide extract (MPPS) and PPD stimulate the production of Interleukin 1 and lymphocyte proliferation. Clin Exp Immunol (1984):*58*;581-586

Exp. Hematol. (suppl. 17) 13:108–109 (1985)
© International Society for Experimental Hematology

The Effects of the Intestinal Microflora of Selectively Decontaminated Patient on the Severity of Acute Graft-Versus-Host Disease of the Gut

A Comparative Study on Selective and Total Decontamination in Patients Undergoing Allogeneic Bone Marrow Transplantation

H. F. L. Guiot[1], J. W. M. van der Meer[1], W. E. Fibbe[2], M. M. de Planque[2], F. E. Zwaan[2], and I. Biemond[3]

[1] Department of Infectious Diseases,
[2] Department of Hematology,
[3] Department of Gastroenterology, University Hospital, Leiden, The Netherlands

INTRODUCTION

Infection prevention in adult granulocytopenic patients is performed in our institute by selective elimination of the aerobic potentially pathogenic micro-organisms from the digestive tract. This procedure has been called selective antimicrobial modulation (SAM) and the efficacy has been proven in a double-blind, placebo-controlled study in patients undergoing chemotherapy for acute myelogenous leukemia (Guiot et al., 1983). Also in allogeneic bone marrow transplantation (BMT), SAM has shown to be effective (Van der Meer et al., 1984).

An unsolved question is whether the large numbers of facultative streptococci and anaerobic bacteria, that are not eliminated from the gut by SAM, increase the risk of acute graft-versus-host disease (aGVHD) in BMT patients in comparison with the risk in patients given antimicrobial drugs with the aim to eliminate all micro-organisms. It has been suggested that bacterial antigens pass through the epithelium of the gut and activate donor lymphocytes that cross-react with antigens on the target tissue, resulting in aGVHD. Although it is likely that in mice the aerobic gram-negative rods (e.g. Enterobacteriaceae) are involved in aGVHD, it is not clear whether extrapolation may be made to patients given SAM, leaving only the facultative streptococci and anaerobic bacteria in the intestines.

With the purpose to investigate whether these persisting bacteria are involved in aGVHD, patients undergoing allogeneic BMT were randomly allocated to receive SAM without -, or SAM with additional antimicrobial drugs active against the micro-organisms usually persisting in patients given SAM (Guiot et al., 1981). The additional antimicrobial drugs were Cephaloridin (CE) and Clindamycin (CL) and therefore the group of patients given this kind of prophylaxis are called SAM-CE/CL.

METHODS

Patients on SAM: From day 14 prior to BMT until the first day of the conditioning regimen, the patients were put on the standard regimen, consisting of a combination of oral polymyxin-B, neomycin, nalidixic acid, and amphotericin-B. During both the conditioning phase and the first weeks after BMT when the patients have difficulties taking oral drugs, cotrimoxazole was administered intravenously to maintain the decontaminated state. As soon as they could take oral drugs again (between day 7 and 14 after BMT), the oral SAM was reinstituted and continued till day 60. Antimicrobial prophylaxis was supported by local antimicrobial treatment in the oral cavity. The patients were nursed in laminar flow rooms, and a diet with a low bacterial content was prescribed. Details have been described by Van der Meer et al., 1984.

Patients on SAM-CE/CL: These patients were given SAM and cotrimoxazole as described above, but in addition they were given Cephaloridin orally, 500 mg twice daily, or if they were not able to swallow the drug, Clindamycin intravenously, 600 mg three times a day, both from day 1 to day 35 after BMT. As soon as possible CL i.v. was replaced by CE orally; if aGVHD occurred within this period, CL or CE was continued until the symptoms of intestinal aGVHD had been diminished or resolved by therapy.

Diagnosis and classification of the severity of aGVHD: The diagnosis of aGVHD was made on clinical symptoms and confirmed by biopsies in most patients. Severity of aGVHD was classified by the grading system according to Thomas (1975). Intestinal protein loss was used to compare the severity of gastrointestinal involvement. Protein loss was calculated from monitoring the albumin concentration of the serum as a function of time and the need of intravenous albumin support to maintain the serum albumin concentration above the level of 40 gr/l. In addition, α_1-antitrypsin clearance was calculated from the concentration found in 24-hour portions of feces and the concentration in the serum measured by radial immunodiffusion in 12 patients once weekly after BMT (Weisdorf et al., 1983).

RESULTS

Until now the results in 14 patients given SAM and 11 patients given SAM-CE/CL can be evaluated. All patients were in complete remission of acute myelogenous leukemia or acute lymphocytic leukemia, or they were in the chronic phase of myelocytic leukemia. These diagnoses were equally distributed over the two groups of patients. All patients had a HLA-identical, MLC nonreactive sibling donor, and the patients characteristics were similar for both groups. The mean age was 32 and 29 years for patients on SAM and SAM-CE/CL, respectively. The patients of the two groups were treated similarly regarding conditioning for BMT, aGVHD prophylaxis (methotrexate, 7 patients on SAM-CE/CL and 8 on SAM; cyclosporin-A, 4 patients on SAM-CE/CL and 6 on SAM) and aGVHD treatment (high dose methylprednisolone). No differences were observed in the incidence of fever and infection.

Acute graft-versus-host disease (aGVHD): Acute GVHD was observed in 8 of 11 patients (73%) given SAM-CE/CL, versus 13 of 14 patients given SAM (93%); the severity of aGVHD in the patients with the disease was lower in the SAM-CE/CL group, with a mean grade of 1.2 versus 2.2 in the SAM group; the differences are borderline statistically significant (p=0.08).

The less severe aGVHD observed in SAM-CE/CL was mainly caused by a lower incidence of aGVHD of the liver, i.e. in 50% of the patients on SAM, the bilirubin concentration was below 60 µg/ml within a period of 60 days after BMT versus 91% of the patients on SAM-CE/CL. Remarkably, the incidence of diarrhea was similar for both groups. Since diarrhea (aspect and volume) is an unreliable parameter for the severity of aGVHD of the gut, the intestinal protein loss was measured. A correlation was observed between protein (albumin) loss and fecal α_1-antitrypsin clearance, and these parameters correlated with the severity of aGVHD classified according to Thomas (r=0.66). A high correlation coefficient (r=0.81) was found after exclusion of 6 patients with aGVHD without gut involvement. By using these data as additional parameters for the measurement of the severity of aGVHD, it was found that in the patients on SAM-CE/CL only one of 11 patients appeared to have aGVHD of the digestive tract, resulting in diarrhea, high albumin loss (> 20 g/day) and liver involvement. In the patients given SAM, 5 of 14 patients fulfilled these criteria. Probably diarrhea in the patients on SAM-CE/CL was primarily caused by disturbance of the osmoregulation in the absence of a normal intestinal micro-flora.

Survival: The tendency of mitigation of aGVHD of the gut and liver by SAM-CE/CL is not reflected in a better survival of the patients evaluable at present. The cause of death was clearly related to aGVHD in only one (7%) patient on SAM and none of the group on SAM-CE/CL. Death might have been indirectly related to aGVHD (e.g., interstitial pneumonitis and infectious pneumonitis with still active aGVHD) in 5 (36%) patients on SAM and 4 (36%) on SAM-CE/CL. Death probably not related to aGVHD (e.g., relapse, infectious hepatitis) occurred in 3 (21%) patients on SAM and 3 (27%) on SAM-CE/CL. The survival was 35% (day 60-770 after BMT) and 36% (day 140-520 after BMT) for the group on SAM and SAM-CE/CL, respectively.

DISCUSSION

At present, there is still no consensus regarding the measures which have to be taken for prevention of infections during allogeneic BMT. The measures taken in the various centers for BMT vary from nearly none to highly sophisticated measures, the latter including laminar air flow isolation, sterile food and antimicrobial drugs to eradicate all micro-organisms (total antibiotic decontamination - TAD). The measures taken in our institute are somewhere in between both extremes, including laminar air flow isolation, a low bacterial diet and SAM. With this strategy, to which was decided as a consequence of previous failures with more strict measures in adult patients (e.g., TAD and a sterile diet), we aimed to have a reasonable cost-complience-benefit ratio. Because both animal experiments and data of results of BMT in man continue to suggest a beneficial effect of gut sterilization on aGVHD (Watson, 1983), a randomised study was started comparing SAM and SAM-CE/CL. The latter regimen should substantially reduce the number of intestinal bacteria (details will be published after termination of the study) and subsequently result in reduction of the incidence and severity of aGVHD, while maintaining a reasonable cost-complience-benefit ratio. The results reveal a clear tendency of reduction of the severity of aGVHD of the gut due to the addition of CE/CL to SAM, which is reflected by the lower intestinal protein loss and a lower incidence of liver involvement. However, until now no effect on survival has been achieved. Of course, it might be that SAM-CE/CL, given during a longer period, or other regimens aiming to result in more complete gut sterilization, will result in better mitigation of aGVHD and subsequently improvement of survival.

REFERENCES

Guiot HFL, Meer JWM van der, Furth R van (1981). Selective antimicrobial modulation of human microbial flora: Infection prevention in patients with decreased host defense mechanisms by selective elimination of potentially pathogenic bacteria. J Infect Dis 143: 644-654.

Guiot HFL, Broek PJ van den, Meer JWM van der, Furth R van (1983). Selective antimicrobial modulation of the intestinal flora of patients with acute nonlymphoblastic leukemia: A doubleblind, placebo-controlled study. J Infect Dis 147:615-623.

Meer JWM van der, Guiot HFL, Broek PJ van den, Furth R van (1984). Infections in bone-marrow transplant recipients. Semin Hematol 21:123-140.

Thomas ED, Storb R, Clift RA, et al. (1975). Bone marrow transplantation. New Eng J Med 292:832-843, and 895-902.

Watson JG (1983). Problems of infection after bone marrow transplantation. J Clin Pathol 36:683-692.

Weisdorf SA, Salati LM, Longsdorf JA, Ramsay NKC, Sharp HL (1983). Graft-versus-host disease of the intestine: a protein losing enteropathy characterized by fecal α_1-antitrypsin. Gastroenterology 85:1076-1081.

Exp. Hematol. (suppl. 17) 13:110 (1985)
© International Society for Experimental Hematology

Factors Associated with Infections After Bone-Marrow Transplantation

T. Paulin, O. Ringdén, B. Lönnqvist, B. Wahren, B. Nilsson, and G. Gahrton

Departments of Clinical Immunology, Transplantation Surgery, Clinical Haematology and Oncology,
Department of Medicine, Huddinge Hospital,
Department of Virology, National Bacteriological Laboratory, and
Department of Cancer Epidemiology, Karolinska Hospital, Stockholm, Sweden

Due to immunoincompetence, infectious complications are major sources of morbidity and mortality following bone marrow transplantation (BMT). We have analysed prognostic factors associated with cytomegalovirus infections and late infections after BMT.

Patients and methods

1975-1983, 73 patients received BMT, of whom 58 had hematological malignancies, 14 had aplastic anemia and one had Gaucher´s disease. Conditioning was mainly according to the Seattle protocol. Attempts to isolate CMV were made before transplantation, weekly during the first 12 weeks after BMT, at least monthly during the first half year, and in addition, whenever an infection was suspected. Antibodies were measured by ELISA. 14 prognostic factors were analysed in relation to CMV infection. Six prognositic factors were studied in relation to major bacterial, fungal and non-CMV hepatitis infections, as well as varicellae zoster, occurring more than one month post-BMT. An infection was considered to have occurred if there was a positive culture and/or isolation and if treatment was given. Each prognostic factor was bivariately analysed using the life table method, and the simultaneous effects of several factors were analysed by regression technique (Cox et al. 1972).

RESULTS

41 patients had an active CMV infection with an actuarial incidence at one year of 68%. CMV serology of the recipient was of utmost importance for the subsequent development of CMV infection (Table 1). Among the prognostic factors that were associated with CMV infection were high recipient age, high donor age and administration of white cells (w.c.). In multivariat analyses, the impact of negative recipient serology was so strong that it obscured the contribution of the other analysed factors to the prognosis for achieving CMV infection. If this factor was controlled for in a stepwise hazard regression analysis, w.c. was highly significant (p=0.005), and if w.c. was controlled for, a low marrow dose predisposed to CMV infection compared to high dose (p=0.03). None of the 14 analysed factors were significantly associated with symptomatic disease. However, the ability to answer with a significant titer rise after BMT was lowered in patients with interstitial pneumonitis (i.p.) compared to patients with other clinical symptoms of the CMV infection (p<0.01; Mann Whitney U test).

Bacterial, fungal, non CMV hepatitis and varicella zoster (v.z.) infections were divided into pulmonary and systemic infections, and also analysed as one group ("total"), with and without v.z. Patients who had been infected in any of these ways had a higher frequency of low marrow cell dose (<3x10^8 cells/kg, p<0.01), had experienced acute GVHD (p<0.001), were splenectomised (p<0.01) and had experienced CMV (p<0.05) when "Total" infections (v.z. excl.) were analysed (Table 2).

Conclusion

A positive patient CMV serology prior to BMT was of utmost importance for the subsequent development of CMV infection. Other predisposing factors were high donor and recipient age, and transfusions of white cells. CMV infection, low marrow cell dose, splenectomy and GVHD all predisposed to late infections.

Table 1. Donor and recipient serology prior to BMT and incidence of subsequent CMV infection

Patient groups	Compared subgroups	No of pat	Actuarial CMV inf, 9 months	p-value
All	Recipient CMV-/CMV+	22/45	35/87	0.0001
All with known donor serology	Donor CMV-/CMV+	23/31	52/80	0.026
CMV- donors	Recipient CMV-/CMV+	14/9	24/100	0.00009
CMV+ donors	Recipient	4/27	25/88	0.03

Table 2. Incidence of bacterial, fungal and non-CMV hepatitis. "Total" infection (v.z. excl.)

Factor	Compared subgroups	No of pat	% with inf at 1 year	p-value
Marrow dose x 10^8/kg	<3/>3	35/32	67/26	0.0006
CMV inf	No/yes	23/44	28/53	0.05
Splenect	No/yes	61/6	41/83	0.006
Acute GVHD	gr 0-I/ II-IV	49/18	37/70	0.0001
Chron GVHD	No/yes	50/17	44/48	0.68

Ref: Cox DR: Regression models and life-tables. JR Stat Soc Series B 34: 187-220, 1972.

Diagnosis of Graft Versus Host Disease

Exp. Hematol. (suppl. 17) 13:111 (1985)
© International Society for Experimental Hematology

Neopterin Levels in Serum After Bone Marrow Transplantation are Possibly Helpful to Estimate the Activity of Graft-Versus-Host-Disease

P. Kalhs [1], M. Fischer [1], R. Dudczak [1], W. Hinterberger [2], B. Volc-Platzer [1], K. Lechner [1], H. Frischauf [1], I. Schwarzinger [1], and E. Deutsch [1]

[1] First Department of Medicine and
[2] First Department of Dermatology, University of Vienna, Austria

Introduction: Neopterin, (Npt, 6-1', 2', 3'-D-erythro-trihydroxy)prop-y-pteridin) is formed from Guanosine-Triphosphate during the biosynthesis of Tetra-hydrobiopterine, a co-factor of aromatic hydroxylation. The biological function of Npt is not yet known. It has been shown, that stimulation of T-lymphocytes in viral infections and malignant disorders may cause elevation of Npt levels in serum and urine (1,2,3,4). The aim of this study was to evaluate the usefulness of regular radioimmunological determinations of serum-Npt levels in human bone marrow graft recipients suffering from GVH-D reactions.

Patients and Methods: 6 patients (1f, 5m, 18-39 years), after receiving allografts for CML (n=3), AML-CR (n=2) and SAA (n=1), were studied. Acute and chronic GVH-D reactions were defined by clinical criteria and histological examinations of the skin (Volc-Platzer, this issue). Npt serum samples were studied on alternate days by means of a commercially available radioimmunoassay-kit (Henning-Berlin). Ingredients from one assay were used throughout each study. Intra- and Interassay variation coefficients at low Npt serum levels were 7.1 and 13.1 %, and at high serum levels 8.5 and 14.6 %, respectively. The mean Npt level in the serum of 12 normal individuals was 1.15+0.37 ng/ml.

Results: 5 of 6 patients developed acute (n=4) and/or chronic (n=3) GVH-D reactions.
Following conditioning with TBI and Cyclophosphamide, baseline Npt levels had decreased by 55±28 %. During periods of acute GVH-D, Npt serum levels ranged from 15-41 ng/ml (peak levels). During chronic GVH-D reactions, peak levels ranged from 4-14 ng/ml. It seemed, that the increase of Npt preceded the clinical and histological manifestations of acute GVH-D (Table 1).

Npt levels returned to normal after successful immunosuppression (example shown in Figure 1). In a few patients who recently passed the first 100 days without GVH-D reactions, no increase of Npt levels during haemo-lymphatic reconstitution was seen.

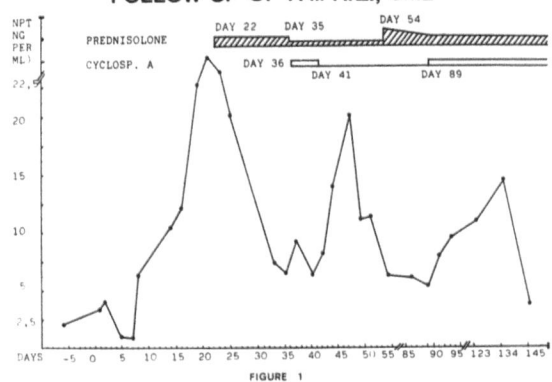

FOLLOW UP OF PAT. H.E., CML

FIGURE 1

Discussion: Decreasing Npt levels during the conditioning procedure seem to confirm the concept that Npt is a sensitive indicator of T-lymphocyte activation (5,6). This concept is further supported by the observation of decreasing Npt levels after successful immunosuppression. We feel that Npt estimations, in the future, may successfully be used to monitor a number of T-cell mediated reactions, such as GVH-D, viral infection and possibly graft rejection. Thus, Npt levels may serve as a sensitive, although not specific, indicator of T-cell activation and may in selected clinical situations support therapeutic decisions.

NPT.-INCREASE AND HISTOLOGICALLY VERIFIED GVHD

PATIENT	NPT.-INCREASE DAY	CUT. HIST. POS. DAY	DIFFERENCE (DAYS)
H.E.,CML	8	12	4
S.F.,AML	13	23	10
U.A.,AML	13	22	9
M.A.,AA	16	24	8
H.J.,CML	26	39	13
x̄ ∓ SD			8,8 ∓ 3,27

References:
1. Wachter et al, Hoppe-Seyler'Zschrft Physiol. Chemie 360, 1957-1960, (1979)
2. Hausen et al, Clin Chim Acta 117, 297-305, (1981).
3. Fuchs et al, in: Chemistry and Biology of Peridines. Eds: Blair, J.A., 885-890, Walter de Gruyter, Berlin, New York (1983).
4. Fink et al, in: Biochemical and Clinical Aspects of Pteridines, Vol 2. Eds: Wachter, H., Curtius, H., Pfleiderer, W., 223-234, Walter de Gruyter, Berlin, New York (1983).
5. Huber et al, Klin. Wschrft. 62, 103-113 (1984).
Huber et al, J.Exp.Med. 160, 310-316 (1984).

Supported by Grant 4100 of the "Fonds zu Förderung der Wissenschaftlichen Forschung in Österreich" and by the "Kommission für Leukämieforschung und Knochenmarktransplantation" of the Austrian Academy of Sciences

Exp. Hematol. (suppl. 17) 13:112–113 (1985)
© International Society for Experimental Hematology

Monoclonal Antibody Purging of Bone Marrow Using CAMPATH 1 and UCHT 1 for Matched and Mismatched Family Allogeneic Bone Marrow Transplantation

R. L. Powles[1], G. D. Goss[1], Ann Barrett[1], J. Millar[1], M. Gore[1], F. Porta[2], P. Pimentel[1], S. Bagnulo[1], and F. Hernandez[1]

[1] The Royal Marsden Hospital, Downs Road, Sutton, Surrey SM2 5PT, Great Britain
[2] Clinica Pediatrica, Universita di Pavia, Pavia, Italy

INTRODUCTION

In a series of 96 matched sibling bone marrow transplants treated for acute leukaemia, in which the sole prophylaxis against graft versus host disease was cyclosporin given for six months after transplant. Fatal graft versus host disease occurred in 5% of patients,[1] although 70% developed the syndrome) and the overall cure rate for this group of patients was approximately 50%.[2] There were two major causes of death. The first was a leukaemic relapse rate of approximately 12%,[1] and the second was a multiorgan failure syndrome characterised by a vascular endothelial lesion leading to fatal pulmonary oedema in many instances (20%).[3] In a series of 35 transplants where the donors were family members mismatched for one haplotype and cyclosporin without purging was used as prophylaxis against graft versus host disease, the incidence of fatal vascular endothelial problems was 35%.[3] In this original series marrow engraftment and graft versus host disease were not a major problem.

Because of the higher incidence of the vascular endothelial problem in mismatched transplant patients, we feel that a factor involved in its aetiology is a form of graft versus host disease. However, there is also evidence to suggest that cyclosporin may be implicated. In an attempt to reduce this problem, five pilot studies using bone marrow purged of immunocompetent lymphocytes prior to transplant have been undertaken. The goal has been to improve the results in our mismatched bone marrow transplant programme, although some of the logistics of using monoclonal antibody purged marrow in our matched programme needed to be worked out. There were ethical considerations that needed to be taken into account when using purged marrow without cyclosporin in matched bone marrow transplants because as we have already shown the cure rate of first remission AML patients under the age of 16 treated with unpurged marrow and cyclosporin is approximately 80%.[2] However, the results from other groups using monoclonal purged marrow suggested that similar results could be obtained without the use of cyclosporin.

Study 1

Our initial study was undertaken between 26 June 1983 and 7 March 1984. Five patients received one haplotype mismatched bone marrow transplants from family members after conditioning with cyclophosphamide and total body irradiation. The marrow prior to infusion was treated with the mouse IgG monoclonal antibody UCHT1 which does not bind complement and has a spectrum of activity similar to OKT_3. The antibody was incubated with a mononuclear cell fraction of the marrow, and the marrow dose for the recipients was 0.33 to 0.8 x 10^9/kg (m 0.66). The marrow was washed and then infused in an attempt to obtain opsonization of antibody bound cells. Cyclosporin was given intravenously for 5 days in a dose of 8 mg/kg from the day prior to BMT and then oral cyclosporin was given thereafter at a dose of 8 mg/kg/day. Of the 5 patients 4 had prompt engraftment, one had failure of graft-take and died at day 21. Three of the other patients developed fatal leaky vascular endothelium with pulmonary oedema, and one died of a cerebral haemorrhage.

Study 2

Because of the many other problems involved in mismatched BMT that make the interpretation of marrow purging difficult a small pilot study involving purged donor marrow from HLA matched siblings was undertaken. Between 14 March 1984 and 30 May 1984 this study involved 8 patients (5 remission AML). A Ficoll metrizoate mononuclear cell preparation of the marrow was made (marrow dose 0.28-0.85 x 10^8/kg (m 0.53) and this was treated with CAMPATH 1 100 µg/ml, at room temperature, without complement lysis and the marrow was then infused. No other immunosuppression was used i.e. these patients did not receive any cyclosporin. Of these 8 patients 5 needed retransplanting, and no patient had a polymorph count of >0.5 x 10^9/l in less than 39 days. Four of the 8 patients have died, 2 of graft failure, one of leukaemia and one of cyclosporin toxicity. In the last patient cyclosporin was used as prophylaxis against GVHD following retransplantation. This was the only patient in this study who developed acute GVHD. Two patients in this study relapsed (one died), one of whom was a first remission AML.

Study 3

In July 1984 a small workshop involving all groups using the monoclonal antibody CAMPATH1 was held in London. Fifty patients were reviewed. It became apparent that the cell dose of bone marrow after CAMPATH treatment was a critical factor and that the use of buffy coat preparation rather than a mononuclear cell preparation prior to the addition of CAMPATH was important. Seven patients were included in this study (6 first remission AML) and the marrow dose given ranged from $1.02-3 \times 10^8$/kg (m 1.92). No patients received cyclosporin after transplantation. Of these 7 patients 2 required retransplantation, and one of these was due to a drop in platelets associated with a viral infection. This patient had a prompt return of a normal blood count within two days after transplant. Six of the 7 patients remain alive and one patient has relapsed. Only one patient in this group developed acute graft versus host disease. The time following transplant to the appearance of 0.5×10^9/l polymorphs in the peripheral blood in this group of patients ranged from 15 - 28 days (m 19).

Study 4

It was felt that the information learnt concerning the purging of marrow in matched transplants could be used in our mismatched bone marrow transplant programme. In this study as in Study 1 cyclosporin plus marrow purging was used. Buffy coat marrow was treated with CAMPATH and cyclosporin was started the day prior to transplant and given for 5 days followed by oral cyclosporin. Two patients were included in the study and the marrow dose was 1.6 and 1.8×10^8/kg. One patient had total failure of engraftment inspite of two further attempts at retransplantation and the other patient had prompt engraftment but cyclosporin was stopped at 10 days, and three weeks after transplant the graft was rejected. Neither of these patients developed acute graft versus host disease.

Study 5

The studies outlined above and our major cyclosporin programme for matched transplant indicated that a factor producing the multi-organ failure due to vascular endothelial damage was the use of high dose intravenous cyclosporin. We also felt that the graft rejection of purged marrow in the mismatched programme was due to inadequate immuno-suppression of the patient. We did not wish to increase the immunosuppression of the patient using further cytotoxic agents during the induction regimen because of the additional toxic consequences. An alternative was to give oral cyclosporin from 21 days prior to transplant so that by the time the marrow was given the cyclosporin would be exerting an immunosuppressive effect on the patient. This would avoid the use of high doses of intravenous cyclosporin, and would be sufficiently immunosuppressive to permit engraftment of a mismatched graft (when coupled with the cyclophosphamide and total body irradiation). Five patients have been

included in this study (4 first remission AML) and obviously follow-up is at present short. The donors were all family members with a one haplotype mismatch with AB and/or CD antigens foreign to the recipient. The marrow dose was $2-3.9 \times 10^8$/kg (m 2.96). The results of these 5 transplants are as follows: the first patient is now 15 weeks since transplant with good engraftment and apart from weight loss and some mild chest symptoms is alive and well. The second patient is 13 weeks after transplant and karyotypic studies have shown that there has been auto-reconstitution. The patient is well without problems. The third patient is 8 weeks from transplant has good engraftment and does not have problems. Of the 2 remaining patients one died of bilateral pneumothoraces (possibly CMV related) three weeks after transplant. Bone marrow biopsy and the blood count showed good engraftment. The fifth patient is now four weeks after transplant, has no evidence of engraftment and is being retransplanted with her own cryo-reserved remission marrow.

The lesson learnt from these five patients is that prompt engraftment within 21 days of transplant occurred in three of the five patients and there has been no evidence of multi-organ failure or vascular endothelial damage. One patient developed grade 2 GVHD. The only valid conclusions that can be drawn from this study at present is that it is ethically justifiable to continue although obviously larger numbers and longer follow-up will be requried before a statement can be made upon its long-term efficacy.

Concluding Remarks

These five pilot studies have shown that CAMPATH purged marrow without cyclosporin in matched transplants is associated with a very low incidence of GVHD (2/21). Also we have shown that the cell inoculum to prevent failure of graft take is important with 5 out of 8 patients requiring retransplantation when buffy coat was used. In addition we feel that intravenous cyclosporin is probably toxic to the endothelium. Lastly, if cyclophosphamide plus TBI are used as the conditioning regimen for mismatched transplants then oral cyclosporin should be given for at least three weeks prior to infusion of the marrow to allow the host to accept the graft.

References

1. Powles RL, Clink HM, Spence D, et al. Cyclosporin A to prevent graft versus host disease in man after allogeneic bone marrow transplantation. Lancet i: 327-329, 1980.

2. Powles RL, Goss GD, Millar J, et al. Prevention of graft versus host disease following allogeneic bone marrow transplantation. Proceedings of Tokai University Symposium on Basic and Clinical Problems in Bone Marrow Transplantation (1984). In Press.

3. Powles RL, Pedrazzini A, Crofts M, et al. Mismatch Family Bone Marrow Transplantation. Sem Haematol XXI; 3: 182-187.

Exp. Hematol. (suppl. 17) 13:114 (1985)
© International Society for Experimental Hematology

T-Cell Depletion with Campath 1 to Prevent GVHD

J. Hows[1], J. Apperley[1], J. Yin[1], G. Hale[2], H. Waldman[2], J. Goldman[1], and E. Gordon-Smith[1]

[1] Department of Haematology, Hammersmith Hospital, London
[2] Department of Immunology, Addenbrooks Hospital, Cambridge, Great Britain

We have transplanted 34 patients using the rat IgM monoclonal antibody Campath 1 (Hale et al 1983) to prevent GVHD by T lymphocyte depletion. Campath 1 has panlymphocyte specificity and is lytic with human complement in vitro.

PATIENTS AND METHODS

Patients transplanted include 24 with chronic granulocytic leukaemia (CGL), 6 with severe acquired aplastic anaemia (SAA) and 4 with Fanconi anaemia (FA). 25 donors were HLA identical siblings, 4 were HLA phenotypic matches and 5 were HLA mismatches for 1 or 2 antigens (Table 1).

Table 1 - Patients transplanted using Campath 1

| Disease | Median age | HLA match donor/recipient | | | |
		Id Sib	Pheno	M/M	Total
CGL	30 (8-45)	20	1	3	24
SAA	16 (7-32)	4	0	2	6
FA	10	1	3	0	4

Pretransplant conditioning was with cyclophosphamide (CP) 50 mg/kg x 4 for SAA, CP 5 mg/kg x 4 and TBI 3 x 200 cGy for FA, CP 60 mg/kg x 2, daunorubicin 60 mg/m², RBI 200 x 5 or 6 cGy and splenic irradiation 500 x 2 cGy for CGL. 30/34 patients received cyclosporine post transplant starting on Day -1. Donor marrow was treated with Campath 1 100 µg/ml and 20-25% v/v donor serum as the complement source.

RESULTS

1. Marrow treatment: The treated marrow contained 1.3-4.4 x 10⁸/kg (mean 2.8 x 10⁸/kg) nucleated cells and 0-1% (mean 0.3%) residual E+ mononuclear cells.
2. Peripheral blood recovery: 20/34 patients regenerated satisfactorily. The mean time to 0.5 x 10⁹/l neutrophils was 19 days (range 10-30). 8 patients did not engraft. This included 5/5 patients transplanted from HLA mismatched donors and 3/4 patients transplanted for SAA from HLA identical sibling donors. One additional patient developed late graft failure on Day +43. Survival of marrow

GM-CFC after Campath treatment was very variable (5-120%) and did not correlate with in vivo engraftment.
3. GVHD: 18/26 evaluable patients had Grade 0-1 acute GVHD, 4/26 had Grade II and 3/26 >Grade II disease. 5/20 evaluable patients have limited chronic GVHD.
4. Survival: The overall survival of patients following BMT with Campath treated marrow is shown in Table 2.

Table 2 - Survival* following BMT using Campath 1

| Disease | HLA match donor/recipient | | |
	Id Sib	Pheno	M/M
CGL	16/20	1/1	0/3
SAA	3/4	-	1/2
FA	1/1	3/3	-
TOTAL	20/25 (75%)	4/4 (100%)	1/5 (20%)

*Follow up 64-881 days post BMT.

CONCLUSIONS

1. Preliminary results of CAMPATH treatment in BMT for CGL and FA from HLA identical or phenotypically matched donors are encouraging. In this group of patients the incidence of severe GVH was low and engraftment was satisfactory.
2. Using current immunosuppressive protocols and CAMPATH treatment, the incidence of graft failure is unacceptably high in patients transplanted from HLA mismatched donors and in patients transplanted for SAA from HLA identical sibling donors. Further work is required to determine the underlying mechanisms for graft failure of T-depleted marrow. More powerful immunosuppressive protocols may be required to reduce the incidence of graft failure in the high risk patient groups defined above.

REFERENCE
Hale G, Bright S, Chumbley et al (1983). Removal of T cells from bone marrow for transplantation. An immodonal antilymphocyte antibody that fixes human complement. Blood 62 873-882.

Exp. Hematol. (suppl. 17) 13:115–116 (1985)
© International Society for Experimental Hematology

T Depletion Using MBG6 and RFT8 Monoclonal Antibody Combination and Complement Lysis Prevents Significant Acute and Chronic GvHD in HLA Matched Allogeneic Marrow Transplants

H. G. Prentice, M. K. Brenner, G. Janossy, M. J. M. L. Gilmore, J. Patterson, J.-P. Grob, K. Ivory, D. Skeggs, S. Graphakos, A. Thomas, and A. V. Hoffbrand

Departments of Haematology, Immunology and Radiotherapy, Royal Free Hospital, London NW3 2QG, Great Britain

INTRODUCTION

Forty-one patients have received marrow from HLA-matched sibling donors with in vitro T-depletion using 2 monoclonal antibodies MBG6 and RFT8 and rabbit complement. No other immunosuppression was given. Engraftment occurred in 39 of 40 evaluable patients. The incidence of acute and chronic GvHD is minimal with a Royal Free acute GvHD score for the group of 0.07. The incidence of viral infections is low with no fatalities. Of the 20 evaluable patients transplanted in 1st CR of AL or 1st CP of CGL, only one patient has had a leukaemic relapse to date (CGL/BT). In poor risk patients who have a high relapse incidence the conditioning has been modified

A further 11 patients have received T-depleted marrow from HLA mismatched donors. In this group the incidence of rejection has been approximately 50%, and conditioning has been modfied in an effort to prevent rejection. Prevention of GvHD in this group is less impressive.

1. HLA MATCHED BMT.

Patient characteristics.

1CR of AL or 1CP	All Others
n = 20 (12 M and 8 F)	n = 21 (12 M and 9 F)
7 AML	8 ALL 2 CR
7 ALL	5 ALL Ref/Rel
6 CGL	2 AML Ref/Rel
$\bar{x}$ age = 25 years	3 CGL AP/BT
	3 Thalassaemia/Aplastic Anaemia/Fanconis Anaemia
	$\bar{x}$ age = 21 years

Marrow Treatment: After harvest (x = 3.4 x 10^8/kg range 1.8-9.1) donor mononuclear cells were incubated with MBG6 (anti-T12) + RFT8 (anti-T8) and rabbit complement (1). A mean of 0.39 x 10^8/kg cells were infused (range 0.14-0.99 x 10^8/kg).

% T-Depletion

	No.
82 - 90%	2
91 - 95%	2
96 - 100%	36
NE	1

The range of T cells infused was 0-0.02 x 10^8 T cells/kg (median of 0.0027 x 10^8/kg).

Engraftment: Engraftment occurred in 39 of 40 evaluable patients (1 patient died at day +8 from cardiac failure). Engraftment has been sustained in all cases. A WBC >1 x 10^9/l was achieved by a mean of 23 days (range 12 to 37) and neutrophils >0.5 x 10^9/l by mean of 27 days (range 13 to 72 days).

GvHD:
Incidence of acute GvHD:

No. T-depleted	Evaluable (60 days+)		Grade				
			0	I	II	III	IV
41	35		26	7	1*	1	0

* SAA.

Chronic GvHD: Chronic GvHD occurred in 4 of 35 evaluable patients, in one case without preceding acute GvHD. It was minimal in three and resolved in all patients with steroids (± Azathioprine).

In vitro and clinical details of 10 patients who developed acute or chronic GvHD.

Status	UPN	Age	% T-Depl.	Abs. No. T cells x 10^8/kg	GvHD		
Rel	73	10	>98.5	<0.0032	I	→	C
AP	91	36	>99	0	I	→	O
1 CR	94	30	99.43	0.001	0	→	C
Rel	99	18	97.77	0.0022	I	→	O
BT	104	39	97.90	0.0027	I	→	O
1 CR	109	42	98.46	0.0018	I	→	C
1 CP	110	31	81.65	0.0191	III	→	C
AA	120	19	88.69	0.02	II	→	O
1 CR	121	21	91.37	0.0191	I	→	O
2 CR	125	12	96.12	0.015	I	→	O

The 2 patients with the most severe grades of GvHD (UPN's 110 and 120, Grade III and II respectively) received the greatest numbers of T cells.

Infections: No fatal viral infections have occurred. Four patients have developed CMV infections, including 2 with pneumonitis. Both patients with pneumonitis recovered on trial hyperimmune CMV immunoglobulin (Biotest). Three of the 4 cases occurred in patients with GvHD.

Leukaemic Relapse: Only one patient transplanted in 1 CR or 1 CP has had a leukaemic relapse with a median follow up of 6.8months (range 0.25 to 20.5 months: (Fig. 1).

116

The quality of life within this group is excellent with a median KS of 100%. However, 12 of 18 patients transplanted beyond 1st CR or 1st CP have subsequently relapsed.

FIGURE 1.

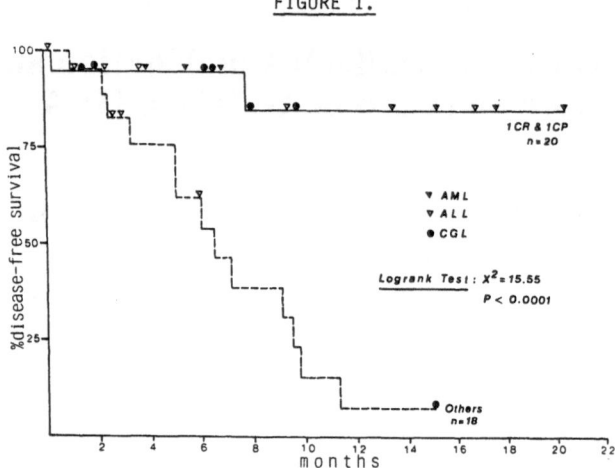

ACTUARIAL DISEASE-FREE SURVIVAL FOR

T-DEPLETED BMT:1CR or 1CP versus Others

Immune Reconstitution: Recipients of T cell depleted grafts do not demonstrate the T8 overshoot usually associated with allogeneic BMT. In addition NK cell activity returns rapidly in these recipients and donor B cell immunity can be adoptively transferred.

2. HLA-mismatched BMT: Eleven patients have received T-depleted marrow from HLA mismatched donors (9 sibling, 2 parental). This was a poorer prognostic group which included: 5 patients in 2 CR (3 AML, 2 ALL), 1 patient in PR of AML, 2 patients with ref/relapsed disease, 2 patients with CGL in 1st CP and 1 in AP. Engraftment occurred after the first BMT, in 6 patients only (55%). (One other patient engrafted after a second infusion of unmanipulated marrow). The 7 patients evaluable for GvHD had a RF GvHD score of 0.32. In an attempt to prevent rejection the conditioning has been modified twice. The first 4 patients were conditioned with single dose radiation and Cyclophosphamide 60mg/kg x 2. Two engrafted, another required a 2nd BMT. The next 6 patients were conditioned with fractionated TBI (950 rads 3 fractions over 3 days) plus Cyclosporin A and Prednisolone. Three patients engrafted. The 11th patient, the first in the new series, received our Wisconsin (modified) protocol: Single fraction TBI (7.5Gy), high dose Ara-C and Cyclophosphamide (see Discussion). This patient engrafted on Day + 18.

DISCUSSION

Conditioning: Of 41 HLA matched patients the first 31 leukaemic patients were conditioned with single dose, fast rate radiation (7.5Gy at 26cGy/min in air) and Cyclophosphamide 60mg/kg x 2 (conditioning differed for the 3 patients with Fanconi's anaemia, aplastic anaemia and thalassaemia). This

conditioning proved excellent for permitting engraftment which occurred in all but 1 patient. However beyond 1st CR or 1st CP this conditioning has not proved adequate for preventing leukaemic relapse for those transplanted other than patients in 1 CR or 1 CP. In this group the incidence of leukaemic relapse is high. Thus for this category of patient we now use the Wisconsin (modified) protocol: Ara-C 3g/m² 12 hrly x 6 Cyclophosphamide 45mg/kg x 2 and single dose TBI 7.5Gy. All 4 patients conditioned with this protocol have engrafted. At only 4 months since its introduction it is too early to know the effect on the incidence of leukaemic relapse. This protocol has also been extended to all HLA mismatched transplants, who receive in addition Cycloporin A (5mg/kg/day) and Prednisolone 1-2mg/kg/day) to prevent rejection.

GvHD: Only ten patients have developed any GvHD. The 2 patients who developed more severe GvHD were amongst the three receiving the highest T cell numbers. However the other patients received small numbers of T cells (0.0-0.019 x 10^8/kg). 3 of our 4 cases of CMV infection have occurred in patients with GvHD. This finding may help clarify the relationship between infection and GvHD.

CONCLUSIONS

HLA matched T-depleted BMT:
1. T cell depletion can be achieved with monoclonal antibodies and rabbit complement but further technical improvements are required.
2. T cell depletion alone prevents significant aGvHD and cGvHD.
3. An apparent reduction in CMV infections may be related to a reduction in the incidence of GvHD.
4. Engraftment occurs with the current conditioning protocols.
5. One patient only transplanted in 1 CR or 1 CP has had leukaemic relapse to date.
6. More intensive anti-leukaemic conditioning may reduce the risk of subsequent relapse in poor risk patients.

HLA-mismatched T depleted BMT.
1. In mismatched BMT T cell depletion may not be adequate to totally prevent GvHD.
2. Graft rejection or "non-take" is a major problem, but data from other centres suggests that more immunosuppressive conditioning may allow us to overcome rejection.

REFERENCES

1. Prentice, HG, Blacklock HA, Janossy G. et al. Depletion of T lymphocytes in donor marrow prevents significant graft versus host disease in matched allogeneic leukaemic marrow transplant recipients. Lancet 1984:472-476.
2. Patterson J, Prentice HG, Gilmore M. et al. Analysis of rejection in HLA matched T depleted bone marrow transplants. (This issue).

Exp. Hematol. (suppl. 17) 13:117 (1985)
© International Society for Experimental Hematology

Analysis of Rejection in HLA Matched T-Depleted Bone Marrow Transplants

J. Patterson[1], H. G. Prentice[1], M. Gilmore[1], H. Blacklock[9], M. K. Brenner[1], G. Janossy[1], D. Skeggs[1], K. Ivory[1],
A. V. Hoffbrand[1], J. Apperley[2], J. Goldman[2], A. Burnett[3], J. Gribben[3], M. Alcorn[3], C. Pearson[3], I. McVickers[3],
I. Hann[4], C. Reid[5], D. Wardle[6], A. Bacigalupo[7], and A. G. Robertson[8]

[1] Royal Free Hospital, London
[2] Hammersmith Hospital, London
[3] Royal Infirmary, Glasgow
[4] Royal Hospital for Sick Children, Glasgow
[5] Northwick Park Hospital, London
[6] Harley St. Clinic, London
[7] Ospedale San Martino, Genova, Italy
[8] Glasgow Institute of Radiotherapeutics and Oncology, Glasgow
[9] G.O.S. Hospital for Sick Children, London

INTRODUCTION

In February 1984 a collaborative trial was begun using the Royal Free (RF) cocktail of MBG6 and RFT8 monoclonal antibodies to T-deplete donor marrow for allogeneic BMT for leukaemia. The trial followed the successful use of the cocktail in 25 patients. A proportion of patients from all centres experienced rejection of the graft. Because of this serious problem, T-depletion was temporarily suspended at the other centres. In the parent institution all but 1 of the subsequent 13 grafts were successful. Rejection occurred in 3 forms : no engraftment at all; partial or complete engraftment followed by early loss of graft, or late loss of graft (at 4 months). Preliminary data from centres using other anti-T cell monoclonal antibodies and from this study strongly implicate the pre-transplant conditioning as being critical to successful, sustained engraftment.

Patients. Nine patients receiving MBG6 and RFT8 T-depleted BMTs have experienced rejection. Only 1 case occurred in 38 (2.6%) patients transplanted at the RF, whereas 8 rejections occurred amongst 13 (62%) patients at participating centres. The 9 patients (4 male, 5 female; age range 2 - 37 years, median 18 years) included 6 with ALL, 2 with CGL and 1 with AML. Three patients were in 1st CR, 4 in 2nd CR and 2 in 1st CP. All were HLA matched with their sibling donors.

CONDITIONING

Chemotherapy. Four regimens of intensive chemotherapy were used. All were based on Cyclophosphamide 60mg/kg x 2 except for one patient who received high dose Melphalan (100mg/m^2).

Radiotherapy. All 8 patients at the participating centres received fractionated TBI 10-12Gy in 5-6 fractions over 3 days, whereas all patients at the parent centre receive single dose TBI (7.5Gy at 26cGy/min in air).

Marrow treatment. Marrow mononuclear cells were incubated with MBG6 and RFT8 and rabbit complement according to the RF in vitro manipulation protocol, (3 of the T depletions were performed by the RF). There was no deviation from the in vitro manipulation protocol at other centres and the degree of T depletion and preservation of CFU-GM were similar at all centres.

Rejection. An increment in P.B. granulocytes or marrow evidence was considered indicative of engraftment. Three patterns of rejection occurred.

Non-engraftment. Three patients did not achieve neutrophils of >0.5 x 10^9/1 and 1 patient had no increment in WBC.

Complete or partial engraftment followed by early loss of graft. Three patients achieved neutrophils >0.5 x 10^9/1 which decreased from day +12 on.

Delayed loss of graft. Two patients lost their grafts at 4 months. Both had engrafted promptly.

Infections. Viral infections occurred in 4 patients, including H. Zoster from day +2 in the 1 patient with no increment.

GvHD. GvHD (skin only, Grade II) occurred in 3 patients.

Regrafting. Regrafting was attempted in 7 patients, 5 with non-manipulated marrow of whom 2 engrafted. Two regrafted with manipulated marrow failed to engraft.

CONCLUSIONS.

The incidence of rejection at other centres following MBG6 and RFT8 T-depleted BMT is 62% c.f. 2.6% at the RF. There was no difference in marrow manipulation and T depletion between centres. The major difference in management between the RF and all other centres was the radiation conditioning, all RF patients receive single dose 7.5Gy TBI at a fast rate (26cGy/min in air) c.f. all other centres used fractionated TBI of 10-12Gys. Thus there appears to be a narrow therapeutic window for TBI where T depletion is used. We conclude that rejection appears to be largely preventable by adequate radiation conditioning.

REFERENCES

1. Prentice, H.G., Brenner, M.K., Janossy, G. et al. Exp. Haem.(This issue).

Exp. Hematol. (suppl. 17) 13:118 (1985)
© International Society for Experimental Hematology

An Immunological Analysis of Three Cases of Bone Marrow Failure Associated with Campath-I-Incubation

D. Bunjes, M. Wiesneth, Th. Schmeiser, R. Arnold, and W. Heit

Department of Internal Medicine III, University of Ulm, D-7900 Ulm, Federal Republic of Germany

Introduction: T-cell purging is effective in preventing GvHD but increases the risk of graft failure (1). We have observed two cases of graft rejection and one episode of reversible bone marrow hypoplasia in three leukaemic patients who had received a HLA-identical graft incubated with Campath-I. An analysis of the mechanism of rejection has been performed using immunological techniques and stem cell culture technology.

Patients and Methods: Patient data are given in Tbl.1

Table 1: Clinical data

Pat.	Dg.	Age sex	Blood group	Clinics	Time post BMT	Marrow dose x $10/kg$
1	CML	35F	D ABRh$^+$ R B Rh$^+$	Pancyt.	d 60	1.6
2	AML	30F	D A Rh$^+$ R O Rh$^+$	graft reject.	d 20	2.2
3	AML	30M	D A Rh$^+$ R O Rh$^+$	graft reject.	d 60	1.6

D=Donor; R=Recipient, Pancyt.=Pancytopenia + BM-hypoplasia

Peripheral blood was drawn from patients during the rejection phase and peripheral blood mononuclear cells (PBMNC) were isolated using a Ficoll-Hypaque gradient. Donor bone marrow mononuclear cells (BMMNC), Ficoll-separated and cryopreserved at the time of transplantation were used as the source of stem cells whenever possible. Ficoll-separated fetal liver cells (FLC) were used as an alternative. Surface marker analysis of patient PBMNC was performed with standard indirect immunofluorescent techniques using the following antibodies: OKT3 (pan-T), OKT8 (T-killer/suppressor), OKT4 (T-helper), Leu7 (NK-cells), OKIa1 (framework DR). Y chromosome analysis and chromosome banding were performed with standard cytogenetic techniques. Patient PBMNC and supernants of these cells (unstimulated) were tested in stem cell assays (BFU-c, CFU-E, CFU-GM) using donor marrow (after incubation) or fetal liver cells as sources of stem cells

Results: The results are given in Table 2 a and b.

a)

Pat. Nr.	Origin of lymphocytes	OKT3	OKT8	OKT4	Leu7	OKIa1
1	n.c.	92%	83%	8%	38%	85%
2	h	88%	82%	34%	17%	73%
3	n.c.	90%	68%	24%	19%	70%

b)

pat.	Inhibition by 10^6 pat.cells$^+$		of supernant$^+$ (30%v/v)	
1	CFU-e$^+$:	89.2	CFU-e$^+$:	n.d.
	CFU-GM$^+$:	48.3	CFU-GM$^+$:	87.7
	BFU-e$^+$:	0	BFU-e$^+$:	0
2	CFU-e$^+$:	76.1	CFU-e$^+$:	27
	CFU-GM$^+$:	43.0	CFU-GM$^+$:	64
	BFU-e$^+$:	0	BFU-e$^+$:	0
3	CFU-e^{++} :	100	CFU-e^{++} :	22
	CFU-GM^{++} :	49,4	CFU-GM^{++} :	68.5
	BFU-e^{++} :	0	BFU-e^{++} :	0

Summary and Conclusions:

1. Graft failure is associated with the presence of presumably host-derived, activated T-killer/suppressor cells.

2. These cells inhibit hemopoietic stem cells in co-culture experiments. CFU-e appear to be more sensitive than CFU-GM, whereas BFU-e are not affected.

3. The inhibitory effect on CFU-GM seems to be mainly factormediated, whereas the effect on CFU-e seems mainly cellmediated.

(1) Martin PJ, Hansen JA, Storb, R, et al. Depletion of T cells in donor marrow for prevention of graft-versus-host disease. Abstracts of the 10th international Congress of the Transplantation Society 1984; 537.6:249

Exp. Hematol. (suppl. 17) 13:119 (1985)
© International Society for Experimental Hematology

The Use of Gradient Separated Stem Cell Grafts in HLA Matched Donor-Recipient Bone Marrow Transplantation

B. Löwenberg, G. Wagemaker, D. W. van Bekkum, W. Sizoo, K. Sintnicolaas, W. D. H. Hendriks, and A. Hagenbeek

The Dr. Daniel den Hoed Cancer, P.O. Box 5201, 3008 AE Rotterdam, The Netherlands

INTRODUCTION AND OBJECTIVE

In order to prevent the occurrence of GvHD (Graft-versus-Host-Disease) following the application of allogeneic bone marrow grafts, several groups have recently undertaken attempts to eliminate T-lymphocytes from the graft. In vitro treatment utilizing T-cell separation principles may also permit the employment of HLA mismatched bone marrow transplants with acceptable risks of GvHD and thus to extend this treatment modality to larger patient groups. Early data in a variety of centers, however, suggest that these advantages are counterbalanced by new problems, which are the direct consequence of the removal of T-cells. These difficulties mainly relate to a higher incidence of take failures. It is therefore conceivable that in "incomplete" removal of T-lymphocytes provides a better balance of GvHD prevention and restorative capacity of bone marrow transplants without compromising take.

We investigated the use of bone marrow stem cell concentrates obtained in a discontinuous albumin gradient from which on the average 90% of mature T-lymphocytes had been eliminated, and evaluated engraftment and the occurrence of GvHD in 9 HLA compatible bone marrow recipients. These patients were also placed on Cyclosporin A post transplantation for 6 months.

RESULTS AND CONCLUSION

The mean cell size and the mean number of T-lymphocytes in the grafts were 2.2×10^7 nucleated cells, 7.4×10^4 CFU-GM and 5×10^6 E rosette positive lymphocytes per kg body weight. Overall survival was in part influenced by the relatively unfavourable prognostic patient group selected for transplantation, in particular second remission AML (n=1), CML-blastic crisis (n=2). Seven of nine patients survived beyond 1 month post grafting and were considered evaluable. Of these, 5/7 patients developed acute GvHD, of which in two cases of moderately severe grade, and in two cases of minimal grade, and the other 2/7 did not show clinical signs of GvHD. Two patients developed histologically confirmed chronic GvHD, one de novo and one after a moderately severe acute GvHD syndrome. Five patients have died, i.e., from pneumococcus meningitis, AML recurrence, pneumonia (2) and interstitial pneumonia. Four patients currently survive at 16+ - 20+ mo in good health and free of leukemia. These data suggest that although GvHD was usually therapeutically manageable, this procedure of partial T-cell separation provides insufficient GvHD profylaxis.

Exp. Hematol. (suppl. 17) 13:120 (1985)
© International Society for Experimental Hematology

Prophylaxis of Graft Versus Host Disease Using Lymphocyte Depleted Marrow Followed by Short Term Immunosuppression

T. de Witte, A. Plas, E. Koekman, B. de Pauw, J. Wessels, and C. Haanen

Division of Hematology, Department of Internal Medicine, University Hospital, 8 Geert Grooteplein, 6525 GA Nijmegen, The Netherlands

Graft versus Host Disease (GVHD) is a major complication after allogeneic bone marrow transplantation (BMT), despite the prophylactic use of methotrexate (MTX) or cyclosporin (Cy). Several approaches have been investigated to reduce the incidence and severity of GVHD, postulating that acute GVHD arises from immunologically competent mature T-lymphocytes present in the graft. We have developed a method to remove lymphocytes from marrow grafts by combining density flotation centrifugation and counterflow centrifugation (1). A limitation till now was the small size of the chamber in the Beckman elutriator rotor, which made 5 to 6 consecutive runs of one hour necessary.

Recently a new set-up was developed containing 4 standard elutriaton chambers (Dijkstra BV, Amsterdam, The Netherlands). Several experiments showed that the separation profiles of the individual chambers was identical. An example with the data from 2 chambers is presented in fig. 1.

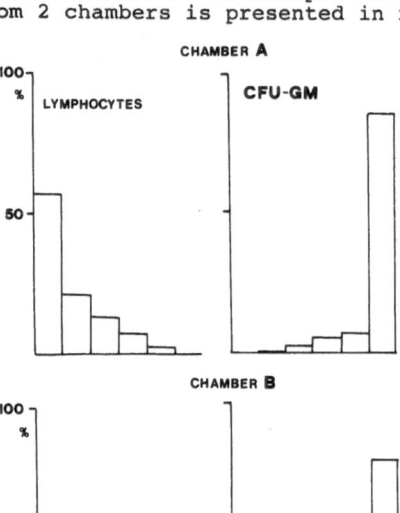

The recovery of the lymphocytes and the CFU-GM in the 6 fractions was identical in both chambers with an almost complete separation of the lymphocytes from the CFU-GM.

29 patients were transplanted with a lymphocyte depleted graft from a histocompatible sibling, as described before (2). Two patients received no prophylaxis after BMT. Both developed acute GVHD. 9 patients received MTX. GVHD was not observed, but 5 patients died from infectious complications (2). 18 patients received Cy (3 mg/kg iv or 9 mg/kg p.o.) for 6 weeks with a gradual tapering off and a discontinuation after 12 weeks; MTX (10 mg/kg iv) was given once weekly in week 5-16 post-BMT. 8 patients had acute leukemia and 10 patients had CML.

Table 1. Recovery (%) in the "stem cell" fraction after CC of BM from 18 donors.

Nucleated cells	11.1± 2.1
Lymphocytes	1.7± 1.4
E-rosette pos. cells	2.0± 1.4
CFU-GM	75.8±30.8
BFU-E	83.3±33.3

Only 2% of the original number of T-lymphocytes were present in the grafts. BM recovery was not impaired: leucocytes(>10*9/1): 13.9 ± 2.1 days; thrombocytes(>20x10*9/1): 18.0±6.6 days. None of the 18 patients developed acute GVHD. Ten patients have completed the GVHD-prophylaxis scheme. Cy was discontinued after 110±17 days and MTX 135±13 days post-BMT. 2 patients developed chronic GVHD of the skin (grade 1), which responded promptly to low dosages of Cy.

Conclusions:1. repopulation capacity after elimination of 98% of the T-lymphocytes by counterflow centrifugation was not impaired. 2. short term immunosuppression after BMT with lymphocyte depleted grafts offers an effective prevention of acute GVHD and severe chronic GVHD. 3. the new elutriation set-up with 4 separation chambers allows a rapid lymphocyte depletion within 2 hours.

References: 1. De Witte T, et al (1984) Transplantation 37: 151
2. De Witte T, et al (1984) Exp Hematol 12(suppl.15): 62

Exp. Hematol. (suppl. 17) 13:121–122 (1985)
© International Society for Experimental Hematology

T Cell Depletion of Marrow for the Prevention of Graft Versus Host Disease

W. Friedrich, S. F. Goldmann, R. Blütters-Sawatzki, W. Ebell, A. Raghavachar, E. Kleihauer, and B. Kubanek

Department of Pediatrics and Department of Transfusion Medicine, University of Ulm, D-7900 Ulm, Federal Republic of Germany

INTRODUCTION

Selective depletion of T cells from marrow grafts is an attractive approach to reduce the incidence and severity of GvHD. Recent studies in man clearly indicate that this approach is valid, opening the way to perform BMT across HLA barriers (1,2,3). However, this initial experience also reveals an increased risk of graft failures after transplantation of T cell depleted marrow, in particular when HLA non-identical donors are used (4). We report similar experience obtained in 24 patients transplanted with in vitro processed marrow from HLA matched and mismatched donors, using lectin agglutination and/or rosetting by sheep red cells for T cell depletion.

MATERIAL AND METHODS

The method of Reisner et al. (5) or a modification of it was used to remove T cells. In the former, marrow cells were agglutinated by soybean agglutinin (Vector Laboratories, Burlingame, California) followed by removal of residual T cells after rosette formation with SRBC treated by neuraminidase. In the latter, modified method, T cells were removed only by rosette formation. In HLA haploidentical BMT, rosetting was repeated as necessary to obtain final fractions completely free of T cells. Sheep red cells were obtained from two individual sheep selected from a flock of animals, screened for reproducibly high rosetting activity of human T cells.

RESULTS

Table 1 shows results obtained by the two procedures for T cell depletion regarding content and recoveries of nucleated marrow cells, CFU-c and T cells. Recoveries of stem cells, as determined by CFU-c, averaged at about 50 % with both procedures. However, a wide range of recoveries is apparent in the lectin method. A total of 24 pediatric patients were given T cell depleted marrow grafts. Underlying diseases were severe combined immunodeficiency (SCID) (n = 15), leukemia (n = 3), severe aplastic anemia (SAA) (n = 2), Wiskott Aldrich Syndrome (WAS) (n = 2), Chediak Higashi Syndrome (n = 1), Osteopetrosis (n = 1). All SCID patients received transplants from HLA haploidentical parents and, with one exception, grafts were processed by the lectin methods (table 2). Eleven patients with SCID survive from 8 to 32 months after BMT and have donor dependent, functioning T cell systems. Complications of GvHD developed in one patient only. In two surviving infants (SCID with ADA deficiency), cytoreductive conditioning treatment was used and was followed by prompt donor dependent hemopoietic reconstitution. In the other surviving patients no conditioning treatment was given and hemopoiesis remains of host type. Also in the latter group, functional B cell reconstitution presently remains with one exception insufficient, as measured by lack of adequate antibody responses following immunizations. Thus, host B cells in B⊕ SCID appeared not to readily

Table 1
Results of Bone Marrow Fractionations for T Cell Depletion

Fractionation Procedure	Final Fraction Used for BMT				T Cell Contamination[2]
	Content of		% Recovery of		
	Nucleated Cells	CFU-c	Nucleated Cells	CFU-c	
E-Rosetting	20×10^8 [1] (9 – 48)	33×10^6 (21 – 46)	9.3 (5 – 21)	61 (31 – 85)	≤ 0.1 %
Lectin Agglutination and E-Rosetting	5.1×10^8 (0.9 – 14)	24×10^6 (3 – 49)	2.4 (0.9 – 5.1)	51 (15 – 96)	0 %

(1) Given numbers represent mean values obtained in 6 fractionation procedures using E-rosetting only and in 20 fractionation procedures using lectin agglutination plus E-rosetting. Numbers in parentheses indicate the ranges.
(2) As measured by T cell specific monoclonal antibody staining and by E-rosetting T cell assay.

Table 2
HLA Nonidentical BMT in Patients with Severe
Combine Immunodeficiency (n = 15)

Donors:	15/15	Haploidentical parents	
Conditioning:	11/15	None	
	3/15	ATG (40 mg/kg x 4)	
		Busulfan (2 mg/kg x 4)	
		Cytoxan (50 mg/kg x 4)	
	1/15	Busulfan (4 mg/kg x 4)	
T Cell Depletion:	14/15	Lectin Aggl. + E-rosetting	
	1/15	E-rosetting (2nd transplant)	
GvHD Prophylaxis after BMT:	15/15	None	
Outcome:	11/15	Alive (8 – 34 months)	
	4/15	Dead 3: Infection	
		1: Lymphoma	
Immune functions in survivors:		T cell (donor) Regular:	9
		Subnormal:	2
		B cell (donor) Regular:	2
		" " (host) Regular:	1
		Weak to absent:	8
GvHd acute:	1/15	(Grade II)*	
chronic:	0/11		

*T cell depletion by E-rosetting only (2nd trans-
plant). Patient died of infection.

gain functions after engraftment of haploidentical
T cells. Also engraftment of donor B cells in non-
conditioned patients (both B⊕ and B⊖ SCID) was not
apparent. The persisting humoral immunodeficiency
is adequately controlled by regular gamma globulin
substitution.

We observed more graft failures in non-SCID
patients. Thus, of four patients given HLA haploidentical bone marrow depleted of T cells by the
lectin method, none developed marrow reconstitution
(2 patients with ALL, 1 with CML, conditioning:
fractionated TBI (1320 rad, 11 fractions) and cyclophosphamide 120 mg/kg; 1 patient with WAS, conditioning: ATG 160 mg/kg, VP-16C 40 mg/kg, Busulfan
16 mg/kg, and cyclophosphamide 200 mg/kg). In addition,
2 pts transplanted from HLA identical siblings after
T cell depletion by E-rosetting failed to show sustained marrow engraftment (pt with Chediak H. Syndrome
and pt with Osteopetrosis, conditioned as pt with
WAS). None of these patients developed signs of GvHD.

Sustained engraftment after haploidentical BMT
was observed in only one patient. This child with
WAS, conditioned as the patients with WAS described
above, received a parental, haploidentical transplant
depleted of T cells by E-rosetting. He, as the only
case in the non-SCID-series, developed grade II GvHD.
The transplant course was complicated by a lympho-
proliferative, EBV induced syndrome, to which the
child succumbed eight weeks after BMT. Two patients
with SAA were successfully treated with T cell
depleted marrow (E-rosetting) obtained from identical
siblings after conditioning with cyclophosphamide
(200 mg/kg) and total lymphnode irradiation (750 rad).
No GvHD developed and patients survive 200 and 380
days after BMT.

In patients with graft failures, these were com-
monly preceded by signs of beginning marrow activities, as evidenced by cellular marrow aspirates.
Shortly later, host type lymphocytes appeared in
peripheral blood, frequently in excess of $5 \times 10^3/\mu l$.
Host origins could be established either by HLA
typing or, in matched BMT, cytogenetically. Repeated
marrow aspirates revealed a total absence of hemopoietic activities. The phenotype of these host cells,
as observed in several patients and determined by
monoclonal antibody staining, suggests a close relationship to NK cells (E-rosette ⊕, OKT 3 ⊕, OKT 4 ⊖,
OKT 8 ⊕, OKT 10 ⊕, Ia ⊕, Leu 7 ⊕).

DISCUSSION

GvHD is preventable when T cells are removed
from marrow grafts. This is clearly documented by
the series of 11 surviving patients with SCID
presented here, where donor dependent T cell recon-
sitution developed after haploidentical BMT without
complications of GvHD. However, in other than SCID
patients, T cells depleted BMT presented major
difficulties, particularly in nonidentical BMT.
Several mechanisms for the observed high rate of
graft failures can be postulated.

Our data would suggest that host factors play
major roles in graft failure. In patients without
primary cellular immunodeficiency, although having
received conditioning treatment adequate to allow
marrow engraftment in standard transplant situations,
host cells reappeared and likely mediated graft
rejection. Studies are underway to determine the
function of these radio-chemotherapy resistant cells
more specifically. In addition, our findings in two
patients with SCID, where BMT was performed after
conditioning and was followed by rapid and complete
donor cell engraftment, also argues that restricted
or impaired development of graft functions is mainly
imposed by host related factors. One could speculate
that by preventing donor T cell mediated alloreactivity by T cell depletion, a possible immunosuppressive
mechanism operative against residual host resistance
is also removed. Of note in this regard is that in
our series the only non-SCID patient, where haploidentical marrow solidly engrafted, developed acute
GvHD.

Our results suggest that more intense and, if
possible, more specific immunoablation is needed to
allow successful reconstitution when using T cell
depleted marrow.

ACKNOWLEDGMENT

This work was supported by the Deutsche
Forschungsgemeinschaft (SFB 112).

REFERENCES

1. O'Reilly RJ, Kirkpatrick D, Kapoor D et al. (1984),
   in: Griscelli C, Vossen J (eds) Progress in Immunodeficiency Research and Therapy. Excerpta
   Medica, Amsterdam, pp 385-392.
2. Friedrich W, Goldmann SF, Vetter U et al. (1984),
   Lancet 1 : 761-764.
3. Prentice HG, Blacklock HJ, Hanossis G et al. (1984),
   Lancet i : 472-475.
4. O'Reilly RJ, Collins NH, Brochstein J et al. (1985),
   Transpl Proceed 13 : 455-459.
5. Reisner Y, Kapoor N, Kirkpatrick D et al. (1983),
   Blood 61 : 34 - 48.

Exp. Hematol. (suppl. 17) 13:123 (1985)
© International Society for Experimental Hematology

Prevention of Graft Versus Host Disease II

The Use of Pan-T Monoclonal Antibodies in ex-vivo for Prevention of Acute GvHD

Clinical Results of Cooperative Pilot Study

E. Racadot[1], P. Herve[1], A. Bernard[4], M. Flesch[1], J. P. Vernant[2], G. Souillet[3], E. Plouvier[1], N. Philippe[3], E. Beaujan[2], A. Ehrsam[3], J. Pico[4], J. Y. Cahn[1], J. L. Touraine[3], B. Rio[5], and G. Andreux[5]

Bone Marrow Transplant Units of Besançon[1], Créteil[2], Lyon-Debrousse[3] and Villejuif[4], Paris, Hotel Dieu[5], France

The following is a report of the clinical results of a cooperative study (5 french centers) for the prevention of Graft-Versus-Host-Disease (GvHD) utilizing a combination of 3 monoclonal antibodies and complement mediated cytolysis for the ex-vivo treatment of the marrow inoculum.

Patients and methods

Twenty six patients, 10 female and 16 male, median age 20.2 yrs (2.5-40) received T-cell depleted allograft matched for 24 pts and mismatched for 2. Of these pts, 10 had ALL (2 CR1, 5 CR2, 3 relapses), 8 had AML (4 CR1,1 CR2, 3 relapses), 5 had CML (2 CP, 3 AP), 1 had Hodgkin's disease. Ten pts were conditioned by fractionated TBI (12 Gy) followed by cytoxan (120 mg/kg), 5 pts by cytoxan followed by fractionated TBI, 9 pts by cytoxan followed by TBIsingle dose (10 gy) and 2 pts by chemotherapy alone.
Conventional post-transplant management with MTX was maintained in 8 pts (group I), stopped at day 6 post BMT in 2 pts (group II) and in 16 pts no post-transplant immunoprophylaxis was administered (group III).

Before ex-vivo treatment the mononucleated marrow cells containing hemopoietic stem cells were isolated from the whole bone marrow. We used 3 MoAbs (kindly provided by A. BERNARD) : CD2/D66 (IgM class) + CD5/A50 (IgG2 class) + CD7/I21 (IgG2 class). The antibody concentration was of 10 ug/1x10^7 nucleated cells. The neonatal rabbit complement was provided either by TEBU Lab. or prepared by the Blood Transfusion Center of Besançon (final dilution = 1 : 1).

Results

The percentage ofT-cells in the harvested marrow was 30.2 % ± 10.5. The removal ofdonor's marrow T-cells was 92.3 % ± 6.9.
Three pts died in early post BMT from infectious complications. Thus 23 pts were evaluable. Of these 4 pts did not achieve engraftment : 2 pts after mismatched BMT and 2 pts after matched BMT. For the 19 pts who achieved engraftment, the time required to reach 0.5 x 10^9 granulocytes per liter was 17.7 days ± 4.18 and to reach 50 x 10^9 platelets per liter, it was 33.6 days ± 20.97.
Nineteen pts were evaluablefor acute GvHD prevention: we observed 2 aGvH grade II in the group I and 1 aGvH grade IV in the group III. For 7 pts with a follow-up of more than 3 months we observed 2 chronic GvH.
Three pts relapsed within 4 months post-BMT (2-4 mo).

Two late graft failures occured at 75 and 60 days after BMT.

Ten pts are alive and well, in complete remission with a short median follow-up of 3 months (1-6 mo).

Discussion

Effective depletion of T-lymphocytes can be accomplished ex-vivo by adding this MoAb pool into the marrow cell suspension.
Thus the pan-T MoAbs and complement mediated cytolysis is an effective approach to prevent acute GvHD.

In this pilot study we met an unexpected problem after T-cell depleted marrow infusion : the unacceptable high percentage (25 %) of graft failure (either no take or late graft failure). The incidence of this complication was variable according to the team and maybe in relation to the conditioning regimen used. However so far one of these teams has never observed marrow graft rejection in matched situations. We can assume that the host residual immunity plays a major role in graft failure (Host versus graft) and all the efforts should be made to obtain a better immunosuppression before BMT to prevent graft rejection.
Lastly heterogeneity of our group of patients should be emphasizedand it is too early to analyse the relapse incidence because of short follow-up so far.

Exp. Hematol. (suppl. 17) 13:124–125 (1985)
© International Society for Experimental Hematology

Ex-vivo Treatment with Pan-T Monoclonal Antibody Combination and Complement for Prevention of Acute GvHD

Pilot Study of 25 Cases

P. Herve[1], M. Flesch[1], E. Racadot[1], E. Plouvier[1], J. Y. Cahn[1], G. Souillet[2], and N. Philippe[2]

Bone Marrow Transplant Unit of Besançon[1] and Lyon-Debrousse[2], France

The following is a report of our clinical experience of the ex-vivo treatment of marrow inoculum for the prevention of acute Graft-Versus-Host Disease (GvHD) using a pan-T monoclonal antibody combination (either CD2/OKT11 + CD3/OKT3 or CD2/D66 + CD5/A50 + CD7/I21) and baby rabbit complement. In pre-clinical experiments on marrow mononuclear cells we determined the optimal conditions for the complement-mediated cytolysis in order to achieve efficient and rapid killing of marrow T-cells (E. RACADOT, 1983).

Patients and methods

Twenty-five pts, 11 female and 14 male, median age 16 yrs (2.5 - 40) received T-depleted allograft matched for 24 pts and mismatched for 1 pt. To assert the "pure" chimerism there were 10 sex-mismatches and 7 major blood group mismatches. Of these pts, 10 had ALL (7 CR2, 1 CR3, 2 relapses), 7 had AML (4 CR1, 2 CR2, 1 relapse), 5 had CML (1 BT, 2 AP, 2 CP), 1 had multiple myeloma, 1 had NHML and 1 had Hodgkin's disease.

Twenty four pts were conditioned by fractionated TBI (12 Gy) followed by cytoxan (120 mg/m^2). Additional chemotherapy such as VP-16 and aracytine were given in 5 pts and the pt with Hodgkin's disease received CBV protocol (cytoxan, BCNU, VP-16) without irradiation. Post-transplant management with MTX or cyclosporin-A was maintained in 7 pts (group I), stopped at day 11 post BMT in 6 pts (group II) and in 12 pts no post-transplant immunoprophylaxis was administered (group III). Fourteen pts received a transplant treated with CD2/OKT11 (IgG2) and CD3/OKT3 (IgG2) purchased from ORTHO-France and 11 pts received a transplant treated with CD2/D66 (IgGM) + CD5/A50 (IgG2) + CD7/I21 (IgG2) kindly provided by A. BERNARD. The neonatal rabbit complement was either provided by TEBU Lab. or prepared by our blood transfusion center. The details of the bone marrow processing and ex-vivo treatment have been previously reported (1).

Results

The percentage of removal of donor's marrow T cells ex-vivo before infusion was 93.7 % ± 4.08. Patients received 0.92 x 10^6 ± 0.61 residual viable T-cells per kg. In terms of efficiency of T-cell killing, we did not observe a significant difference between the 2 Mo Ab associations. Four pts having received additional chemotherapy in the preparative regimen died in early post-BMT due to therapy-related complications. Twenty-one pts were evaluable. Engraftment was achieved in all matched BMT. Overall the time required to reach

0.5 x 10^9 granulocytes per liter was 21.7 days ± 4.7 and to reach 50 x 10^9 plts per liter was 29.8 days ± 8.13. We observed one mixed chimerism without evidence of leukemic relapse 1 yr post-BMT. The pt grafted in mismatched situation (first cousin) showed evidence of graft failure. Engraftment was achieved after a 3rd graft from the haplo-identical father. No acute GvHD (< grade I) was observed in the 3 groups of pts. Until now no pt has developed chronic GvHD (for 12 pts the follow up is longer than 6 mo).

Six pts relapsed within 6 months post BMT (2 - 6 mo); 15 pts are alive and well in CR with a median follow up of 13.1 mo (7 - 19), 13.9 mo (12 - 16), 3.5 mo (1-8) for pts in group I, II, III respectively. Until now no B-lymphoproliferative disorders have been described in our pts.

Discussion

These 2 pan-T MoAb "cocktails" can be used for effective removal of T-cells from the marrow without affecting marrow engraftment. Their efficiency in T-cell lysis was equivalent although the antibody concentration per 1.10^7 nucleated cells was 10 fold higher for the D66 - A50 - I21 in comparison to the OKT3 - OKT11 combination.

DIAGNOSIS	HLA COMPAT.	T-CELL DEPLE-TION(%)	CONDIT. REGIMEN	STAND GvH PROPH.	ENGRAFT MENT	OUTCOME
AML	mm	99	CTX TBI	MTX	NO TAKE	DIED POST 3rd GRAFT
AML	mm	95.3	CTX TBI	MTX	NO TAKE	DIED POST 3rd GRAFT
AML	m	97.5	HDM	NO	REJECT. DAY 60	DIED POST 2nd GRAFT
ALL	m	99	CTX f.TBI	NO	AUTOLOG. RECON-STITUT. DAY 42	A & W
AA	m	73	CTX f.TBI	NO	NO TAKE	DIED POST 2nd GRAFT
LMC	m	94.6	CTX TBI	MTX	REJECT. DAY 75	2nd GRAFT PLANED

Table 1 - Effects of ex-vivo T-cell depletion on engraftment. Clinical data of patients with graft failure.

No graft failure was observed in the group of matched BMT. Our results differ from another clinical assay having reported a 20 % graft failure after T-cell depleted BMT. We can assume that the residual viable T-cells in our marrow inoculum could limit the host versus graft reaction. Obviously the choice of preparative regimen plays a prominent part in the fate of T-cell depleted graft, the lowest possible level of the host residual immunity must be reached.

An important practical outcome of this clinical study is that T-cell depletion by ex-vivo treatment may prevent the sometimes fatal GvHD related complications. For all our pts their general physical condition is excellent. An efficient method of ex-vivo T-cell depletion should prove cost effective when compared to prolonged courses of post-transplant GvH prophylaxis.

References

1. Hervé P, Flesch M, Cahn JY et al. Removal of marrow T-cells with OKT3-OKT11 MoAbs and complement to prevent acute GvHD. A pilot study in 10 patients. Transplantation (in Press).

Exp. Hematol. (suppl. 17) 13:126 (1985)
© International Society for Experimental Hematology

Experience with 100 Allogeneic Marrow Grafts Using Cyclosporin-A (CYA) for Prophylaxis Against GVHD

B. Speck[1], A. Gratwohl[1], B. Osterwalder[1], C. Nissen[1], and E. Signer[2]

[1] Kantonsspital Basel, [2] Kinderspital Basel, Switzerland

Of the 100 patients 29 had AML, 30 ALL, 24 CML and 17 SAA. Median age was 28 years (4-42). Median follow up is 26 months (7-55). Patients with leukemia were conditioned with Cy 2x60 mg/kg and 10 Gy TBI. Patients with SAA were given Cy 4x50 mg/kg and donor buffy coat from 4 units of blood on 5 successive days after BMT. 95 patients had an HLA-identical sibling donor. 5 times an HLA-haploidentical family member served as a donor. The CyA protocol was changed three times (1). We always started with a parenteral application on day -1 and later changed to oral CyA 12.5 mg/kg in a single daily dose up to 6 months and then gradually reduced and stopped at one year. The dose was adjusted primarly to the serum creatinine level but to some extent also to the blood CyA through level. Patients developing grade II or greater GvHD were treated with bolus methylprednisolone in addition. I g was given as a 24-hour infusion on the first day, followed by 500 mg on the second day. Then the dose was reduced to 0.5 mg/kg. Compared to our previous experience with MTX, CyA did not influence the incidence of GvHD, but decreased its severity. In patients who died from transplant related mortality it was often difficult to distinguish between GvHD and/or viral infections. 29 of 51 patients transplanted for acute leukemia in first remission and CML in chronic phase became long term disease free survivors (57%). Only 8 of 32 patients transplanted in later stages of the disease survived (25%) without evidence of leukemia. In the first group relapse was the cause of death in 15 %, in the second one in 85 %. Fatal transplant related complications were comparable in both groups: ± 15 % with an unusally low incidence of interstitial pneumonia of 4 %. In 16 patients with SAA BMT was the primary treatment of their disease. 10 of them are living and well (62.5%) without any chronic problems. Of the 6 deaths 3 were due to acute GvHD, 1 to cardiac failure, 1 to CMV-infection and one to rejection. One patient with SAA had ALG as primary treatment. He had many transfusions from family members. His conditioning consisted of 10 Gy TBI. This patient never showed any evidence of engraftment and died. The 5 patients with haploidentical transplants all had leukemia. They did rather poorly: only 1 became a long term disease free survivor: 3 died of acute GvHD, one of leukemic relapse after having had severe GvHD. Several side effects of CyA were seen. They proved to be reversible and subsided upon dose reduction. Renal insufficiency, mild hepatic dysfunction, facial edema, tremor and anorexia were the most frequent ones. 4 patients had fits that responded to antiepileptic therapy and 2 had reversible facial nerve palsies. Reversible cotton wool lesions in the retina were seen in 5 patients. Upon stopping CyA at one year 40 % of the patients developed signs of acute GvHD which subsided upon resumption of the drug, proving its therapeutic efficacy in the treatment of GvHD. Only one patient has severe chronic GvHD. It is restricted to the liver and presents like primary biliary cirrhosis. From this experience we conclude that CyA has markedly reduced our transplant related mortality in particular from interstitial pneumonia. In our study age did not play an important role for transplant related mortality between the age of 10 and 40 years. Leukemic relapse remains a major problem in particular in patients transplanted in late stages of leukemia, In our limited experience with HLA-haploidentical BMT CyA proved to be of little or no value in preventing severe GvHD. No chronic renal insufficiency or other serious long term side effects of CyA were observed.

Ref. 1) Speck B et al:
Allogeneic bone marrow transplantation: The Basel trial with Cyclosporine
Transpl Proc 15 (Suppl 1): 2617-9, 1983

Exp. Hematol. (suppl. 17) 13:127 (1985)
© International Society for Experimental Hematology

Impact of Mismatching for Minor Histocompatibility Antigens on the Occurrence of Graft-Versus-Host Disease

E. Goulmy[1], E. Blokland[1], J. W. Gratama[1], F. E. Zwaan[2], J. M. J. J. Vossen[3], B. Speck[4], and J. J. van Rood[1]

[1] Department of Immunohaematology and Blood Bank, University Hospital, Leiden, The Netherlands
[2] Isolation Pavilion, University Hospital, Leiden, The Netherlands
[3] Department of Pediatrics, University Hospital, Leiden, The Netherlands
[4] Kantonsspital Basel, Switzerland

The results in human bone marrow transplantation are still not fully satisfactory. Despite the selection of HLA identical siblings as bone marrow donors for patients with severe aplastic anemia or hematologic malignancies, Graft-versus-Host Disease (GvHD) occurs in approximately 20-70% of the patients depending on their age. This complication can be caused by disparity for the products of minor Histocompatibility (minor H) systems.

Previously, we reported on the presence of cytotoxic T lymphocytes (CTLs) in a patient suffering from severe chronic GvHD. Those CTLs, which were demonstrated from two months after bone marrow grafting onwards, were directed against patient's own pre-transplant lymphocytes. Analysis of the in vitro cytotoxic activity of the patient's post-transplant lymphocytes demonstrated the presence of a minor H antigen of which the recognition was HLA restricted (Goulmy et al. 1982).

This observation prompted us to continue our search for minor H antigens and their role in bone marrow transplantation. We investigated post-transplant lymphocytes from a series (n=19) of recipients of HLA identical bone marrow grafts for the presence of anti-host cytotoxic activity. Such CTL activity could be detected post bone marrow transplant in five patients suffering from GvHD, but was absent in patients without GvHD (for review see: Goulmy 1985). Further analysis of the cytotoxic activity patterns of the post-transplant lymhocytes of the latter five patients, revealed five different CTL populations each directed against different minor H antigens. Four of the five minor H antignes were recognized in an HLA restricted fashion (Goulmy 1985). Expansion of the five CTL populations provided us with large amounts of cellular typing reagents specific for these minor H antigens.

In order to obtain information about the relevance of minor H antigens in the pathogenesis of GvHD, we performed an retrospective typing analysis for these five different minor H antigens, on a series of HLA identical bone marrow donor/recipient combinations (n=47).

The results of this analysis (see table) demonstrate that incompatibilities for one (or more) minor H antigens between HLA identical donor and recipient were found in the group of patients suffering from GvHD. Consequently, when more than one bone marrow donor is available, cellular typing for minor H antigens may be helpful in avoiding one of the risk factors for GvHD.

Table. Cellular typing of human minor H antigens with minor H antigen specific CTLs.

Donor/recipient pairs	Typing for 5 minor H antigens	
	identical	non-identical
recipients without GvHD	13	1
recipients with acute GvHD	16	3
recipients with chronic GvHD	6	8

p= 0.0045

References.

- Goulmy E, Gratama J.W., Blokland E, Zwaan F.E. & Van Rood J.J. (1982).
Recognition of an -as yet unknown-minor transplantation antigen by post-transplant lymphocytes from an AML patient. Exp. Hemat. 10: 127-129.

- Goulmy E. (1985).
Class I restricted human cytotoxic T lymphocytes directed against minor transplantation antigens and their possible role in organ transplantation. Prog. Allergy 36: 44-72.

Supported in part by the Dutch Foundation for Medical Research (FUNGO) which is subsidized by the Dutch Organization for the Advancement of Pure Research (ZWO), the J.A. Cohen Institute for Radiopathology and Radiation Protection (IRS).

Exp. Hematol. (suppl. 17) 13:128–130 (1985)
© International Society for Experimental Hematology

The Biology of Chronic Graft-Versus-Host Disease

H. J. Deeg

Fred Hutchinson Cancer Research Center and the University of Washington School of Medicine, Seattle, Washington, USA

Chronic graft-versus-host (GVHD) disease occurs in as many as 30-50% of long-term survivors after allogeneic marrow transplantation, even when the donor was an HLA genotypically identical sibling (1,2). Because of severe morbidity and mortality associated with this syndrome, it has a major effect on long-term results of clinical marrow transplantation (3). Chronic GVHD generally develops within 3 months to one year after transplantation. Three forms of onset have been recognized (4): 1) Progressive chronic GVHD, i.e. as a continuation of acute GVHD, 2) quiescent chronic GVHD, i.e. after a disease-free, asymptomatic interval following acute GVHD, and 3) de novo chronic GVHD in patients who never had any clinical manifestation of acute GVHD. The prognosis is the worst for patients with progressive chronic GVHD, intermediate with quiescent, and best with de novo chronic GVHD.

The target organs of chronic GVHD include skin liver, mucous membranes, eyes, exocrine glands, esophagus, gastrointestinal tract, serous membranes, muscoskeletal system, and the lungs. The disease can either be limited, i.e. only one or two target organs, usually skin and liver, are involved - this form occurs in about 15-20% of patients with chronic GVHD and has a favorable prognosis - or the disease can be extensive, a form observed in about 80 to 85% of patients, with involvement of numerous organs and an unfavorable prognosis. The clinical findings of chronic GVHD are summarized in Table 1. In addition, patients can develop a severe wasting syndrome and are extremely susceptible to infections. In fact, chronic GVHD is the most significant risk factor for the development of late infections after marrow transplantation (5). Other problems, such as autoimmune hemolytic anemia and thrombocytopenia, have also been recognized (6).

Laboratory findings associated with chronic GVHD are summarized in Table 2. Most important for the clinical course appears to be a complex immunodeficiency involving both T helper and B lymphocytes (7). Patients with chronic GVHD tend to have circulating nonspecific suppressor cells (suppressing proliferative responses of donor lymphocytes to unrelated stimulators) and lack specific suppressor cells (specific for host cells), whereas patients without GVHD generally have specific but not nonspecific suppressor cells (8).

Table 1. Clinical findings of chronic GVHD

SKIN	--	Erythema, dyspigmentation, scleroderma, contractures, alopecia, dystrophic nails, photosensitivity
LIVER	--	Icterus, hepatomegaly, enzyme elevation
MUCOSA	--	Stomatitis, Sicca, lichen planus, vaginitis, synechiae, stenosis
EYES	--	Keratoconjunctivitis sicca
ESOPHAGUS	--	Esophagitis, stenosis
GI TRACT	--	Enteritis
SEROSA	--	Polyserositis
MUSCULOSKELETAL	-	Polymyositis, synovitis, tendinitis, eosinophilic fasciitis
LUNGS	--	Restrictive/obstructive changes, impaired diffusion, bronchiolitis

Table 2. Laboratory findings of chronic GVHD

Autoantibodies

Hypergammaglobulinemia (with selective Ig deficiencies)

Immune Complexes

Eosinophilia

Lymphocytotoxic antibodies

T and B Cell Defects

Dermo-epidermal Immunoglobulin + C' Deposits

Anemia

Thrombocytopenia

The pathology of chronic GVHD has been described extensively (9). One can summarize the findings as follows: Initially there are cellular infiltrates in the various target organs leading to the appearance of hypertrophy and resulting in tissue necrosis. In response to that, repair mechanisms are initiated, possibly involving the production of abnormal collagens or abnormal amounts thereof which results in tissue fibrosis rather than regeneration of the specific functional organ tissue. This in turn is associated with a loss of function.

At least three risk factors for the development of chronic GVHD have been recognized (3) (Table 3).

Table 3. Risk factors for chronic GVHD

Acute GVHD

Age

Infusion of Donor Buffy Coat Cells

The presence of acute GVHD appears to have an overwhelming effect. Whereas only 20% of patients with aplastic anemia without acute GVHD develop chronic GVHD, approximately 80% of those with acute GVHD Grades II-IV do. Those with Grade I acute GVHD have an intermediate incidence. One can assume, therefore, that risk factors for acute GVHD, for example the presence of certain histocompatible antigens (10,11) may also be risk factors for chronic GVHD. This correlation between acute and chronic GVHD and the observed responses to immunosuppressive therapy suggest that chronic GVHD similar to acute GVHD is the result of a reaction of immunocompetent donor cells (T lymphocytes) to host antigens. The second factor, age, is particularly important for the development of de novo GVHD. Whether this is related to thymic involution with increasing age remains speculative (12). Efforts at boosting thymic function by thymic tissue fragment implantation and the administration of thymosine Fraction V have not been successful (13). Infusion of donor buffy coat cells is a significant risk factor for chronic GVHD in patients with aplastic anemia (3). More recent observations indicate that this also applies for patients with hemopoietic malignancies. In addition, evidence has been presented that infection with or reactivation of cytomegalovirus (14) or a positive cytomegalovirus immune status of the donor (this symposium) may predispose patients to an increased risk of chronic GVHD.

The diagnostic criteria for chronic GVHD and the use of early screening studies have been described in detail previously (1,4) and in the present symposium. Patients with overt chronic GVHD generally are found to have abnormal skin biopsies and decreased tear production. This may also be present, however, in patients with subclinical chronic GVHD who are asymptomatic at the time of examination and only subsequently develop their disease.

Attempts at therapy of chronic GVHD in the early and mid 70's were generally unsuccessful. It was found subsequently that treatment with a combination of prednisone and a cytotoxic agent, generally azathioprine, may be quite successful in preventing the disease progressive and, in fact, resulted in complete arrest of the disease in the majority of patients (4). More recently, we and others have found that cyclosporine is a useful agent for the treatment of chronic GVHD.

The only benefit of GVHD that has been observed so far is possibly an antileukemic effect (15). It had been observed already in the mid 50's in mice that transplantation of marrow might destroy residual leukemic cells in lethally irradiated recipient mice. More recent clinical studies indicate that both acute and chronic GVHD in the clinical setting also may have an antileukemic effect and lead to improved long-term survival in patients transplanted for hemopoietic malignancies.

In summary, chronic GVHD is a complication of allogeneic marrow transplantation occurring in 30-50% of patients given nonmanipulated HLA-identical marrow grafts. The incidence is increased in patients who have acute GVHD, in older patients, and in patients who are given viable donor buffy coat cells in addition to the marrow. The clinical picture resembles (but is different from) collagen vascular diseases. Chronic GVHD is a multi-organ syndrome that can lead to severe dysfunction and most importantly to significant immunodysregulation, making the patient extremely susceptible to viral, bacterial, and fungal infections. In vitro studies show that patients with chronic GVHD have host-reactive lymphocytes and nonspecific suppressor cells but lack specific suppressor cells which are present in patients who have no manifestations of chronic GVHD. So far, attempts at prophylaxis of chronic GVHD with early administration of steroids have not been uniformly successful.

REFERENCES

1. Sullivan KM, Parkman R. The pathophysiology and treatment of graft-versus-host disease. In: Clinics in Haematology, 12: 775-789, 1983.

2. Deeg HJ, Storb R. Graft-versus-host disease: Pathophysiological and clinical aspects. Ann Rev Med 35: 11-24, 1984.

3. Storb R, Prentice RL, Sullivan KM, et al. Predictive factors in chronic graft-versus-host disease in patients with aplastic anemia treated by marrow transplantation from HLA-identical siblings. Ann Intern Med 98: 461-466, 1983.

4. Sullivan KM, Shulman HM, Storb R, et al. Chronic graft-versus-host disease in 52 patients: Adverse natural course and successful treatment with combination immunosuppression. Blood 57: 267-276, 1981.

5. Atkinson K, Farewell V, Storb R, et al. Analysis of late infections after human bone marrow transplantation: Role of genotypic nonidentity between marrow donor and recipient and of nonspecific suppressor cells in patients with chronic graft-versus-host disease. Blood 60: 714-720, 1982.

6. Graze PR, Gale RP. Chronic graft versus host disease: A syndrome of disordered immunity. Am J Med 66: 611-619, 1979.

7. Witherspoon RP, Lum LG, Storb R. Immunologic reconstitution after human marrow grafting. Semin Hematol 21: 2-10, 1984.

8. Tsoi M-S. Immunological mechanisms of graft-versus-host disease in man. Transplantation 33: 459-464, 1982.

9. The Pathology of Bone Marrow Transplantation, Sale GE, Shulman HM (eds). New York, Masson Publishing USA, Inc., 1984.

10. Storb R, Prentice RL, Hansen JA, et al. An association between HLA-B antigens and acute graft-versus-host disease. Lancet 2: 816-819, 1983.

11. Bross DS, Tutschka PJ, Farmer ER, et al. Predictive factors for acute graft-versus-host disease in patients transplanted with HLA-identical bone marrow. Blood 63: 1265-1270, 1984.

130

12. Storb R, Thomas ED. Allogeneic bone-marrow transplantation. Immunol Rev 71: 77-102, 1983.

13. Atkinson K, Storb R, Ochs HD, et al. Thymus transplantation after allogeneic bone marrow graft to prevent chronic graft-versus-host disease in humans. Transplantation 33: 168-173, 1982.

14. Lonnqvist B, Ringden O, Wahren B, et al. Cytomegalovirus infection associated with and preceding chronic graft-versus-host disease. Transplantation 38: 465-468, 1984.

15. Weiden PL, Sullivan KM, Flournoy MS, et al. Antileukemic effect of chronic graft-versus-host disease. Contribution to improved survival after allogeneic marrow transplantation. N Engl J Med 304: 1529-1533, 1981.

Supported by grants CA 18221, CA 30924, CA 18029, CA 15704 awarded by the National Institute of Health, DHHS.

Exp. Hematol. (suppl. 17) 13:131–132 (1985)
© International Society for Experimental Hematology

Role of Lymphokines in the Induction of Graft-Versus-Host Disease

D. Niederwieser[1], J. Troppmaier[1], G. Adolph[3], R. Margreiter[2], and C. Huber[1]

[1] Clinical Immunobiology, Department of Internal Medicine, University of Innsbruck
[2] Department of Surgery I, University of Innsbruck
[3] The Boehringer Institute, Vienna, Austria

INTRODUCTION
It is now generally accepted that acute graft-versus-host disease (GvH-D) is mediated by alloreactive T cells (1). Surprisingly, evidence accumulates that this alloresponsiveness can be amplified by exposure to environmental antigens: the relative resistance of gnotobiotic animals to (2) and the association of cytomegalovirus (CMV) disease with GvH-D (3) represent examples of this relationship. The hypothesis presented here implies that T cells stimulated by environmental antigens release excessive amounts of lymphokines, which enhance alloreactivity. As far as interleukin-2 (IL-2) and its capacity to mediate clonal expansion and generation of alloreactive T killer cells is concerned, a vast body of information has been published (4). In this respect, only little is known about the impact of interferon-gamma (IFN-γ), the other well characterized lymphokine released by activated T cells. This article presents experimental evidence in support of the above hypothesis. In detail, we demonstrate that (i) IFN-γ enhances alloreactivity by virtue of its capacity to induce the expression of functional MHC class II antigens; (ii) endogenous interferon release is dramatically increased around the time of hemopoietic reconstitution and preceded clinical manifestation of GvH-D; (iii) this burst of endogenous cytokine production takes place independent of the presence of histocompatability barriers.

MATERIALS AND METHODS
MLC cultures were established as previously described (5) using allogeneic peripheral blood mononuclear cells (pbmc) stimulators. Simultaneously, the HLA-DR+ cells were removed from the stimulators by means of complement dependent lysis with the monoclonal antibody Q5/13. These cells were also reinduced to express HLA-DR antigens by preincubation for three hours with 100 U/ml of rhu IFN-γ (Genentech, USA).

In 13 leukemia or tumor patients transplanted with MHC identical allogeneic, two patients with autologous and one with a syngeneic bone marrow graft, urinary neopterin excretion was measured using standard techniques (6). Serum IFN-levels were obtained by growth inhibition of mouse EMC virus tested on lung cell carcinoma cells.

RESULTS
1. IFN-γ enhances alloreactivity by virtue of its capacity to induce the expression of functional MHC class II antigens on stimulator cells:
While much is known about the essential role the lymphokine IL-2 plays in the proliferation and the

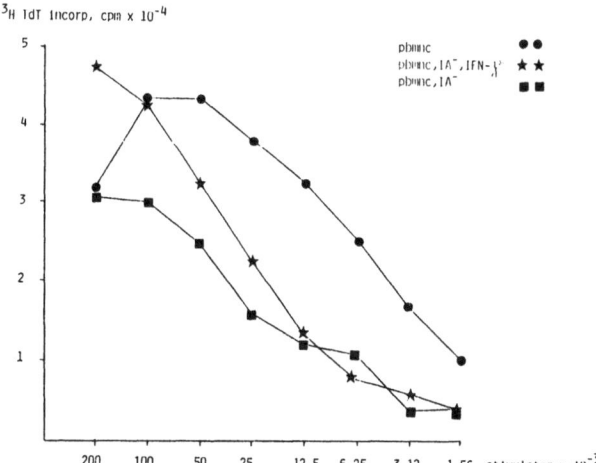

Fig 1: Stimulatory capacity of pbmc before and after depletion from HLA-DR+ cells and of HLA-DR+ depleted pbmc preincubated with IFN-γ in the mixed lymphocyte culture.

generation of alloreactive cytotoxic T-lymphocytes (CTL), only limited information is available concerning IFN-γ. An example illustrating the capacity of IFN-γ to amplify alloantigen responses at the level of the stimulator cell is depicted in Fig. 1. As shown, preincubation of pbmc depleted of HLA-DR+ cells with IFN-γ restores their stimulatory capacity.

2. Endogenous IFN release is increased around the time of hemopoietic reconstitution in human bone marrow transplant recipients:
Our attempts to measure changes of serum IFN levels in BMT recipients between total body irradiation and the time of hemopoietic reconstitution remained relatively unsuccessful. Only levels below 3 U/ml were detected. When, however, neopterin, a molecule released from macrophages under control of interferons (7), was evaluated, dramatic changes occurred (8).

The summary in Table 1 shows that almost twice as much neopterin was excreted at the time of hemopoietic recovery as compared with pretreatment levels. We take this as evidence of markedly increased endogenous IFN production. With respect to this pattern, autologous and syngeneic transplants did not differ from allogeneic combinations. This rules out the

TABLE 1: Summary of the normalized excretion values of 16 bone marrow transplant recipients from the time before transplantation until hemopoietic reconstitution[+]

	Before cyclo-phosphamide	total body irradiation	at leuco-cyte nadir	at time of hemo-poietic reconst.
neopterin excretion (mean ± SD of normalized values)*	100 ± 0	257 ± 270	72 ± 44	193 ± 82
no. of patients	16	14	16	16
day before (-) or after (+) transplan-tation (mean ± SD)	-5	-1	+7 ± 1	+15 ± 4
statistical analysis**		p <0.05	p <0.02	p <0.001

*urinary neopterin values were normalized by setting the pretransplant levels at 100%. The absolute levels on day -5 were 397 ± 203 µmol neo-pterin/mol creatinine (mean ± SD)

**Student's t-test

[+]results quoted from ref. (8).

possibility that stimulation by histocompatibility antigens is responsible for the cytokine burst observed; rather, it suggested, but by no means proved, the involvement of environmental antigens.

3. Enhanced endogenous IFN release precedes clinical manifestation of GvH-D:

After hemopoietic reconstitution, seven patients (two autologous, one syngeneic, four allogeneic) revealed falling neopterin values. Nine further patients developed acute GvH-D subsequent to hemopoie-tic recovery. In all of them, continuously increasing neopterin levels preceded manifestation of clinical disease. Results are summarized in Table 2.

TABLE 2: Increase of neopterin preceding the clinical manifestation of graft-versus-host disease[+]

	days before clinical diagnosis of graft-versus-host disease		
	-2 days	-1 day	day 0
neopterin excretion* (mean ± SD of normalized values)	51 ± 13	77 ± 25	100 ± 0
number of patients	9	9	9
statistical analysis**	p< 0.02	p< 0.02	

*urinary neopterin values were normalized by setting the levels on the day of clinical diagnosis of GvH-D at 100%. The absolute levels on day 0 were 875 ± 405 µmol neopterin/mol creatinine (mean ± SD)

**Student's t-test

[+]results quoted from ref. (8)

DISCUSSION

In this paper a hypothesis is presented which helps to explain the intimate relationship between exposure to infectious pathogens and induction of GvH-D. The hypothesis implies that lymphokines, such as IL-2 and IFN-γ are produced by T cells stimulated by infec-tious agents. These lymphokines at the site of re-lease can then enhance generation of alloreactive effector T cells mediating GvH-D. In support of this view the following experimental findings are pre-sented: (i) around the time of hemopoietic reconsti-tution the excretion of neopterin, a marker molecule produced by gamma interferon-stimulated macrophages, is noticeably increased. We take this as evidence of enhanced endogenous IFN production. Since induction

of IFN-γ is invariably associated with induction of IL-2, we further conclude that both these crucial lymphokines are produced at increased rates around the time of hemopoietic recovery. (ii) The fact that IL-2 in vitro amplifies generation of alloreactive T cells is now well established. We present in vitro evidence that IFN-γ enhanced recognition of alloanti-gens, although not on the level of the effector cells but on the level of target cells. It seemed very likely that both these lymphokines released in vivo would act in the same manner. (iii) Although no direct proof for the role of infectious agents in inducing increased lymphokine levels has been ob-tained, they represent the most likely candidates for stimulating antigens. Results in autologous and syn-geneic combinations clearly excluded the participa-tion of major or minor histocompatibility antigens.

Although antigens are essential for initiating activa-tion of immune cells, their further growth and func-tional differentiation is controlled by antigen-unspecific mediators such as lymphokines. We feel that more attention should be paid to understanding the pathogenic significance of these unspecific ampli-fication mechanisms. Should the news presented here prove correct, attempts to develop a prophylaxis against stimulation with infectious pathogens and to inhibit lymphokine release by pharmacological or immunological means should be intensified.

This work was supported by the Austrian Research Fund "Zur Förderung der Wissenschaftlichen Forschung", project no. 5288.

REFERENCES
1. Korngold R, Sprent J. Lethal GvH-D across minor histocompatibility barriers: nature of the effector cells and role of the H2-complex. Immunol. Rev (1983) 71; 5.
2. Pollard M, Chang LF, Srivstava KK. The role of microflora in development of graft versus host disease. Transplant. Proc. (1976) 8; 533.
3. Lönnqvist B, Ringden O, Wahren B, Gahrton G, Lundgren G. Cytomegatovirus infection associated with and preceding chronic graft versus host disease. Transplantation (1984) 38; 465.
4. Wagner H, Hardt C, Heeg K, Pfizenmeier K, Solbach W, Bartlett R, Stockinger H, Röllinghoff M. T-cell interactions during cytotoxic T-lymphocyte responses: T-cell derived helper factor (IL-2) as a probe to analyse CTL responsiveness and thymic maturation of CTL progenitors. Immunol. Rev. (1980) 51; 215.
5. Huber C, Merkenschlager M, Gattringer C, Royston I, Fink U, Braunsteiner H. Human autologous mixed lymphocyte reactivity is primarily specific for xenoprotein determinants adsorbed to antigen-presenting cells during rosett formation with sheep erythrocytes. J. Exp. Med. (1982) 155; 1222.
6. Hausen A, Fuchs D, König K, Wachter H. Determina-tion of neopterin in human urine by reversed phase high performance liquid chromatography. J. Chromatogr. (1982) 227; 61.
7. Huber C, Batchelor J, Fuchs D, Hausen A, Lang A, Niederwieser D, Reibnegger G, Swetly P, Tropp-mair J, Wachter H. Immune response-associated production of neopterin. J. Exp. Med. (1984) 160; 310.
8. Niederwieser D, Huber C, Gratwohl A, Bannert P, Fuchs D, Hausen A, Reibnegger G, Speck B, Wach-ter H. Neopterin as a new biochemical marker in the clinical monitoring of bone marrow transplant recipients. Transplantation (1984) 38; 497.

Exp. Hematol. (suppl. 17) 13:133 (1985)
© International Society for Experimental Hematology

Lymphocyte Reactivity After Cytomegalovirus Infection May Predict Development of Chronic Graft Versus Host Disease

P. Ljungman[1,2], G. Gahrton[2], B. Lönnqvist[2], O. Ringdén[3,4], and B. Wahren[1]

[1] Department of Virology, National Bacteriological Laboratory, Stockholm, Sweden
[2] Department of Medicine, Huddinge Hospital, Huddinge, Sweden
[3] Department of Transplantation Surgery, Huddinge Hospital, Huddinge, Sweden
[4] Department of Clinical Immunology, Huddinge Hospital, Huddinge, Sweden

It has been shown that a preceding CMV infection was more common in BMT recipients who did develop chronic GVHD than in those who did not (1). The aim of this study was to study lymphocyte responses after CMV infection and development of chronic GVHD.

METHODS

Lymphocytes from 46 patients were studied before and repeatedly after BMT. Lymphocyte stimulation was performed with cytomegalovirus (CMV) antigen (2). Separate cultures were stimulated with phytohemagglutinin (PHA). A net count was calculated by subtracting the mean cpm from triplicate cultures with control antigen from the mean of cpm from virus stimulated cultures. A net cpm >10000 was regarded as a positive response. Loss of response was defined as a positive test followed by 2 or more negative tests. Variable response was defined as a lost response followed by one or more positive responses.

Viral IgG and IgM antibodies to CMV were determined by enzyme-linked immunosorbent assay (ELISA), performed with serum taken at the time of stimulation tests. The diagnosis of a viral infection was made by virus isolation or by either of the following serological criteria: specific IgM production, seroconversion or a 5-fold specific IgG increase in the absence of blood transfusions.

RESULTS

The occurrence of CMV infections was analysed in relation to pretransplant serology for donor and recipient (Table 1)

Table 1:

CMV-serology		Number of		
Donor	Recipient	Patients	CMV-inf.	%
Positive	Positive	18	14	78
Positive	Negative	6	2	33
Negative	Positive	9	7	78
Negative	Negative	13	1	8

The first 12 weeks after BMT the recipient lymphocytes rarely reacted with CMV; usually the reactivity did not return until a CMV infection had occurred. This was seen in all three groups where the donor, the recipient or both were seropositive.

Twenty-four of the 46 recipients developed a CMV infection after BMT. In 68% of these cases, CMV infection was followed by a specific CMV lymphocyte stimulation response. Eight responses came within 3 months from the diagnosis of the CMV infection, 5 later (3-6 months). A lymphocyte stimulation response to CMV anti-

gen was better correlated to CMV isolation than the appearance of CMV-specific IgM (p=0.01). No significant difference was seen between lymphocyte stimulation response and 5-fold specific IgG increase (p=0.07).

Table 2:
Stimulation responses following CMV infection and chronic GVHD

Stimulation response to CMV	No. of patients chronic GVHD	
	Yes	No
Early (<3 months)	1	7
Late (>3 months)	5	0
Absent (repeated tests)	2	0
	p=0.002	

Eight out of the 15 patients with CMV infection that survived >6 months after BMT developed CH GVHD (Table 2). An early lymphocyte response to CMV was present mainly in patients who later did not develop CH GVHD (p=0.002; Fishers's exact 2-tailed test). Patients who did subsequently develop chronic GVHD had either a late or no lymphocyte response at all to CMV. There was no difference in the incidence or severity of acute GVHD between the recipients with or without an early lymphocyte response to CMV.

At follow-up more than 6 months after the CMV infection, the CMV lymphocyte reactivity was still present in 6/7 recipients without chronic GVHD, while it was lost, variable or repeatedly negative in recipients with chronic GVHD (p=0.005).

CONLUSION

In this study we have found that the recipients with an early response (up to 3 months) to CMV antigen after the CMV infection were less prone to develop chronic graft versus host disease (GVHD) than those who responded later or not at all. After the CMV infection, the increased lymphocyte CMV reactivity remained in recipients without chronic GVHD, while recipients with chronic GVHD often lost their reactivity. The results suggest that it may be possible to predict which patients that are going to develop chronic GVHD by studying lymphocyte responses to CMV infections.

LITERATURE CITED

1. Lönnqvist B, Ringdén O, Wahren B, Gahrton G, Lundgren G. Cytomegalovirus infection associated with and preceding chronic graft-versus-host disease. Transplantation, in press.
2. Wahren B, Robèrt K-H, Nordlund S (1981) Conditions for cytomegalovirus stimulation of lymphocytes. Scand J Immunol:13, 581.

Exp. Hematol. (suppl. 17) 13:134 (1985)

Donor Cytomegalovirus Immunity is a Risk Factor for Chronic Graft-Versus-Host Disease (GvHD) After Allogeneic Bone Marrow Transplantation

Niels Jacobsen[1], Peter Skinhøj[1], H. Kerzel Andersen[2], Lars Ryder[3], and Per Platz[3]

[1] Department of Infectious Diseases,
[2] Tissue Typing Laboratory, Rigshospitalet, Copenhagen
[3] Institute of Medical Microbiology, Århus University, Denmark

Introduction

Chronic Graft-versus-host disease (GvHD) develops in approximately 3o% of patients after allogenic bone marrow transplantation, presumably mediated by an immunologic reaction of transplanted donor cells against recipient antigens. Recipient age and previous acute GvHD have been found to predispose for this complication[1]. More recently, it has been reported that the onset of chronic GvHD frequently is preceded by a cytomegalovirus (CMV) infection[2]. We hypothesised that an immunologic reaction of donor cells against CMV infected recipient cells could be involved in the pathogenesis of chronic GvHD. We therefore decided to analyse the effect of donor pretransplant CMV immunity on the incidence of chronic GvHD.

Materials and methods

Between 198o and 1984, 54 patients were treated with allogenic bone marrow transplantation. Forty-three patients survived ≥ 1oo days after transplantation and were considered at risk for developing chronic GvHD. Of the latter group of patients, six had severe aplastic anaemia and 37 had haematologic malignancies. They were conditioned with total body irradiation and/or cyclophosphamide prior to infusion of unseparated bone marrow cells obtained from HLA identical (36 patients) or haploidentical, MLC compatible (7 patients) family donors. Patients were treated germ-free using total decontamination in laminar-air-flow cabinets. Cyclosporin and/or metotrexate were given as prophylaxis against acute GvHD. CMV antibodies in donor and recipient serum were determined by complement fixation (CF) test prior to transplantation. A titer ≥ 4 was considered positive. Posttransplant four fold recipient CF-titer increase and/or CMV excretion as determined by culture were taken as evidence of CMV infection. All cases of chronic GvHD were confirmed by biopsies. Cumulative incidence of CMV infection and GvHD were calculated by product-limit estimates.

Results

Eight of 15 recipients with a CMV CF-titer positive donor developed chronic GvHD in contrast to only 3 of 28 patients with a negative donor (Table 1).

Table 1

Donor pretransplant CMV immunity	N	Chronic GvHD	Cumulative incidence
positive	15	8	55%
negative	28	3[x]	16%

[x]$P_{2\alpha} = o.o1$, Fisher's test

No similar effect of recipient pretransplant CMV immunity on the incidence of chronic GvHD was observed. Thirty-four of the 43 patients had posttransplant CMV infection. Of the 34 patients with posttransplant CMV infection, 12 were transplanted with cells from CMV immune donors and 7 developed chronic GvHD, in contrast to only 3 of 22 with non-immune donors. Donor CMV immune status had no influence on the incidence or severity of acute GvHD or posttransplant CMV infection. The ratio of CMV immune donors increased markedly with donor age. Thus, of 3o donors < 3o years, only 5 were immune. In contrast, 1o of 13 donors >3o years were immune. Furthermore, since most donor-recipient pairs were siblings of approximately the same age, the proportion of immune donors also increased with recipient age. Donor CMV immunity was associated with increased incidence of chronic GvHD regardless of recipient and donor age per se. No significant influence of HLA mis-match on the incidence of chronic GvHD was observed.

Discussion and conclusion

The present results demonstate a correlation between donor pretransplant CMV immunity and chronic GvHD after allogenic bone marrow transplantation. Posttransplant CMV infection was associated with a low incidence of chronic GvHD when the donor was non-immune. The effect of donor immunity was not mediated through an increase in the incidence of acute GvHD or posttransplant CMV infection. Donor CMV immunity may be the determinant that predisposes older patients for chronic GvHD. This study suggests that an immunologic reaction of preimmunized donor cells against CMV plays a pathogenic role in chronic GvHD.

References

1. Storb R et al: Ann Int Med 1983;98:461-6
2. Lönquist B et al: Transplantation 1984;38:465-68

Clinical Management

Exp. Hematol. (suppl. 17) 13:135–136 (1985)
© International Society for Experimental Hematology

The Treatment of Chronic Graft Versus Host Disease

A. J. Barrett

Haematology Department, Charing Cross and Westminster Medical School, Westminster Hospital, Dean Ryle Street, London SW1, Great Britain

INTRODUCTION

Chronic Graft Versus Host Disease (C-GVHD) represents a significant cause of continued morbidity and mortality persisting for many months after an otherwise successful bone marrow transplant. Its manifestations are extremely variable both in its severity and in its organ involvement. At one end of the spectrum Lichen planus plaques on the skin and in the mouth are relatively easily managed, while severe progressing scleroderma, lung involvement and profound immune suppression remain difficult and serious complications.

Historically, C-GVHD was not well recognised and today the pathophysiology is still not well understood. The first treatment study from Seattle therefore concentrated on the basic question of whether treatment was effective[1]. There have been suprisingly few surveys of the management of C-GVHD since this time, possibly because of a gradual improvement in the evolution of this condition due to better management. In this paper prophylaxis of C-GVHD and the management of intractible multisystem C-GVHD will be discussed.

The Seattle Study
In 1981 Sullivan and co-workers analysed 175 marrow transplants for leukaemia and aplastic anaemia. 52 developed chronic GVHD. They were allocated to receive (a) no treatment, (b) Prednisolone or ATG, (c) Prednisolone and Cyclophosphamide · or Azathioprine. The no treatment group fared significantly worse with over 80% of patients progressing to multisystem GVHD and half dying with C-GVHD. The treatment group receiving Azathioprine or Cyclophosphamide in addition to prednisolone fared best with less than 20% developing disablement or dying from C-GVHD, azathioprine having the advantage over cyclophosphamide that it did not provoke haemorrhagic cystitis. This study clearly showed that immunosuppressive treatment could modify progress of the disease, that azathioprine and prednisolone was very effective, but that prolonged treatment was necessary.

Prevention of C-GVHD
The possibility of preventing C-GVHD by eradicating acute GVHD is an attractive one supported by the fact that about a third of patients develop C-GVHD as a progression from acute GVHD and only a small proportion develop C-GVHD de novo. Since neither MTX nor Cyclosporin prevent acute GVHD it is not surprising to find no obvious reduction in the frequency of C-GVHD in Cyclosporin treated patients. The almost complete elimination of acute GVHD by T Cell depletion of donor marrow with monoclonal antibodies allows this hypothesis to be tested. In a series of ALL patients transplanted by the Westminster Group the acute GVHD incidence has fallen from 65% in 63 cyclosporin treated patients to 5% in 17 Campath 1 + Cyclosporin treated patients. Similarly, the incidence of C-GVHD has fallen from 48% of survivors beyond 100 days to less than 20% of Campath 1 treated patients.

Another approach to preventing C-GVHD has been to use continuous low dose Prednisolone from the time of the BMT[2,3]. The results of two studies are conflicting and at best show only a modest effect on the eventual development of C-GVHD.

Treatment of progressive GVHD
Despite early treatment with azathioprine and prednisolone, some patients progress to lethal immune deficiency, sclerosis and pulmonary complications. In an analysis of 63 patients given cyclosporin GVHD prophylaxis by the Westminster Group 26/54 survivors developed C-GVHD and 3 of these died, one from infection and multisystem GVHD and 2 from progressive sclerosis. Several agents were used to treat refractory patients, (a) cyclosporin, (b) Penicillamine[4], (c) plasma exchange[5]. In addition, in four patients relapsing with leukaemia the effect of chemotherapy treatment was observed

Cyclosporin:
of 5 patients developing progressive sclerosis three improved dramatically with reintroduction of cyclosporin while two patients showed no response.

Penicillamine:
following a case report where penicillamine produced improvement in a patient with GVHD, we used it on three patients with sclerosis with no response.

Plasma exchange:
last year we reported a transient benefit from plasma exchange in one patient with severe sclerosis. The rationale was to remove circulating fibroblast stimulating factor and retard progression of sclerosis

136

Antileukaemia treatment: Four patients with active C-GVHD at time of relapse showed improvement of GVHD after receiving treatment for relapsed leukaemia. Two received a multiple agent reinduction schedule including Ara-C, Daunorubicin, prednisolone, VM26, and vincristine. Two Patients received high dose single agents - Ara-C or methotrexate. One patient with obstructive bronchiolitis had a dramatic and sustained improvement. Three others had rapid improvement of skin and liver C-GVHD.

Other supportive measures

Certain simple measures can help the quality of life of the patient with multisystem C-GVHD. Artificial tears and saliva help the patient with sicca syndrome. Regular physiotherapy and exercise can be useful in patients with sclerosis. It seems appropriate to use septrin or penicillin as long term prophylaxis against infections and the prophylactic role of regular immunoglobulin infusions has not been fully explored. Psychologically, C-GVHD can be one of the worst sequelae to an otherwise successful marrow transplant, and a positive and energetic attitude to treatment is very important.

CONCLUSIONS

The incidence and severity of C-GVHD has diminished in the last few years, partly because of better prevention of severe acute GVHD and partly because of the early use of prednisolone and azathioprine. The data indicates that prompt and continued treatment of mild C-GVHD is vital in preventing progression to multisystem GVHD. In patients who do progress to life threatening immune deficiency, lung disease and sclerosis, reintroduction of cyclosporin and high dose chemotherapy should be tried together with other supportive measures.

REFERENCES

1. Sullivan K M, Shulman H M, Storb R et al. Chronic graft versus host disease in 52 patients: adverse natural course and successful treatment with combination immunosuppression. Blood 57, 267, 1981

2. Ringden O, Lonnqvist B, Lundgren G et al. Experience with a co-operative bone marrow transplantation programme in Stockholm. Transplantation 33, 500, 1982

3. Blume K G, Beutler E, Bross K J et al. Bone marrow ablation and allogeneic marrow transplantation in acute leukaemia. N.Eng.J.Med. 302,1091, 1980.

4. Summerfield G P, Bellingham A J, Bunch C, Woodrow J C. Case report: successful treatment of chronic cutaneous graft versus host disease (GVHD) with penicillamine. J.Clin. and Lab.Haem. 5, 313-318, 1983

5. Barrett A J, Adams J A, Giangrande P L F. Fibroblast colony stimulation in chronic cutaneous graft versus host disease. Exp.Haem.12 (Sup.15) 53-4, 1984

Exp. Hematol. (suppl. 17) 13:137 (1985)
© International Society for Experimental Hematology

Treatment of Active Chronic Graft Versus Host Disease of the Skin with Monoclonal Antibody OKT3.Pan

W. E. Fibbe[1], J. W. Gratama[2], R. G. C. Teepe[3], G. Goldstein[4], and F. E. Zwaan[1]

[1] Departments of Haematology-Bone-Marrow Transplant Unit,
[2] Immunohaematology and
[3] Dermatology, University Medical Centre, Leiden, The Netherlands
[4] Ortho Pharmaceutical Corporation, Raritan, NJ, USA

INTRODUCTION

Monoclonal anti-T-cell antibodies are being used for the *in-vitro* removal of T cells from allogeneic bone marrow grafts, in order to prevent acute graft-versus-host disease (aGVHD). The antibodies are also being used for the *in-vivo* treatment of aGVHD. Previously, we have reported a complete response in 4 of 8 patients with aGVHD, treated for 14 days with the murine anti-T-cell monoclonal antibody OKT3 (Gratama et al., 1984). We now report on the use of OKT3 in 2 patients with active chronic GVHD of the skin that was resistent to conventional immunosuppressive therapy.

PATIENTS

Two male patients, 32 and 33 years old, received a bone marrow transplant from an HLA-identical, MLR-nonreactive sibling donor. Patient 1 suffered from severe aplastic anemia and was conditioned with cyclophosphamide (50 mg/kg x4) and total lymph node irradiation (7.5 Gy in one session). Patient 2 suffered from myelogenous leukemia and was prepared with cyclophosphamide (50 mg/kg x2) and total body irradiation (8 Gy). Methotrexate was given as prophylaxis for aGVHD. Patient 1 developed grade II GVHD of the skin on day 18, which was treated with high dose methylprednisolone. On day 57, a lichenoid pattern developed; histologically, lichen planus-like changes in dermis and epidermis were seen. Nine months post-BMT generalized sclerosis was present, with edema, bullae formation and severe ulcerations. Patient 2 developed an exfoliative erythroderma involving large areas of the body, 2 months post-BMT. From that time on severe desquamation and erythroderma persisted. Treatment with prednisone, azathioprine and cyclosporin-A was unsuccessful in both patients.

RESULTS

Administration and side effects of OKT3. After documentation of a negative skin test, 5 ml of filter sterilized (0.22 μ) OKT3 (Ortho Pharmaceutical Corporation, Raritan, N.J.) per day was slowly injected for 14 days. The first injection was preceded by prednisolone, 1 mg/kg i.v. In patient 1, a severe transien hypotensive reaction occurred, accompanied by spiking fever and oliguria.

Effect of OKT3 therapy on circulating T cells. T cells were enumerated within one hour after OKT3 injection, as described previously (Gratama et al., 1984). After the first OKT3 injection the number of circulating $T3^+$, $T4^+$, and $T8^+$ cells decreased to almost zero. During the next 4 days the number of $T4^+$ and $T8^+$ cells gradually increased to $200/mm^3$, whereas the number of $T3^+$ remained low, suggesting modulation of the T3 antigen. The ratio between $T4^+$ and $T8^+$ T cells did not change significantly during or following therapy. The number of $T3^+$ cells reached pretreatment levels 3-4 weeks after cessation of therapy. In patient 2, a transient overshoot of $T3^+$ cells was seen.

Effect of OKT3 therapy on skin GVHD. In patient 1, the skin lesions remained unchanged clinically, although a temporary decrease in redness of the papules did occur. In patient 2, a slight, but temporary reduction of erythroderma was noted clinically. Control skin biopsies from both patients did not reveal significant reduction of the lympho-histiocytic infiltration.

DISCUSSION

The effect of a 10-day course of daily injections of OKT3 on chronic skin GVHD was studied in 2 patients with severe, active, chronic skin GVHD. Although in both patients temporary reduction of erythroderma occurred, the improvement was of no clinical significance. Furthermore, post-treatment skin histology did not reveal significant reduction of inflammatory infiltration as compared to pretreatment biopsies. A severe adverse reaction was seen in patient 1, in spite of pretreatment with corticosteroids.

Following the first injection of OKT3, virtually all circulating $T3^+$ cells were removed from the circulation, indicating that the dose of the antibody was sufficient. In spite of this, no significant reduction of the inflammatory infiltration was seen in control skin biopsies. Modulation of the T3 antigen was demonstrated in both patients. This is not an explanation for the lack of response, as it also occurred in patients with aGVHD who did respond to OKT3 (Gratama et al.). Furthermore, the role of T cells in mediating chronic GVHD is far less clear than in acute GVHD.

In summary, these case reports suggest that no long-term beneficial effect of OKT3 treatment can be expected in patients with chronic GVHD of the skin.

REFERENCES

Gratama JW, Jansen J, Lipovich RA, Tanke HJ, Goldstein G, & Zwaan FE: Treatment of acute graft-versus-host disease with monoclonal antibody OKT3.PAN. Transplantation 38:469-474, 1984.

Exp. Hematol. (suppl. 17) 13:138 (1985)
© International Society for Experimental Hematology

Comparative Value of Clinical Examination, Lip Biopsy and Salivary Scintigraphy for Detecting Sjogren-Like Syndrome in Bone Marrow Transplanted Patients

A. Janin-Mercier[1], A. Devergie[2], J. P. Arrago[3], C. Brocheriou[4], F. Lemarchand-Venencie[2], J. D. Rain[1], and E. Gluckman[2]

[1] Departement of Pathology, F-63000 Clermont-Ferrand
[2] BMT Unit, Hôpital Saint-Louis, Paris
[3] Department of Nuclear Medicine,
[4] Departement of Pathology, Hôpital Saint-Louis, Paris, France

INTRODUCTION

Sjögren-like syndrome (SLS) is one of the criteria used to diagnose extensive chronic graft versus host disease (CGVHD) (1) and it contributes to malnutrition and recurrent local infections in grafted patients (2,3). We compared the diagnostic value of 3 types of examination for detecting SLS : clinical examination, lip biopsy, salivary scintiscan.

MATERIAL AND METHODS

60 patients with allogeneic BMT (25 leukemia, 35 aplastic anemia) and 8 patients with syngeneic BMT (7 leukemia, 1 aplastic anemia) had at Day 100 and one year after the graft 1) a clinical examination of mouth and eyes, a Schirmer test and a slip lamp examination, 2) a lip biopsy graded according to Sale (4), 3) a salivary scintigraphy with functional analysis (5).

RESULTS

On Day 100, all patients had oral dryness. 13 patients had SLS with ocular and oral dryness, grade II lip biopsies and grade III or IV salivary scintiscan. 9 patients had a disturbed Schirmer test, a grade II scintiscan, a grade II lip biopsy. They later developped SLS.
20 allogeneic patients and 7 syngeneic patients had oral dryness without ocular involvement, asymetrical grade III or IV scintiscans and normal lip biopsies. They all had received 10 Gy TBI before the graft. The 3 examinations were normal in 7 allogeneic and 1 syngeneic patients.
The 11 other patients had no SLS but mild CGVHD and a grade I lip biopsy.

DISCUSSION

The diagnostic value of our 3 tests is not the same clinically the detection of SLS on Day 100 was easy when SLS was complete (13 patients). It was then associated with extensive CGVHD. Isolated oral dryness is not a good diagnostic criterion for SLS at Day 100 since it can be a consequence or radiotherapy. Ocular involvement is a more reliable diagnostic criterion for SLS but it sometimes needs to be detected by Schirmer test at Day 100.
Salivary scintiscan is a non-invasive method which can be repeated. It was sensitive for detecting early salivary gland involvement for 9 patients who later progressed to SLS. Its functional analysis allows a distinction between sequelae of radiotherapy.
(well analysed in syngeneic patients) and early or confirmed SLS where scintiscan involvement is homogeneous for the 4 major salivary glands. Lip biopsy cannot be graded on focus score used for isolated Sjögren syndrome since no voluminous lymphocytic aggregate is observed in SLS (4). It is a sensitive method for detecting SLS since the patients with radiotherapy sequelae had a normal lip biopsy. It has a predictive value since in our series of 24 patients with SLS only one had a normal lip biopsy at Day 100.
Ocular involvement salivary scintiscan and lip biopsy ara valuable tools for detecting SLS at Day 100. Since SLS is different from idiopathic Sjögren "syndrome" and radiotherapy-induced damage it might be a separate type of salivary gland lesion related to immune disorders of CGVHD.

1 - SHULMAN H.M., SULLIVAN K.M., WEIDEN P.L., Mc DONALD C.B., STRIKER G.E.,SALE G.E., HACKMAN R., TSOI M.S., STORB R., THOMAS E.D. : A long term clinicopathologic study of 20 Seattle patients. Am. J. Med. 1980, 69 : 204-217

2 - RODU B., GOCKERMAN J.P. : Oral manifestations of the chronic graft-versus-host reaction. J.A.M.A. 1983, 249 : 504-507

3 - SCHUBERT M.M., SULLIVAN K.M., MORTON T.H., IZUTSU K.T., PETERSON D.E., FLOURMOY N., TRUELOVE E.L., SALE G.E., BUCKNER C.D., STORB R., THOMAS E.D. : Oral manifestations of chronic graft versus host disease. Arch. Int. Med. 1984, 144 : 1591-1595

4 - SALE G.E., SHULMAN H.M., SULLIVAN K.M., KOPECKY K.J., HACKMAN R.C., MORTON T.H., STORB R., THOMAS E.D. : Oral and ophtalmologic pathology of graft versus host disease in man : predictive value of the lip biopsy. Hum. Pathol. 1981, 12 : 1022-1030

5 - ARRAGO J.P., RAIN J.D., ROCHER F., VIGNERON N., PECKING A., NAJEAN Y. : Syndrome de Gougerot-Sjögren. Etude fonctionnelle des glandes salivaires par la scintigraphie. Presse Med. 1984, 13 : 209-213

Exp. Hematol. (suppl. 17) 13:139–141 (1985)
© International Society for Experimental Hematology

The Spectrum of Cutaneous Graft Versus Host Disease

Georg Stingl, Beatrix Volc-Platzer, Klemens Rappersberger, Klaus Konrad, Wolfgang Hinterberger, Klaus Lechner, and Klaus Wolff

Department of Dermatology I, Department of Internal Medicine I, University of Vienna, Vienna, Austria

INTRODUCTION:
Cutaneous graft-versus-host disease (GVHD) is the sequela of a graft-versus-host reaction (GVHR) affecting the skin and its appendages. The skin is a primary target organ for GVHD and the recognition of the cutaneous GVHD is important for several reasons: (I) Since cutaneous symptoms are occasionally the first indicators of an ongoing GVHR, their recognition should result in prompt confirmation of the diagnosis and in the initiation of appropriate therapeutic measures. (II) Cutaneous GVHD can occasionally be a life-threatening or a disabling condition. (III) Cutaneous GVHD may serve as a biological model for the elucidation of patho-mechanisms operative in skin diseases displaying similar clinical and/or histopathological features.

OCCURRENCE OF CUTANEOUS GVHD:
The requirements for the occurrence of a cutaneous GVHD are defined by the term GVHR, i.e. immunocompetent cells within the graft, immunosuppression of the host, and, possibly, histocompatibility differences between the graft and the host. These requirements are met (I) when an immunodeficient fetus receives maternal lymphocytes via the placental barriere, (II) when neonates and infants with primary immunodeficiency or immunosuppressed individuals (malignancy, cytotoxic drugs) receive leukocyte-rich blood transfusions, and (III), most importantly, when an immunosuppressed patient receives an allogeneic bone marrow transplant (BMT) for the treatment of hematological, metabolical or immunological disorders. In this report, we will describe the spectrum of human cutaneous GVHD rather than the respective animal models and in the context of this meeting - we will restrict this discussion to patients receiving allogeneic BMT.

CLINICAL MANIFESTATIONS OF CUTANEOUS GVHD:
Cutaneous GVHD is not a single disorder but rather composed of two separate phases, acute and chronic, each having different clinical manifestations (1) and possibly a different pathogenesis (2).

Acute cutaneous GVHD:
Acute cutaneous GVHD usually develops 7 - 40 days after BMT. Mild localized or generalized pruritus, pressure pain on palms and soles, and a distinctive auricular and/or periungual erythema occasionally precede the appearance of a maculopapular and/or scarlatiniform eruption. This rash involves the cheeks, neck, upper trunk, hands, and feet, particularly the palms and soles. In mild cases or after prompt initiation of therapy, respectively, this eruption may subside at this point. Alterna-

tively, the eruption may progress to involve large portions of the integument and may finally become generalized (erythroderma). Occasionally, wide-spread epidermal necrosis ensues as evidenced by frank blister formation and sloughing of epidermal sheets from the skin (= toxic epidermal necrolysis, TEN) (3). TEN is the most severe manifestation of acute cutaneous GVHD and is associated with high mortality.

Chronic cutaneous GVHD:
Chronic cutaneous GVHD occurs months to years after BMT and may or may not be preceded by acute cutaneous GVHD. In most patients, two phases of chronic cutaneous GVHD are observed: the early chronic phase that resembles lichen planus (4), and the late chronic phase in which poikiloderma and scleroderma-like features predominate (5,6).

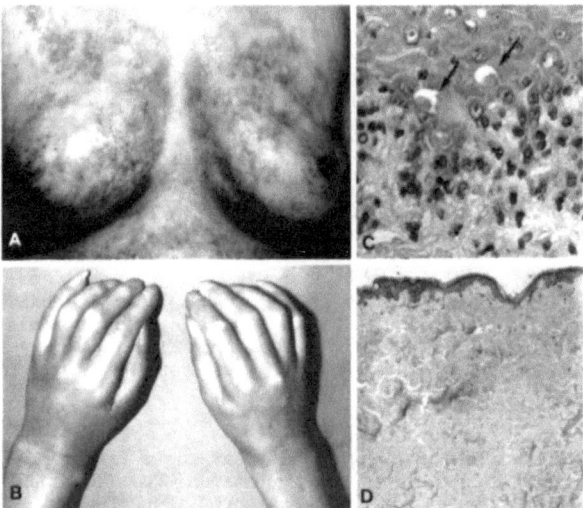

Fig.1: Clinical and histopathological features of chronic cutaneous GVHD. A. Long-standing lichenoid eruption with signs of poikiloderma (pigmentary changes, atrophy) and incipient sclerosis. B. Fully developed sclerodermoid GVHD affecting both hands. C. Lichenoid GVHD. Note dyskeratotic keratinocytes (arrows) and the presence of a mainly lymphocytic infiltrate partially masking the dermal-epidermal junction. D. Sclerodermoid GVHD. The dermis is greatly thickened and consists of tightly packed collagen bundles.

The lichenoid cutaneous GVHD may mimic the entire spectrum of lichen planus, i.e. the appearance of violaceous lichenoid papules on both trunk and extremities and the emergence of whitish plaques on the oral mucosa. The lichenoid eruption localizes frequently to the hair follicles (lichen plano-pilaris) whereas nail involvement is only rarely seen. After resolution the eruption leaves behind a macular or reticular grayish-brownish hyperpigmentation with signs of atrophy and poikiloderma (Fig.1A). In certain patients, the character of the lesions slowly changes to result in either localized or generalized sclerosis (Fig.1B). Individual morphealike lesions (1 - 10 cm) may coalesce to form large confluent sclerotic plaques. The involvement of skin and mucosal appendages is manifested by irreversible alopecia, diminished sweating and sicca syndrome.

HISTOPATHOLOGY OF CUTANEOUS GVHD:

Acute cutaneous GVHD:

The earliest histopathologic abnormalities occasionally precede a clinically detectable eruption for one or two days and consist of focal vacuolar changes in the basement membrane zone of the epidermis and hair follicle epithelium. Caution, however, is warranted not to overinterpret this finding since it may also represent a sequela of conditioning regimens (7). In the case of GVHD, these changes are usually accompanied by a predominantly mononuclear cell infiltrate in the upper dermis. As the reaction progresses, the vacuolar changes become more pronounced, intercellular edema is observed and individual dyskeratotic cells appear in the lower epidermis. These distinctive cells with homogeneous bright eosinophilic cytoplasm, small pyknotic nuclei, and surrounding clear halo or lacunae have been termed "mummified" cells. Occasionally, mononuclear cells may be seen in close apposition to the dyskeratotic cells, the so-called satellite lymphocytes (8). If the disease progresses, the vacuoles coalesce to form subepidermal clefts and the epidermis undergoes widespread necrosis.

Chronic cutaneous GVHD:

Biopsy specimens from patients exhibiting lichenoid cutaneous GVHD greatly resemble those obtained from the patients with idiopathic lichen planus (Fig.1C). The epidermal pathology includes hyperkeratosis, hypergranulosis, acanthosis and basal cell vacuolization. The dermal changes, however, differ from those seen in lichen planus: instead of a band-like mononuclear cell infiltrate along the dermal-epidermal junction, one usually observes a mild perivascular infiltrate composed of lymphocytes, histiocytes, melanophages, and rarely a few plasma cells or eosinophils. Biopsy specimens from sclerodermoid lesions exhibit a thickened reticular dermis composed of hypertrophic, densely packed, brightly eosinophilic collagen bundles (Fig.1D). These changes are paralleled by a progressive reduction of the appendage structures and by a sparse perivascular infiltrate.

ULTRASTRUCTURE OF CUTANEOUS GVHD:

Acute cutaneous GVHD:

The pathognomonic significance of the ultrastructural changes seen in acute cutaneous GVHD (rev.in 9) have to be evaluated with the proviso that patients have received conditioning treatment. Alterations are discrete and focal and consist (I) of intracellular edema of occasional basal cells, (II) of intercellular edema and the occasional occurrence of condensed keratinocytes, densely packed with tonofilaments, pyknotic nuclei with condensed chromatin and devoid of desmosomes - thus resembling dyskeratotic or apoptotic cells -, (III) a numerical reduction of Langerhans cells and (IV) the occasional

occurrence of intraepidermal lymphocytes.

Chronic cutaneous GVHD:

In the lichenoid phase of chronic cutaneous GVHD (10) alterations are again focal and consist of widening of the intercellular spaces of the epidermis, cytoplasmic vacuolization and irregular aggregation of tonofilaments within basal keratinocytes. In fully developed lesions, basal keratinocytes focally exhibit severe damage such as clumping of tonofilaments, condensation of cytoplasm and pyknotic nuclei (Fig.2). There is also frank necrosis of keratinocytes and occasionally, lymphocytes are found in close apposition to these damaged cells which represents the "satellite cell necrosis" seen by light microscopy.

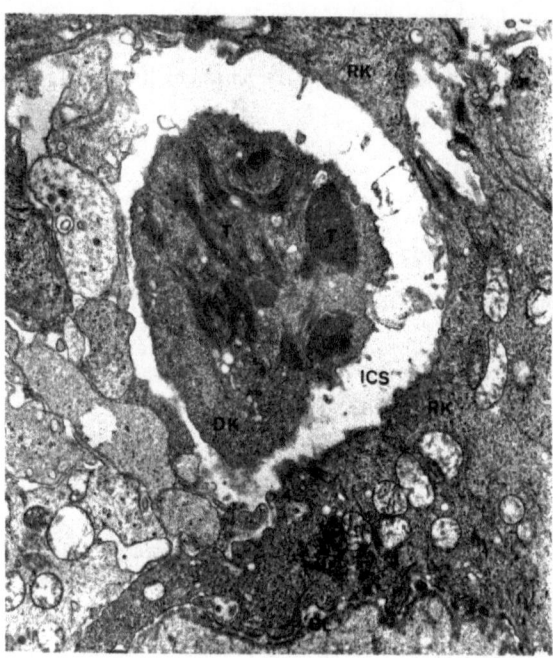

Fig.2: Epidermal ultrastructure of chronic cutaneous GVHD-lichenoid phase. A dyskeratotic keratinocyte (DK) exhibits clumped tonofilaments (T), a condensed cytoplasm and is devoid of desmosomes. The intercellular space (ICS) is greatly widened; neighbouring keratinocytes exhibit signs of regeneration (RK). BL: basal lamina; x 19,000.

In addition, focal keratinocytes with abundant cytoplasm, numerous free ribosomes and occasional mitotic activity indicate cell regeneration (Fig. 2). There are multiple reduplications of the basal lamina and a considerable number of Langerhans cells and melanocytes exhibit massive intracellular edema and intense swelling of the cell-organelles and show features of cytolysis.

The most prominent ultrastructural changes in sclerodermoid cutaneous GVHD consist of broad bundles of densely packed collagen fibres with reduction of interbundle spaces. Normal periodicity and structure of collagen fibres and numerous active fibroblasts in the upper parts of the dermis distinguish GVHD from scleroderma (11).

IMMUNOHISTOLOGY OF CUTANEOUS GVHD:

Apart from conflicting reports about the deposition of immunoglobulins and/or complement components along the dermal-epidermal junction, there is now ample evidence that the expression pattern of MHC-encoded alloantigens in cutaneous GVHD differs from that seen in normal skin. Within normal human epidermis, dendritic Langerhans cells are the only cells to synthesize and to express HLA-D region-encoded alloantigens (11); in cutaneous GVHD, however, class II alloantigens can be readily detected not only on Langerhans cells, but also on a large portion of keratinocytes (12). The demonstration of keratinocyte-bound class II alloantigens represents an important diagnostic tool for cutaneous GVHD, since it usually precedes the clinical and histopathological manifestations of this disease but, on the other hand, is never seen in patients receiving allogeneic BMT without development of cutaneous GVHD (see Volc-Platzer et al., this volume). In vitro studies suggest that HLA-DR expression by keratinocytes results from lymphokine-triggered induction of HLA-DR biosynthesis by keratinocytes; it has been shown that IFN-γ is the major, if not the only lymphokine responsible for the occurrence of such an event (13); a potentially important finding is the recent observation that cells bearing the phenotype of NK cells (Leu-7) populate the epidermis in cutaneous GVHD (Volc-Platzer, et al., this volume). It is tempting to speculate that GVHD-induced increased IFN-γ production leads to the emergence, and possibly maturation, of NK cells which would then lethally injure epidermal targets. This hypothesis gains support from experiments conducted in rodent animals which have shown that the occurrence of murine GVHD can be prevented by pretreating the host with monoclonal antibodies against an antigenic determinant primarily expressed on NK cells (asialo-GM1) (14).

DIFFERENTIAL DIAGNOSIS OF CUTANEOUS GVHD:
The differential diagnosis of an erythematous maculopapular eruption that develops within the first 2 1/2 months after successful BMT includes acute cutaneous GVHD, drug reaction and viral exanthem. Even in those cases without extracutaneous symptoms and without the characteristic histopathological changes of GVHD, the demonstration of class II alloantigens on keratinocyte surfaces strongly favors the diagnosis of cutaneous GVHD. Chronic cutaneous GVHD must be differentiated from lichen planus, lichenoid drug reaction, scleroderma, and poikiloderma. By clinical as well as (immuno)histological grounds, both the lichenoid and sclerodermoid lesions of cutaneous GVHD may greatly resemble their respective idiopathic counterparts. The diagnosis is therefore established by the development of such lesions at least 3 to 6 months following successful marrow transplantation.

TREATMENT OF CUTANEOUS GVHD:
Preventive and therapeutic measures for cutaneous GVHD are those used for prevention and treatment of systemic GVHD (see chapter ...., this volume). In chronic cutaneous GVHD, conventional therapeutic efforts (corticosteroids, azathioprine, cyclosporine A, etc.) occasionally yield only poor results; interestingly several workers have reported on the beneficial effect of UV-phototherapy for chronic cutaneous GVHD (15); due to possible late adverse effects of UV radiation on the immune system, it seems premature to generally recommend this treatment modality.

REFERENCES:
1. Glucksberg, H., Storb, R., Fefer, A., Buckner, C.D., Neiman, P.E., Clift, R.A., Lerner, K.G., Thomas, E.D. Clinical manifestations of graft-versus-host disease in human recipients of marrow from HLA-matched sibling donors. Transplantation, 1974, 18: 295.
2. Parkman, R., Rappeport, J., Rosen F. Human graft-versus-host disease. J.Invest.Dermatol., 1980, 74: 276.
3. Peck, G.L., Herzig, G.P., Elias, P.M., Toxic epidermal necrolysis in a patient with graft-versus-host reaction. Arch.Derm., 1972, 105: 561.
4. Saurat, J.H., Didier-Jean, L., Gluckman, E., Bussel, A. Graft versus host reaction and lichen planus like eruption in man. Br.J.Dermatol., 1975, 92: 591.
5. Siimes, M.A., Johansson, E., Rapola, J. Scleroderma-like graft-versus-host disease as late consequence of bone marrow grafting. Lancet, 1977, II: 831.
6. Lawley, T.J., Peck, G.L., Moutsopoulos, H.M., Gratwohl, A.A., Deisseroth, A.B. Scleroderma, Sjögren-like syndrome, and chronic graft-versus-host disease. Ann.Int.Med., 1977, 87: 707.
7. Sale, G.E., Lerner, K.G., Barker, E.A., Shulman, H.M., Thomas, E.D. The skin biopsy in the diagnosis of acute graft-versus-host disease in man. Am.J.Pathol., 1977, 89: 621.
8. Woodruff, J.M., Eltringham, J.R., Casey, H.W. Early secondary disease in the Rhesus monkey. I. A comparative histopathologic study. Lab. Invest., 1969, 20: 499.
9. De Dobbeleer, G.D., Ledoux-Corbusier, M.H., Achten, G.A. Graft-versus-host reaction. An ultrastructural study. Arch.Dermatol., 1975, 111: 1597.
10. Janin-Mercier, A., Saurat, J.H., Bourges, M., Sohier, J., Didier-Jean, L., Gluckman, E., The lichen planus-like and sclerotic phases of the graft-versus-host disease in man. An ultrastructural study of six cases. Acta Dermatovenerol. (Stockholm), 1981, 61: 187.
11. Rowden, G., Lewis, M.G., Sullivan, A.K. Ia antigen expression on human epidermal Langerhans cells. Nature, 1977, 268: 247.
12. Lampert, J.A., Janossy, G., Suitters, A.J., Bofill, M., Palmer, S., Gordon-Smith, E., Prentice, H.G., Thomas, J.A. Immunological analysis of the skin in graft-versus-host disease. Clin.Exp.Immunol., 1982, 50: 123.
13. Volc-Platzer, B., Leibl, H., Luger, T., Zahn, G., Stingl, G. Human epidermal cells synthesize HLA-DR alloantigens in vitro upon stimulation with γ-interferon. J.Invest.Dermatol., 1985, in press.
14. Charley, M.R., Mikhael, A., Benvett, M., Gilliam, J.N. Sontheimer, R.D. Prevention of lethal, minor-determinate graft-versus-host disease in mice by the in vivo administration of anti-asialo GM_1. J.Immunol., 1983, 131: 2101.
15. Hymes, S.R., Morison, W.L., Farmer, E.R., Walters, L.L., Tutschka, P.J., Santos, G.W. Methoxsalen and ultraviolet A radiation in treatment of chronic cutaneous graft-versus-host reaction. J.Am.Acad.Dermatol., 1985, 12: 30.

Exp. Hematol. (suppl. 17) 13:142−144 (1985)
© International Society for Experimental Hematology

Ocular Manifestations of Graft-Versus-Host Disease Following Bone Marrow Transplantation

G. Grabner[1], W. Hinterberger[2], M. Fischer[2], B. Volc-Platzer[3], M. Stur[1], and V. Huber-Spitzy[1]

[1] Department of Ophthalmology II,
[2] Department of Medicine I, and
[3] Department of Dermatology I, University of Vienna, Vienna, Austria

Graft-versus-host disease (GVHD) is a major complication following allogeneic bone marrow transplantation (BMT) and occurs in 50-70 % of the patients (1,2). It may begin weeks (acute GVHD) or months (chronic GVHD) following the transplantation, the target organ most frequently being the skin, liver and gastrointestinal tract (3). The many life-threatening complications encountered in these patients and the usually late presentation of severe ocular problems may explain their sparse documentation in the ophthalmic literature (4,5,7). Ocular manifestations, however, occur in a high percentage of patients suffering from GVHD and can on occasion severely affect their vision in spite of vigorous treatment.

Twenty-five patients undergoing BMT were examined prior to transplantation and followed thereafter in regular intervals for periods ranging from 6 weeks to 36 months. The eye exam included the standard Schirmer's test without anesthesia, fundoscopy, slit-lamp examination, tonometry, visual acuity (with correction), whenever feasible, and computer-perimetry, as well as fluorescein-angiography, whenever warranted.

Pertinent patient data are given in Table 1, details of the preparative regimen and medical follow-up have been published elsewhere (8,9).

Table 1. Patient data.

Type of BMT	Nr. of patients	Follow-up (after BMT)	Diagn.	Ocular pathol.
allogeneic	18	1.5-36 mo (av.17 mo)	SAA(8) CML(6) AML(4)	14/18 (=78%)
	5	26 - 99 d (av.49 d)	CML(3) AML(1) HD (1)	0
syngeneic	1	30 mo	SAA	0
autologous	1	15 mo	IL	0
total	25			

(11 female,14 male,age at BMT:15-38 y,aver.age:26.5 y) SAA:severe aplastic anemia,CML:chronic myelogenous leukemia,AML:acute myelogenous leukemia,IL:immunoblastic lymphoma (CR),HD:Hodgkin's disease, d:days,mo: months, y:years, Diagn.:diagnosis, Ocular pathol.: pathological ocular findings.

Neither the five patients succumbing within 100 days after BMT nor the two patients receiving an autologous or syngeneic transplant presented any ocular manifestations of the previous disease, GVHD, and/or treatment following BMT. In contrast, 14 / 18 patients (= 78 %) that survived allogeneic BMT for 1.5 to 36 months (aver.: 17 months) showed signs of eye involvement. The ocular findings and incidence of GVHD in our patients are detailed in Table 2.

Table 2. Ocular Findings and Incidence of GVHD.

Prior to BMT	Day 1 - 100 following BMT (Nr.of acute GVHD)	Over day 100 following BMT (Nr.of chronic GVHD)
2/25 retinal hem. 2/25	2/25 (2/2) subconj. hem. 1/25 (1/1) conjunctivitis	11/17 (11/11) reduced tear flow 5/17 (5/5) cataract 6/17 (4/6) blepharitis/conjunct. 1/17 (1/1) chorioretinitis
4/25 = 16%	2/25=8%(9/25=36%)	14/17=82% (13/17=76%)

The retinal hemorrhage observed in two patients prior to BMT resolved without sequelae, the central chorioretinal scars (of unknown origin) seen in two other patients remained unchanged during the observation period, causing a minor reduction of central vision.

Except for a subconjunctival hemorrhage in two patients with acute GVHD (as well as a Candida-conjunctivitis and dermatitis in one of them) the patients were remarkably free of ocular manifestations during the period immediatly following BMT (up to day 100), although acute GVHD was diagnosed in 9 out of 25 cases.

In contrast, 11/13 (=85%) of the patients with chronic GVHD (after day 100) had a reduced tear flow as measured by Schirmer's test on multiple occasions. Six of these were graded as severe keratoconjunctivitis sicca. Two female patients developed sterile corneal ulcerations. Whereas vigorous topical treatment (hourly application of tear substitutes and moist chamber) was sufficient in one of these patients to promote complete healing, the ulcerations progressed to bilateral corneal perforations in a 37-year old woman transplantated for SAA. In spite of maximal topical treatment and multiple corneal surgery (conjunctival flaps, tissue adhesive, corneal transplants, and conjunctival grafts from her donor sister) vision in both eyes was finally reduced to perception of light. Both, the corneal scarring (closely resembling mucous membrane pemphigoid) (6) and the dense bilateral cataracts, possibly caused by intraocular inflammation or long-term steroid-therapy, contibuted to this desastrous outcome (Fig. 1A and 1B). The epithelial cells of the corneal button obtained at the time of surgery for treatment of her corneal perforation displayed HLA-DR α/β -chains on their cell surface (Fig. 2A) and HLA-DR γ -chains within their cytoplasm (Fig. 2B). This finding has not, to the best of our knowledge, been previously reported in any other eye disease. Normal corneal epithelial cells- similar to keratinocytes- are uniformly class II alloantigen negative under normal conditions (10).

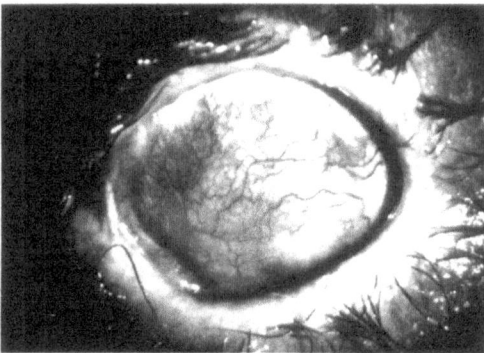

Fig. 1A. Right eye of 37y old woman with severe chronic GVHD following two corneal transplants with conjunctival graft from her donor sister. Symblephara and dense corneal vascularization.

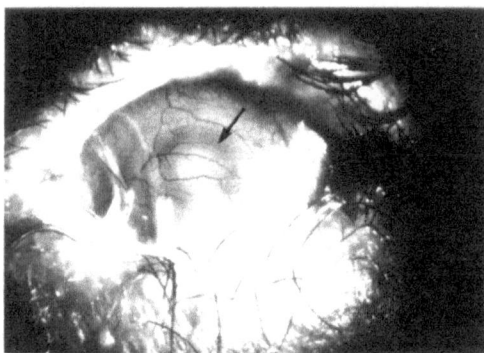

Fig. 1B. Left eye of same patient following one corneal transplant. Trichiasis, symblephara, corneal vascularization and thinning, and cataract (arrow).

Five out of 17 patients displayed bilateral cataracts, in one of the two clinically relevant cases possibly secondary to corneal surgery and intraocular inflammation. The second patient, requiring bilateral cataract extraction, displayed a dense posterior subcapsular cataract, as did the other three patients to a considerably lesser degree. The etiology, although debatable, seems rather related to long-term steroid treatment (used in all patients) than total body irradiation, since only 3/5 patients had received radiation pretreatment.
Pronounced blepharitis and/or conjunctivitis was observed in 4 patients with chronic GVHD, one patient developed an acute conjunctivitis 17 months after BMT, another a mild blepharitis, both without concurrent GVHD. The pigmentary changes in the skin of the eyelids closely correlated with the more widespread skin changes typical of GVHD (11).

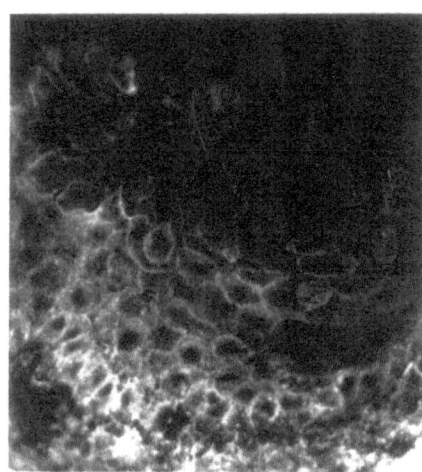

Fig. 2A. Demonstration of surface-bound HLA-DR α/β -complexes on the epithelial cells of the corneal button of the patient shown in Fig.1A. Technical details are given in ref. 10.

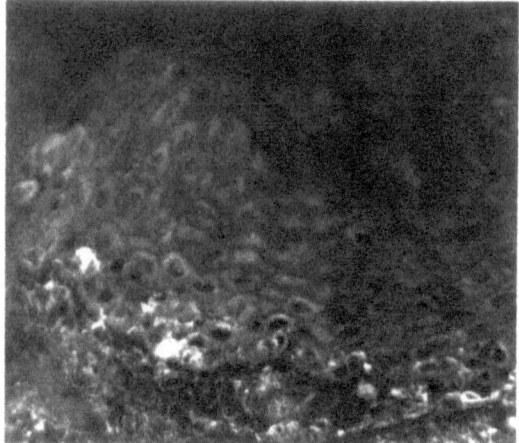

Fig. 2B. Demonstration of intracytoplasmic HLA-DR γ -chain within the epithelial cells of the corneal button obtained from the patient shown in Fig. 1A. Staining is apparent in all cell layers.

Furthermore we observed a bilateral, multifocal, recurrent chorioretinitis with panuveitis in a 21 year old male patient with severe chronic GVHD following BMT for AML (Fig. 3A and 3B). Following multiple recurrences the visual acuity in his right eye dropped to 20/100 (after successful cataract-surgery) and in his left eye to 20/800 (with best possible correction). All test for ocular Toxoplasmosis (including tests for antibodies, Toxoplasma antigen and specific immune-complexes in the aqueous humor) were negative. The fundus lesions appeared several months after BMT (before initiation of cyclosporin A-therapy), and showed several recurrences during systemic steroid treatment. The clinical picture mimics ocular histoplasmosis in some regards, a large series of similar cases has recently been reviewed by Dreyer and Gass(12).

Our observations parallel the findings of others (Table 3):
Severe ocular problems during acute GVHD appear to be rare and responsive to treatment.
Chronic GVHD, however, occasionally threatens the patients vision because of extremely severe keratoconjunctivitis sicca hardly amendable to

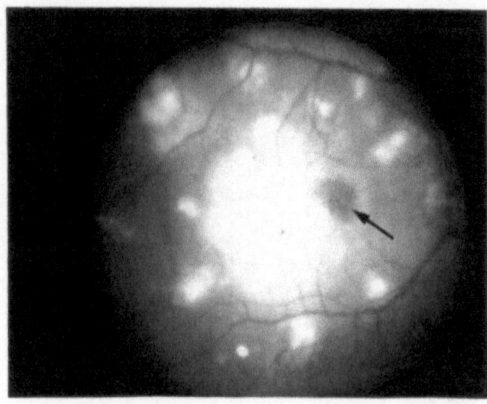

Fig. 3A. Right fundus of patient with multifocal, recurrent chorioretinitis of unknown etiology. Arrow shows submacular hemorrhage in the macular area.

conservative or surgical treatment, the end stage of the disease closely resembling severe mucous membrane pemphigoid. Furthermore, in our series, bilateral cataract (possibly steroid-induced) developed in 5 patients with chronic GVHD. Patients who survive BMT without substantial GVHD have generally been free of ocular problems.

The frequent and potentially severe ocular problems make an intense ophthalmic surveillance mandatory in all allogeneic bone marrow recipients.

Table 3. Ocular Manifestations of GVHD and/or Treatment.

Acute GVHD

Hemorrhagic or pseudomembranous conjunctivitis, conjunctival ulcers
Filiform keratitis, loss of corneal epithelium
Subconjunctival, vitreal, retinal hemorrhage
Dermatitis of the lids

Chronic GVHD

Dermatitis of the lids, ectropium, entropium, madarosis, trichiasis, pigmentary changes
Keratoconjunctivitis sicca, corneal ulceration, perforation and vascularization
Cataract
Iritis, iridocyclitis, chorioretinitis

References:

1. Glucksberg H.,Storb R.,Fefer A. et al.: Clinical manifestations of graft-versus-host disease in human recipients of marrow from HL-A-matched sibling donors.
   Transplantation 1974; 18:295-304.

2. Santos G.W.: Bone marrow transplantation.
   Adv. Intern. Med. 1979; 24:157-182.

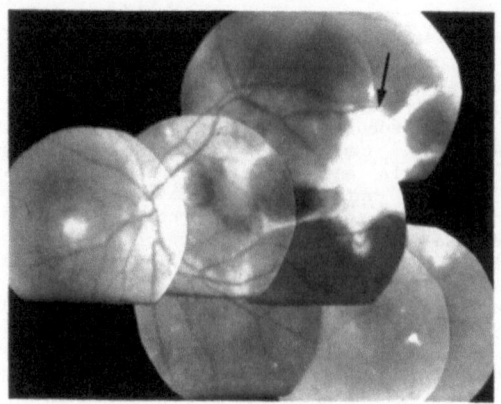

Fig. 3B. Composite photograph of the left fundus of the patient described in the text showing a massive sub- and epiretinal fibrosis (arrow) and multiple chorioretinal lesions.

3. Shulman H.M.,Sullivan K.M.,Weiden P.L. et al.: Chronic graft-versus-host syndrome in man. A long-term clinicopathologic study of 20 Seattle patients Am. J. Med. 1980; 69:204-217.

4. Franklin R.M.,Kenyon K.R.,Tutschka P.J. et al.: Ocular manifestations of graft-vs-host disease. Ophthalmology 1983; 90:4-13.

5. Hirst L.W.,Jabs D.A.,Tutschka P.J.,Green W.R.et al.: The eye in bone marrow transplantation.I. Clinical study.

Ref.(cont.):
   Arch.Ophthalmol. 1983; 101:580-584.

6. Jabs D.A.,Hirst L.W.,Green W.R.,Tutschka P.J.et al.: The eye in bone marrow transplantation.II. Histopathology.
   Arch.Ophthalmol. 1983; 101:585-590.

7. Jack M.K.,Jack G.M.,Sale G.E.,Shulman H.M. et al.: Ocular manifestations of graft-v-host disease. Arch.Ophthalmol. 1983; 101:1080-1084.

8. Schmidmeier W. et al.: this issue.

9. Hinterberger W. et al.: this issue.

10. Volc-Platzer B.,Majdic O.,Knapp W.,Wolff K. et al.: Evidence of HLA-DR antigen biosynthesis by human keratinocytes in disease.
    J. Exp. Med. 1984; 159:1784-1789.

11. Stingl G.: this issue.

12. Dreyer R.F.,Gass J.D.M.: Multifocal choroiditis and panuveitis. A syndrome that mimics ocular histoplasmosis.
    Arch.Ophthalmol. 1984; 102:1776-1784.

This investigation was supported in part by the Fonds zur Förderung der wissenschaftlichen Forschung,Vienna, Austria (Project-Nr.:P 5100).

Exp. Hematol. (suppl. 17) 13:145 (1985)
© International Society for Experimental Hematology

Pulmonary Follow-Up in Patients with Bone Marrow Transplantation (BMT) and Graft-Versus-Host Disease (GVHD)

R. Rodriguez-Roisin, J. Roca, P. Marín, A. Grañena, A. Agustí-Vidal, and C. Rozman

Departament de Medicina (Servei de Pneumologia: Escola d'Hematologia "Farreras Valenti"), Hospital Clínic, Facultat de Medicina, Universitat de Barcelona, Barcelona, Spain

INTRODUCTION

Pulmonary complications have emerged as one of the major problems of allogeneic bone marrow transplantation (BMT). Interstitial pneumonitis is the most well-known complication; however, there is also increasing evidence to support the view that obstructive lung disease can be present in BMT recipients (Rodriguez-Roisín et al, 1984; Ralph et al, 1984; Wyatt et al, 1984). We report here the main pulmonary clinical and functional findings observed in 25 consecutive patients submitted to BMT during an 18 month-period, 20 of whom associated some form of acute and/or chronic graft-versus-host disease (GVHD).

PATIENTS AND METHODS

There were 18 females and 7 males, aged 8–44 yrs. BMT was made in 16 patients for acute leukemia (AL), in 1 for chronic myelogenous leukemia (CML), in 7 for severe aplastic anemia (AA) and in another one for paroxysmal nocturnal hemoglobinuria (PNH). All donors were HLA identical, myxed lymphocyte culture (MLC) negative siblings. Before BMT, AL patients were conditioned with cyclophosphamide (CY) (120 mg/kg) plus total body irradiation (TBI) (1,000 rads), while 4 patients AA received CY (200 mg/kg) plus thoraco-abdominal irradiation (600 rads) with lung shielding. The remaining 4 patients (3 with AA and 1 with PNH) were treated with CY (200 mg/kg) alone.

Respiratory assessment was sequentially recorded before and each 30 days, during the first quarter, and then each 3 months, following BMT. Pulmonary evaluation included a clinical questionnaire, physical examination, chest-x-ray films, and conventional pulmonary function tests (PFT's). Survivors were followed up to 27 months.

RESULTS

Pre-BMT Manifestations. None of the 25 patients had respiratory symptoms and/or signs before BMT; chest-x-ray films were all normal. In all but 2 patients there was no previous respiratory disease. In contrast, 19 showed some functional abnormality. Thus, 12 exhibited impaired gas exchange (low diffusing capacity, DLCO, and/or low PaO_2), 3 an obstructive profile (obstructive ventilatory defect, and/or air trapping, and/or bronchial hyperreactivity, and/or increased airways resistance) and 4 others had both an obstructive profile and impaired gas exchange. There was no restrictive ventilatory impairment.

Post-BMT Manifestations. Following BMT, all the patients developed abnormal PFT's. In GVHD patients these abnormalities were as follows: 5 had an obstructive profile alone, 4 a restrictive pattern alone, 8 a mixed defect, 1 restriction plus obstruction and the remaining one associated a mixed pattern with restriction. Most of these patients (17 cases) also showed impaired gas exchange, present in 10 patients before BMT. One patient had a normal ventilatory capacity and a low DLCO. All together, there were 15 patients with airway dysfunction (present in 3 before BMT) and 14 with a restrictive defect. In all but one case abnormal PFT's were permanent. They were mostly subclinical and not related to the development of the few clinical problems.

In the 8 alive patients, 6 showed transient clinical manifestations. Only 1 patient presented an irreversible disease, consistent with obliterative bronchiolitis. In all but 3 subjects, abnormal PFT's were detected after the onset of GVHD. Major causes of death in 8 of the 12 patients who died were interstitial pneumonitis and bacterial pneumonias. The 5 patients without GVHD also exhibited abnormal PFT's: 3 a mixed ventilatory pattern, 1 both a restrictive and an obstructive one, and the last patient a restrictive defect followed by a mixed one (in 4 cases there was obstruction before BMT); 4 of these patients also had impaired gas exchange, present in 3 before BMT. In 3 of these patients, functional abnormalities were temporarily clinical. Serological testing and cultures from the respiratory tract were only positive in 4 out of the 15 patients with clinical disorders.

DISCUSSION

Our results show that all BMT patients exhibit early pulmonary functional abnormalities, regardless of the presence or absence of GVHD. Among longterm survivors, these abnormal PFT's were clinical in all but one patient, although only chronic and severely irreversible in one (diagnosed of obliterative bronchiolitis). There was a high incidence of both obstructive and restrictive ventilatory defects in GVHD patients; impaired gas exchange was also very frequent, although in most cases it was already present before BMT. The most likely etiology of airflow obstruction seems to be repeated subclinical respiratory tract infections, caused by bacterial and/or viral agents, in an immunosupressed host with or without an immunological mechanism related to the GVH reaction. In summary, our data suggest that the obstructive lung disorders recently reported in BMT patients with GVHD may well be related to the presence of GVHD per se alike the restrictive ones. We therefore postulate the use of repeated conventional PFT's before and after BMT for an early detection of such abnormalities. An early diagnosis would facilitate a therapeutic intervention to reverse or ameliorate the later development of advanced respiratory impairment.

REFERENCES

Ralph DD, Springmeyer SC, Sullivan KM, Hackman RC, Storb R, Thomas ED (1984). Rapidly progressive air-flow obstruction in marrow transplant recipients. Possible association between obliterative bronchiolitis and chronic graft-versus-host disease. Am Rev Respir Dis, 129: 641–44.

Rodriguez-Roisín R, Roca J, Grañena A, Agustí-Vidal A, Rozman C (1984). Obliterative bronchiolitis: a distinct pathophysiological form of pulmonary involvement in bone marrow transplantation. Exp Hematol, 12 (Suppl 15): 12–14.

Wyatt SE, Nunn P, Hows JM, et al (1984). Airways obstruction associated with graft versus host disease after bone marrow transplantation. Thorax; 39: 887–894

Supported by Grants FISS 83/0819 and AR 82/2-124.

T-Cell Depletion

Exp. Hematol. (suppl. 17) 13:146 (1985)
© International Society for Experimental Hematology

Prevention of Acute GvHD in Allogeneic Bone Marrow Transplantation by in vitro Treatment with the Monoclonal Anti-Lymphocyte Antibody Campath-1

M. Wiesneth[1], D. Bunjes[1], R. Arnold[1], Th. Schmeiser[1], G. Hale[2], H. Heimpel[1], and W. Heit[1]

[1] Bone Marrow Transplantation Unit, Department of Internal Medicine, University of Ulm, D-7900 Ulm, Federal Republic of Germany
[2] Department of Pathology, University of Cambridge, Cambridge, Great Britain

INTRODUCTION

One of the major problems in allogeneic bone marrow transplantation (BMT) is acute graft-versus-host disease (aGvHD) because of its high rate of incidence (30%-70%) and lethality (10%-20%) despite posttransplant immunosuppression (3). Animal studies and previous clinical experience have indicated that the elimination of mature T-lymphocytes from the allograft effectively prevents aGvHD (2, 4).

Preliminary results of a single incubation with the monoclonal antilymphocyte antibody Campath-1 (1) and autologous complement as the sole aGvHD prophylaxis are reported.

PATIENTS AND METHODS

16 patients (11 AL, 4 CML, 1 NHL) received a bone marrow transplant from a HLA-identical sibling. The mononuclear bone marrow cells were concentrated using the Haemonetics V50 to reduce the volume for antibody incubation and the number of red cells for ABO-incompatible transplantation. Incubation with Campath-1 (100 µg/ml) and autologous complement (15% v/v) reduces the percentage of E-rosetting cells from a mean of 36% (range 29%-49%) to 1% (range 0%-2%) without significantly affecting stem cell recovery (BFU-E 77%, CFU-GM 103%).

RESULTS

Marrow engraftment and haemopoietic recovery were not impaired in comparison to a historical control group (Table). Acute GvHD of the skin was observed in two patients (grade I-II). Two patients rejected their grafts on day 20 and day 60 post BMT respectively and were regrafted successfully with unpurged bone marrow. Both patients and another two patients died of CMV-pneumonia and one patient of an intraabdominal haemorrhage. 11 out of the 16 patients (69%) are currently alive and well with no evidence of acute or chronic GvHD. So far no relapse has occurred (5 weeks to 12 months post BMT).

CONCLUSIONS

T-lymphocytes can be effectively removed from the allograft using a single incubation with Campath-1 and autologous complement. Marrow engraftment and haemopoietic recovery are not impaired by purging the bone marrow. T-cell depletion alone reduces the incidence and severity of aGvHD. More extensive long-term studies are necessary to evaluate the problem of whether a weaker graft-versus-leukaemia effect due to effective GvHD prophylaxis will result in a higher relapse rate. Similarly the long-term effects of T-cell purging on permanent engraftment and immunoreconstitution require further investigation.

REFERENCES

1. Hale G, Bright S, Chumbley G, et al. Blood 62: 873-882 (1983)
2. Prentice HG, Blacklock H, Janossy G, et al. Exp. Hematol 12 (Suppl 15): 57-58 (1984)
3. Ramsey N, Kersey JH, Robinson LL, et al. N Engl J Med 306: 392-397 (1982)
4. Waldmann H, Hale G, Cividalli G, et al. Lancet 483-486 (1984)

TABLE: Comparison of acute GvHD prophylaxis in HLA-matched bone marrow transplantation

aGvHD prophylaxis	Incubation Campath-1 Complement	Post-transplant Methotrexate Immunosuppression
Patients	16 (11 AL, 4 CML, 1 NHL)	23 (19 AL, 4 CML)
E-rosetting cells ($\bar{x}$)	1%	36%
Engraftment	16/16	23/23
Haemopoietic Recovery	=	=
a GvHD grade I-II	2/16 (13%)	8/23 (35%)
grade II-IV	0/16	5/23 (22%)
Graft rejection	2/16	0/23
Relapse	0/16	2/23

Exp. Hematol. (suppl. 17) 13:147 (1985)
© International Society for Experimental Hematology

In vitro Treatment of Marrow with ATCG or Campath-1 for Prophylaxis of GVHD

Results of the AG-KMT München

H. J. Kolb, H. Rodt, B. Netzel, G. Hale, R. J. Haas, Ch. Bender-Götze, W. Wilmanns, H. Waldmann, and S. Thierfelder

III. Medizinische Klinik, Kinderklinik, Kinderpoliklinik der Universität München, Gesellschaft für Strahlen- und Umweltforschung, Institut für Hämatologie, München, Federal Republic of Germany
Department of Pathology, University of Cambridge, Great Britain

Graft-versus-host disease (GVHD) is a major obstacle of allogeneic bone marrow transplantation. Presumably mature T-lymphocytes in the marrow graft are responsible for the GVH reaction resulting in GVHD. We have studied removal of T-lymphocytes by treatment of the marrow with absorbed antithymocyte globulin (ATCG) and recently monoclonal antibodies for prevention of GVHD in mice, dogs and man (Rodt et al. 1972, Kolb et al. 1979, Thierfelder et al. 1984). Crossreacting antibodies against hemopoietic stem cells were removed by absorption with liver, kidney, red cells and B-lymphocytes. Campath 1 is a monoclonal antibody produced in a rat hybridoma that reacts against all human lymphocytes and fixes human complement (Hale et al.1983).

Canine ATCG had a complement fixing titer of 1:512, did not suppress the growth of CFU-GM nor delay the engraftment of autologous marrow treated with concentrations of 1:25-100. DLA-heterozygous recipients of marrow from DLA-homozygous littermates (AA'into AB) died of GVHD within 4 weeks when conditioned with 9 Gy total body irradiation (TBI) and given untreated marrow. Treatment of the marrow with ATCG at a titer of 1:200 (v:v) prevented fatal GVHD in 10 out of 13 dogs. At a higher concentration (1:100) graft failure and rejection was observed in some dogs, lower concentrations (1:400-800) did not control GVHD. Engraftment of marrow from DLA-haploidentical littermates was successful after preparation with 18 Gy fractionated TBI and prophylactic administration of methotrexate (MTX), but dogs died with GVHD within 53 days of grafting (AB into AC). Treatment of the marrow with ATCG in this combination led to graft failure at 1:200 and failed to prevent GVHD at 1:400. Thus GVHD across major histocompatibility barriers could only be prevented in donor recipient combinations with weak host-versus-graft reactions.

Human ATCG was produced in analogy to the canine ATCG in rabbits, absorbed and added to the marrow at a concentration of 1:200 for 30 min at 4°C without addition of complement. Campath 1 was used in a concentration of 100 μL/ml, incubated for 10 min at room temperature and after addition of 20vol% donor serum as complement for 45 min at 37°C. Prior to antibody treatment the marrow was separated from plasma and red cells to a volume of 200-250 ml. Antibody treated marrow was administered via a transfusion set after pretreatment of the patient with prednisolone. Four groups of patients with leukemia were compared retrospectively. They were conditioned with chemotherapy and TBI and grafted with marrow from HLA-identical siblings. Twenty patients received ATCG-treated marrow and MTX postgrafting as compared to 14 patients treated with MTX only, 8 pat-

ients were given Campath 1 treated marrow and cyclosporin A (CSA) as compared to 7 patients treated with CSA only. Only patients with engraftment were evaluable for GVHD and patients grafted in an advanced stage of leukemia and surviving more than 3 months were evaluable for leukemic recurrence.

Graft-versus-host disease, relapse of leukemia and survival after antibody treatment of the graft.

Regimen	No.of patients with GVHD = II per No. evaluable	rec. leukemia per No. evaluable	surviving
MTX	6/10	2/7	4
MTX + ATCG	4/18	6/11	5
CSA	7/7	1/4	6
CSA + Camp 1	0/8	4/4	5 (3 with rel)
MTX + Camp 1	1 without engraftment		
CSA + ATCG	1/1	-/-	1

GVHD was less frequent in patients given ATCG-treated marrow and GVHD of grade = II was not seen in patients given Camp 1 treated marrow. Mild GVHD of the skin was seen in two patients of the latter group and another patient succumbed to a Lyell-syndrome. However survival was not improved by antibody treatment of the graft. In part graft failures (2/9 given Camp 1 treated marrow) and relapse of leukemia may be responsible. Retransplantation was not successful in both patients. In patients with successful engraftment the time until recovery of blood counts was not delayed in antibody treated groups with the exception of reticulocytes rising 4 days later after ATCG-treatment of the marrow. The duration of pancytopenia was shorter in patients treated with CSA than in those treated with MTX.

In conclusion prophylaxis of GVHD was improved by the treatment of the graft with anti-T-cell and antilymphocyte antibodies, but survival was not improved. In part ahigher rate of recurrent leukemia may account for this discrepancy. Rejection is a serious problem of T-cell depleted grafts in dogs and man. Improved immunosuppressive and antileukemic conditioning regimens may solve both problems.

References: Rodt H. et al. Blut 25: 385, 1972
                Kolb H.J.et al. Transplant.
                        27: 242, 1979
                Thierfelder S. et al. Exp. Hematol.
                        12: 373,1984
                Hale G. et al. Blood 62: 873, 1983

Exp. Hematol. (suppl. 17) 13:148 (1985)
© International Society for Experimental Hematology

T Cell Recovery in T-ALL After Transplantation of Autologous BM Purged with Anti-T(WT1)-Coupled to Ricin

G. C. de Gast[2], F. W. M. B. Preyers[2], Th. de Witte[2], P. J. A. Capel[2], L. F. Verdonck[1], and E. J. E. G. Bast[1]

[1] Department of Haematology and Clinical Immunology, University Hospital Utrecht
[2] Department of Haematology and Nephrology, University Hospital Nijmegen, The Netherlands

INTRODUCTION

Patients with a T-ALL and hyperleukocytosis have a bad prognosis, which may be improved by consolidation by high dose chemo/radiotherapy and autologous BMT. To minimize the chance of returning leukemic T cells, the bone-marrow graft can be treated with immunotoxines such as ricin A coupled monoclonal antibodies. The effect of this procedure on T cell recovery and relapse is not known. In this case report T cell recovery appeared to be normal in such a patient.

PATIENT

A 27 yrs old man was treated for acute T-lymphoblastic leukemia with hyperleukocytosis with OP-DOP (remission induction) and intermediate dose ara-C + Cy (consolidation) and subsequently with Cy + TBI (8 Gy) + Auto-BMT. CNS prophylaxis was done with 4x MTX intra-thecally.

T-ALL typing

CD 1+ (OKT6), CD2+ (E_s), CD3+ (Leu 4), CD5+ (Leu 1) WT1+, TdT weak+, CD4+ CD8±. Chromosomal translocation 7/14, 12p-, 11q-.

Bone marrow purging

Purging of BM in 1st CR was performed with WT-1 coupled to ricin A after testing the effect on PB leukemic T cells. The effect was checked by phenotyping the lymphocytes before and after purging and by ^{3}H-leucine incorporation.

Recovery of T cells.

Recovery of T cells was studied in PB with monoclonal antibodies and by functional tests (mitogen- and antigen induced lymphocyte sitmulation).

RESULTS

In vitro treatment with WT-1 Ricin A antibodies:Leukemic T cells from PB treated with WT 1- Ricin A and NH4Cl showed a strong decrease in protein synthesis. BM from a control and from the patient showed no inhibition of CFU-GM. Marker studies before and after treatment of patient BM (in CR) showed no decrease of the T cell markers Leu 1, CD4 and CD 8 and only WT 1 (also present on normal BM cells) disappeared, CD1+ (OKT6) positive cells were not present above the limit of detection (1:10,000) in IF.

Recovery of T cells after BMT

T cells recovered rapidly to normal ranges after BMT with a preponderance of CD8+ T cells. Later on CD8+ T cells decreased, whereas CD4+ T cells remained low. No T cells with the malignant phenotype (WT1+, CD1+) appeared in the first 3 months.

T cell function after BMT

PHA-induced lymphocyte stimulation was greatly depressed after BMT and recovered only gradually. PMW-induced T cell help for B cell differentiation showed a better recovery (up to 32% of normal after 3m). Lymphocyte stimulation by herpes simplex virus (HSV) was higher after BMT (S.I. 33.7 at 1 month) than before BMT (S.I. 13.2). Lymphocyte stimulation by tetanus toxoid was present before (SI 33.8) and after BMT (SI 13.1) but decreased gradually.

Follow-up of patient.

Six months after BMT a relapse of the T-ALL was noted with hyperleukocytosis and the patient died 2 weeks later (therapy was not given). Phenotyping of the malignant T-cells showed the same phenotype as initially (e.g. WT1+ CD1+, CD2+, CD3+, CD5+, CD4+, CD8±, TdT+).

SUMMARY AND DISCUSSION

By WT1-Ricin antibody treatment, WT 1 expression on leukemic T cells disappeared and protein synthesis was inhibited, but CFU-GM in BM were not affected. In the treated 1st CR BM, where cells with the malignant phenotype were absent (1:10,000), other T cell antigens were still detected. After BMT T cells recovered rapidly with a preponderance of CD8+ T cells. T cell reactivity to mitogens remained low, but reactivity to viral antigens as HSV was high, indicating that sensitized T cells were present in a very early stage (1 month after BMT).
Despite purging with WT1 antibody, the relapse leukomic cells were WT1+ with exactly the same phenotype as initially. The origin of the relapse is unclear; the purged BM or the residual leukemic cells in the body.

Exp. Hematol. (suppl. 17) 13:149 (1985)
© International Society for Experimental Hematology

A Clinicopathological Study of Bone-Marrow Transplant Associated Pulmonary Disease

Th. Schmeiser, B. Heymer, R. Arnold, M. Wiesneth, H. Heimpel, and W. Heit

BMT-Unit, Department of Internal Medicine and Department of Pathology, University of Ulm, D-7900 Ulm, Federal Republic of Germany

INTRODUCTION

Survival of patients treated with bone marrow transplantation (BMT) is mainly determined by pulmonary complications (1, 2).
In 21 of 38 consecutively transplanted patients pulmonary complications occurred. These complications were analysed clinically and histologically.

MATERIALS AND METHODS

Between 5/1980 and 2/1984 a BMT was performed in 38 adult patients (aplastic anaemia (AA) n=10, acute leukaemia (AL) n=24, chronic granulocytic leukaemia (CGL) n=4). Thirty-six patients were transplanted with HLA-identical and MLC-negative sibling bone marrow grafts, one patient with a HLA-identical and MLC-positive sibling graft and one patient with a graft from his identical twin. All patients received antimicrobial prophylaxis. Graft-versus-host disease (GvHD)-prophylaxis was given in 37 patients (Methotrexate n=33), Cyclosporin A n=1, monoclonal antibody n=3). Eight patients were treated with Cytomegalovirus (CMV)-hyperimmunoglobulin for prevention of CMV-infection or CMV-reactivation and all patients received a Pneumocystis carinii-prophylaxis. Before BMT conditioning therapy was given (Cyclophosphamide in patients with AA or Cyclophosphamide and total body irradiation (TBI) in patients with AL or CGL). Engraftment was demonstrable in all patients. The diagnosis and the grade of GvHD were established clinically and histologically. Pulmonary complications after BMT were analysed clinically (physical investigation, lung function tests, blood gas analysis, microbiology), radiologically and - when ever possible - histologically.

RESULTS

In this group of patients with BMT pulmonary complications occurred frequently (55%) and were associated with a high lethality (65%). In 67% of the patients the pulmonary complication appeared early (<day +100 after BMT), in 33% of the patients late (>day +100 after BMT). The majority of the patients (65%) developed infectious pulmonary complications, non-infectious pulmonary complications were less common (35%). Often there was an association of GvHD and pulmonary complication.

Patients with AA had fewer pulmonary complications (30%) as compared with patients with AL or CGL (64%). Only patients with AL or CGL developed interstitial pneumonia. All interstitial pneumonias led to death. Seven out of 8 interstitial pneumonias were caused by CMV. In all patients with CMV-pneumonia the viral infection was generalized with a high incidence of infection of the liver and gut, whereas the pancreas and other salivary glands were only rarely affected. The majority of patients with histologically confirmed CMV-infection developed bacterial and/or fungal superinfections. Two patients died of CMV-pneumonia whilst on CMV-prophylaxis with CMV-hyperimmunoglobulin. Four patients with non-infectious pulmonary complications showed dyspnoea, emphysema and a severe restrictive and obstructive disorder in lung function tests. All four patients had active chronic GvHD at the same time, two died of respiratory insufficiency and two are alive. The overall survival of patients with AA was 80% as compared with 43% in patients with AL or CGL. Survival of patients with pulmonary complications was 35% whereas 83% of patients without pulmonary complications survived.

CONCLUSIONS

The frequent incidence of lethal pulmonary complications - especially of interstitial pneumonia - early after BMT in patients with AL or CGL explains the lower survival rate as compared with patients with AA, whereas both groups showed no difference in the incidence of GvHD. In patients with AL or CGL the frequency of severe pulmonary infections is probably induced by the immunosuppressive effect of TBI. In 14 out of 15 patients who died of pulmonary complications respiratory failure was the immediate cause of death.

REFERENCES

1. Buckner CD, Meyers JD, Springmeyer SC, et al. (1984) Pulmonary complications of marrow transplantation. Exp Hematol 12 Suppl 15: 1-5.
2. Sloan JP, Depledge MH, Powles RL (1983) Histopathology of the lung after BMT. J Clin Pathol 36: 546-554.

Exp. Hematol. (suppl. 17) 13:150 (1985)
© International Society for Experimental Hematology

Transvenous Liver Studies of the Hepatic Disturbances After Bone Marrow Transplantation

A. Grañena, E. Carreras, C. Rozman, J. Bosch, M. Bruguera, R. Mastai, J. Bruix, and P. Marin

Postgraduate School of Haematology and Liver Unit, Hospital Clinic, University of Barcelona, Barcelona, Spain

INTRODUCCION

Different liver disorders complicating BMT, such as GvHD, drug toxicity, viral hepatitis, total parenteral nutrition-associated liver disorder and venocclusive disease (VOD) can share a common clinical syndrome. In order to establish an accurate diagnosis, histologic examination of the liver is usually required. However, transparietal liver biopsy frequently cannot be carried out due to the coexistent haemostatic impairment. To overcome this difficulty, we use the transjugular catheterization of the hepatic vein with 2 aims: a) to measure both wedged and free hepatic venous pressure as complement to VOD diagnosis; b) to safely perform the liver biopsy.

PATIENTS AND METHODS

Eleven studies were performed in 8 patients, 3 with ALL, 3 with ANLL and the remaining 2 with SAA (Table).

RESULTS

In 5 instances (4 patients), the venous gradient measurement yielded clear-cut increased values (higher than 10 mmHg). Histologic diagnoses were distributed as follows: VOD 2, VOD + GvHD 1, GvHD alone 2, hepatitis 2, MHI 3, biopsy not done 1.
The gradient was clearly increased in 3 instances of histologically-proven VOD (once associated with GvHD), and in one case (UPN 81) with strong clinical suspicion of VOD. The gradient was normal in all instances of MHI or isolated GvHD and in the remaining case of hepatitis.

DISCUSSION

An accurate differential diagnosis between liver disorders post-BMT is difficult unless the histopathological examination is carried out. It has generally been accepted that the association of

UPN	DIAG	ONSET SYMPTOMS	DAY STUDY	BILIRRUBIN mg/dl	ALAT/ASAT UI/L	HEPATOM cm	ASCITIS ↑WEIGHT	GvHD	GRADIENT mmHg	HISTOLOGY
55	ALL	+ 23	+ 26	3.8	41/58	3	YES	NO	4	MHI
			+ 78	3.7	93/114	5	NO	Mild	6	MHI
81	ALL	+ 20	+ 27	3.9	114/325	6	YES	NO	10.5	NOT DONE*
95	ALL	+ 12	+ 19	3.6	363/715	3	YES	NO	24	VOD
			+ 50	31.8	110/313	4	YES	Mild	16	VOD + GvHD
88	ANLL	+ 143	+ 151	4.1	30/85	1	NO	Severe	3	GvHD
			+ 250	36.3	173/485	3	YES	Severe	4	GvHD
98	ANLL	+ 16	+ 34	3.1	250/310	3	YES	Mild	11	VOD
98	ANLL	+ 50	+ 68	1	340/1410	1	NO	Mild	11	HEPATITIS
74	SAA	+ 15	+ 47	2.2	250/272	2	NO	NO	5	HEPATITIS
91	SAA	+ 20	+ 38	2.2	29/34	2	YES	NO	4.5	MHI

* (to small vein caliber).

All had less than 40 x 10^9/l platelets. Three patients were studied twice because of persisting hepatic disfunction several weeks after the first examination. In 6 instances (5 patients) GvHD was present at the time of the study.
Hepatic vein catheterization was performed with a preshaped catheter through the right internal jugular vein. After measuring the wedged (WHVP) and free hepatic venous pressure (FHVP), as an estimation of portal pressure which is reported as the gradient between WHVP and FWVP (normal values less than 5 mmHg, clearly abnormal more than 10 mmHg), transvenous liver biopsy was obtained with a modified Ross needle (1).
Histologic diagnosis was based on following criteria: a) VOD-occlusion of centrolobular veins by subintimal proliferation of connective tissue; b) GvHD- Dysplastic lesions of bile duct epithelium associated with lobular changes, particularly cholestasis and hepatocellular damage; c) Hepatitis- Cell degeneration and inflammatory changes predominanting in the lobules; d) Mild hepatocellular injury (MHI)- This term was applied to cases showing ballooning of liver cells without necrosis or inflammation.

jaundice, development of hepatomegaly and/or ascitis strongly suggest VOD, when appearing early postransplant (2). From our studies it is clearly evident that based on clinical criteria only, VOD would be overdiagnosed.
Transjugular approach offers at least two advantages over the usual management of these patients. Firstly, it enables the clinician to obtain histological liver sample in spite of the haemostatic impairment. Secondly, the measurement of hepatic venous gradient permits to further characterize VOD.

REFERENCES

1.- Lebrec D, Goldfarb G, Degott C, Rueff B and Benhamou JP.(1982) Transvenous liver biopsy. Gastroenterology 83: 338-340.
2.- MacDonald GB, Sharma P, Matthews DE, Shulman HM and Thomas D. (1984) Venocclusive disease of the liver after bone marrow transplatation: Diagnosis, incidence and predisposing factors. Hepatology 4: 116-122.

Exp. Hematol. (suppl. 17) 13:151 (1985)
© International Society for Experimental Hematology

Patients with Aplastic Anemia Frequently are Histocompatible (HLA-DR, MLC) with Their Mothers

A. Hajek-Rosenmayr[1], W. Hinterberger[2], W. Schmidmeier[3], C. Urban[4], and W. R. Mayr[1]

[1] Institute for Blood Group Serology, University of Vienna
[2] I. Department of Medicine, University of Vienna
[3] St. Anna Children Hospital, Vienna
[4] Department of Pediatrics, University of Graz, Austria

The real cause of Aplastic Anemia (AA) still is unknown. Some imbalances in the distribution of the HLA-antigens, however, have been reported in families of AA patients (1) (2), but none of them definitely could be confirmed.

In the course of HLA typing and MLC (Mixed Lymphocyte Culture) testing of 22 AA patients and their families for bone marrow transplantation, we recently encountered not only a high number of HLA -DR and -D homozygous persons (3) (4), but also a high number of parents sharing a HLA-DR and -D antigen

Parents who have one HLA-DR antigen in common or are HLA-DR homozygous frequently have children HLA-DR identical with parents and sibs. MLC response between these HLA-DR identical, but HLA-A,-B,-C haplodifferent family members usually is very low.

Comparing the HLA-DR and MLC compatibility of mother and child pairs in healthy and in AA families a significant excess of HLA-DR identical or "one way compatible" (one HLA-DR homozygous and nonstimulating in MLC) Mother child combinations could be observed in AA families, as is shown in table 1:

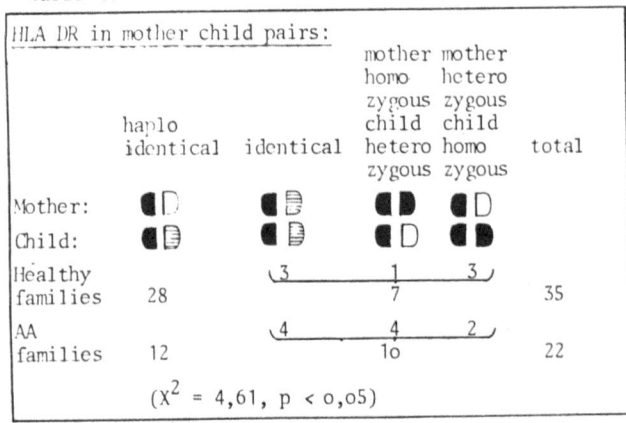

HLA DR in mother child pairs:

	haplo identical	identical	mother homo zygous child hetero zygous	mother hetero zygous child homo zygous	total
Mother:					
Child:					
Healthy families	28		3 / 7	1 / \ 3	35
AA families	12		4 / 10	4 / \ 2	22

$$(x^2 = 4,61, \ p < 0,05)$$

In 1o of 22 AA families, (21 austrian and one hungarian family) a more or less complete HLA-DR and MLC compatibility exists between mother and children. In one exceptional case, however, the diseased child is fully haplodifferent with his mother, but two healthy siblings are HLA-DR identical and MLC compatible with their mother.

Figure 1 shows that MLC reactions between mother and child are much lower in AA families than

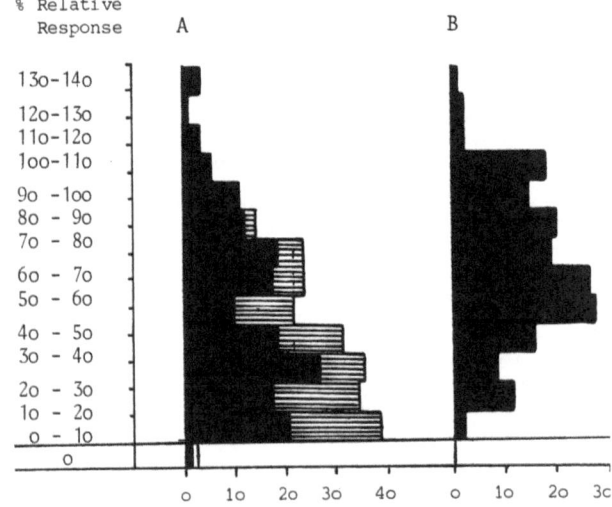

% Relative Response

Number of MLC reactions

A   Aplastic Anemia families:
▤ MLC reactions between mother and AA child
■ MLC reactions between mother and healthy children
B   Healthy families:
■ MLC reactions between mother and healthy children
The two groups of MLC reactions differ significantly. (■ A - ■ B, p < o,oo1; □ A - ■ B, p < o,ooo1; ▤ A - ■ B, p < o,ooo1, Student's T-Test)

Our results show, that HLA-DR and MLC compatibility between mother and child might have an influence on the development of Aplastic Anemia.

In several cases of Severe Combined Immunodeficiency, it recently has been prooved, that the cause of the disease is a materno-fetal transfusion followed by graft versus host disease in the child (5).

We suggest, that a similar mechanism, promoted by the high compatibility between mother and child is at the bottom of Aplastic Anemia as well.

References: 1) Transplantation 23,366 (1977)
2) Tissue Antigens 13,3o7 (1979)
3) Experimental Hematology 4,13,57 (83)
4) Blood, in press
5) N.E.J.Med., 3o7,662 (1982)

Exp. Hematol. (suppl. 17) 13:152 (1985)
© International Society for Experimental Hematology

The Mixed Epidermal Cell Lymphocyte Reaction Allows the Detection of Alloreactivities Before Graft in HLA Identical Siblings

M. Bagot[1], C. Cordonnier[2], M. Heslan[1], A. F. Tilkin[3], L. Dubertret[1], J. P. Vernant[2], and J. P. Levy[3]

[1] Dermatology Department, Hôpital Henri Mondor, Créteil
[2] Hematology Department, Hôpital Henri Mondor, Créteil
[3] INSERM U 152, Hôpital Cochin, Paris, France

INTRODUCTION

Graft-Versus-Host-Disease (GVHD) remains a major clinical problem, sometimes leading to life threatening complications in patients treated by marrow transplantation from HLA identical siblings. Cutaneous signs are both the earliest and the most constant manifestations in acute GVHD, suggesting that epidermal cells (EC) could be a preferential target of this reaction. It has been shown that human EC induce greater proliferations of allogeneic lymphocytes in the mixed-epidermal-cell-lymphocyte-reaction (MECLR) than the same number of peripheral blood lymphocytes (PBL) in the mixed-lymphocyte-reaction (MLR) (Sontheimer et al., 1983). Moreover, EC could allow the detection of weak proliferative responses not found in MLR, especially in primary reactions (Bagot et al., 1985). In this study, we tested the ability of MECLR to detect alloreactivities before graft in HLA identical MLR negative siblings and to predict the patients' evolution after grafting.

MATERIALS AND METHODS

21 patients were studied before grafting with a genotypically HLA identical sibling : 7 acute lymphocytic leukemia, 8 acute non lymphocytic leukemia, 5 chronic myelogenous leukemia and 1 lymphoblastic lymphoma. EC were obtained from the recipients by trypsin disaggregation of a suction blister top. Donor lymphocytes were cultured in microtiter plates with either EC or PBL of the recipient. Tritiated thymidine incorporation was measured after 6 days of culture.

RESULTS

Our results show a frequent dissociation between MLR, which was constantly negative, and MECLR, which was positive in 11/21 cases. Among two HLA identical siblings of the recipient, one can be MECLR+ and the other MECLR- . Moreover, the positivity of the MECLR is correlated with the incidence of acute GVHD, as shown by the following results.

Clinical GVHD Grade	0	1	2-4	Total
MECLR+	3	3	5	11
MECLR-	8	2	0	10
Total	11	5	5	21

DISCUSSION

In patients grafted with bone marrow from HLA identical siblings GVHD is thought to be initiated by incompatibilities for minor histocompatibility antigens (Goulmy, 1985). Some minor histocompatibility antigens could be tissue specific, as already reported in mice for several epidermal alloantigens (Steinmuller, 1984). Since our results demonstrate that the MECLR is able to detect alloreactivities in HLA identical siblings, one could hypothesize that this reaction is directed against skin- or epithelia-specific minor histocompatibility antigens. However, as EC have been shown to be more efficient antigen presenting cells in primary reactions, it is also possible that the discrepancy found between MLR and MECLR could be a quantitative one. In both cases, the MECLR could represent a useful tool to improve the selection of bone marrow graft donors and a predictive test to identify patients with a high risk to develop GVHD. A large scale study is however needed to definitely establish this point.

REFERENCES

BAGOT M, HESLAN M, DUBERTRET L, ROUJEAU JC, LEVY JP (1985) Antigen presenting properties of human epidermal cells compared to peripheral blood mononuclear cells. Br J Dermatol (in press).

GOULMY E (1985) Class I-restricted human cytotoxic T lymphocytes directed against minor transplantation antigens and their possible role in organ transplantation. Prog Allergy 36, 44-72 (in press).

SONTHEIMER RD (1983) The mixed-epidermal-cell-lymphocyte-reaction. I. Human epidermal cells elicit a greater allogeneic lymphocyte response than do autologous peripheral blood lymphoid cells. J Immunol, 130, 2612-2614.

STEINMULLER D (1984) Tissue-specific and tissue-restricted histocompatibility antigens. Immunol Today, 5, 8, 234-240.

Exp. Hematol. (suppl. 17) 13:153 (1985)
© International Society for Experimental Hematology

Cyclophosphamide (CP) Pharmacokinetics and Metabolism After Repeated High Dose Administration in BMT

G. Ehninger, U. Schuler, T. Wagner, and P. Ostendorf

Medizinische Universitätsklinik Tübingen and Medizinische Hochschule Lübeck, Federal Republic of Germany

INTRODUCTION

The cancer chemotherapeutic activities of CP are mediated by metabolites produced by activation in hepatic microsomes by mixed function oxidases (Brock 1976).

Several authors (Tardiff 1969, Gurtoo 1976, Marinello 1981) observed an inhibition of hepatic microsomal enzymes after CP. On the other hand a significant decrease in CP half-life after repeated doses (Sladek 1980, Graham 1983, Bagley 1973, D'Incalci 1979) was measured.

Our study was designed to answer following questions: 1. Is the decrease of CP half-life caused by an impairment of renal reabsorption of CP due to damage by prior dose ? 2. How do these observations of enzyme inhibition and pharmacokinetic alteration relate to blood levels and AUC of activated metabolites (4-hydroxy-CP and the tautomeric aldophosphamide) ? 3. Is the pharmacokinetic of CP changed after repeated high doses ?

METHODS

Eleven patients with severe aplastic anemia (50mg/kgx4) or leukemia (60mg/kgx2) were transplanted according the Seattle protocol. 12 mg/kg mesna was administered prior and 0, 3, 6, 9, 12, 15, 18 hours after CP. CP blood and urine levels were measured by N/P-flame ionization gas chromatography after extraction with dichloromethane and derivatization with heptafluorobutyric acid. Aktivated CP-metabolites (4-HO-CP and aldophosphamide) were determined in blood by liberation of acrolein and its fluorometric determination (Wagner 1981, 1984). Pharmakokinetic analysis was performed with the NONLIN program.

RESULTS

In patients with SAA CP half-life decreased from 7.3+1.1 hrs at day 1 to 4.33 + 0.4 hrs at day 4. In leukemic patients half-life decreased from 4.7 + 1.3 hrs at day 1 to 3.0 + 0.4 hrs at day 2. The drug exposure (AUC) to activated metabolites increased from 17.1 µmol*hrs/L at day 1 to 39.6 µmol*hrs/L at day 4 and from 20.1 to 28.7 µmol*hrs/L respectively. Urinary excretion of CP did not change significantly but tended to decrease after pretreatment.

DISCUSSION

Our results regarding the decrease of CP half-lives in blood after repeated high doses are in accordance with several other publications. The suggestion of Graham (1983) that these changes might be accounted for by an impaired renal reabsorption is ruled out by our observation of a decrease of urinary excretion of CP. Several animal studies showed an inhibition of microsomal enzymes. The relevance of these observations for clinical treatment regimens has never been determined. In our study the activation of CP was not inhibited by prior administration and the AUC of metabolites increased. Two mechanisms may play an important role, firstly an accumulation of 4-hydroxy-CP and aldophosphamide due to an inhibition of their degradation enzymes, secondly a saturation of protein binding sites. Voelcker (1978) could still demonstrate a protein bound fraction of 4-hydroxy-CP up to 48 hours after CP administration, at a time when the free fraction was below the detection limit.

Therefore different conditioning protocols with the same total CP dose in different schedules e.g. 120 mg/kg on day 1 or 60 mg/kg on day 1 and 2 might cause different exposition to cytotoxic metabolites and in clinical terms could influence the relapse rate.

References

Bagley CM et al. (1973) Cancer Res 33:226
Brock N (1976) Cancer Treat Rep 60:301
D'Incalci M et al (1979) Eur J Cancer 15:7
Graham MI et al. (1983)
    Cancer Chemother Pharmacol 10:192
Gurtoo HL et al. (1976)
    Cancer Treat Rep 60: 1285
Marinello AJ et al. (1981)
    Biochem Biophys Res Comm 99:399
Sladek NE et al. (1980)
    Cancer Treat Rep 64:1061
Tardiff RG, Dubois KP (1969)
    Arch Int Pharmacodyn 177:445
Voelcker G et al. (1978)
    Z Krebsforsch 21:127
Wagner T et al. (1981)
    J Cancer Res Clin Onc 100:95
Wagner T, Fenneberg K (1984)
    Eur J Clin Pharmacology 26: 269

Exp. Hematol. (suppl. 17) 13:154 (1985)
© International Society for Experimental Hematology

Marrow Transplantation for Advanced Leukemia in Patients Over 30 Years with Fractionated TBI

A Randomized Trial of MTX and Cyclosporine

C. Irle*, H. J. Deeg, C. D. Buckner, M. Kennedy, R. Storb, R. A. Clift, and E. D. Thomas

Division of Oncology, The Fred Hutchinson Cancer Research Center
The Swedish Hospital Medical Center
The Seattle Veterans Administration Hospital
The University of Washington School of Medicine Seattle, WA, USA, for the Seattle Transplant Team

Bone marrow transplantation(BMT)for leukemia in relapse is often complicated by severe transplant-related toxicities,which are increasing with age ,and result in a high mortality.Among the surviving patients,the relapse frequency is elevated (1,2).The present study was designed to determine the effects of fractionated total body irradiation (TBI, 7 fractions of 2.25 Gy delivered at a rate of 6.5 cGy/min over 7 conscutive days)and Methotrexate (MTX) or Cyclosporine(CSP)immunosuppression,on the outcome of BMT in 56 consecutive patients over 3o years of age with relapsed leukemia.

Immunosuppression was assigned by randomized permutation,3o patients were given MTX,and 26 received CSP.All were conditioned with cyclophosphamide , followed by the fractionated TBI, as well as pre-BMT and post-BMT iT MTX injections, exactely as described else - where (3).

In the present study , patients on MTX had an actuarial relapse rate of 37 % versus 7o % observed in the CSP group. After excluding 5 patients with CGL in remission of blast crisis , and 3 patients transplanted before any treatment for hypoplastic leukemia was given, because of their possibly lower risk of relapse , the "corrected" relapse rate in the MTX group was 47% ,which was not significantly different from the 7o% in the CSP group. These results are comparable to those obtained in a previous study of relapsed ANL patients given loGy TBI in a single session,and MTX (I).Therefore, the increase of TBI from lo Gy to 15.75 Gy in fractionated doses did not have a major impact on disease recurrence in these patients.

The non-leukemic mortality in this study was 51 % , which is slightly less than the 65 % previously reported in relapsed patients given lo Gy.,despite an increase of 1½ decades of the median age in the present study .

Idiopathic intersticial pneumonia (IIP) occured in 13 % ,and fatal intersticial pneumonia mainly secondary to CMV ,occured in 18 % of the patients. These results support previous findings that fractionated TBI may result in a decreased incidence of IIP , but not of IP secondary to CMV(4). The incidence of VOD was 55%. This compares to an incidence of 2o -5o% in patients on concurrent studies receiving 6 daily fractions of 2.ocGy TBI. Age and disease status were found to be the most important risk factors in a multivariate analysis in a previous study.These results indicate that factors other than TBI influence the diagnosis of VOD(5).The actuarial incidence of graft-versus-host disease(GvHD) was 71 % in the MTX arm , and 45 % in the CSP arm. In addition , patients on CSP had a more rapid engraftment, less severe mucositis ,and fewer non-intersticial pulmonnary complications. However, more(transient)renal failures,hypertension, mental depression , and seizures were found in the CSP group.The overall survival of the patients on CSP was not different from those on MTX. The relapse rate in the CSP group may be higher .

In conclusion , no major improvement of the overall survival could be detected when comparing the results of this study to a previous one,differing by age,radiotherapy,and when comparing MTX and CSP immunosuppression.

1.Appelbaum F.R.,Clift R.A.,Buckner C.D.et al Blood 61, 949 (1983)
2.Buckner C.D.,Clift R.A.,Thomas E.D.,et al Leuk.Res.6,389 (1982)
3.Irlé C.,Deeg H.J.,Buckner C.D. et al. Leuk.Res., in press.
4.Meyers J.D.,Flournoy N.,Wade J.C.,Hackman R.C. et al. In:Gale RP ed. Recent Advances in Bone Marrow Transplantation 405 (1983).
5. McDonald G.B., Sharma P.,Matthews D.E. et al. Hepatology 4, 116 (1984).

---

* Present address: Transplantation Immunology Unit, Division of Immunology and Allergology, Department of Medicine, University of Geneva Medical School, Geneva, Switzerland